Barrett's Esophagus

Editors

PRASAD G. IYER
NAVTEJ S. BUTTAR

GASTROENTEROLOGY
CLINICS OF NORTH AMERICA

www.gastro.theclinics.com

Consulting Editor
GARY W. FALK

June 2015 • Volume 44 • Number 2

ELSEVIER

1600 John F. Kennedy Boulevard • Suite 1800 • Philadelphia, Pennsylvania, 19103-2899
http://www.theclinics.com

GASTROENTEROLOGY CLINICS OF NORTH AMERICA Volume 44, Number 2
June 2015 ISSN 0889-8553, ISBN-13: 978-0-323-38888-7

Editor: Kerry Holland
Developmental Editor: Susan Showalter

Gastroenterology Clinics of North America (ISSN 0889-8553) is published quarterly by Elsevier Inc., 360 Park Avenue South, New York, NY 10010-1710. Months of issue are March, June, September, and December. Business and Editorial Offices: 1600 John F. Kennedy Blvd., Suite 1800, Philadelphia, PA 19103-2899. Customer Service Office: 6277 Sea Harbor Drive, Orlando, FL 32887-4800. Periodicals postage paid at New York, NY and additional mailing offices. Subscription prices are $320.00 per year (US individuals), $160.00 per year (US students), $530.00 per year (US institutions), $350.00 per year (Canadian individuals), $651.00 per year (Canadian institutions), $445.00 per year (international individuals), $220.00 per year (international students), and $651.00 per year (international institutions). Foreign air speed delivery is included in all *Clinics* subscription prices. All prices are subject to change without notice. **POSTMASTER:** Send address changes to *Gastroenterology Clinics of North America*, Elsevier Health Sciences Division, Subscription Customer Service, 3251 Riverport Lane, Maryland Heights, MO 63043. **Telephone: 1-800-654-2452 (U.S. and Canada); 314-447-8871 (outside U.S. and Canada). Fax: 314-447-8029. E-mail: journalscustomerservice-usa@elsevier.com (for print support); journalsonlinesupport-usa@elsevier.com (for online support).**

Reprints. For copies of 100 or more, of articles in this publication, please contact the Commercial Reprints Department, Elsevier Inc., 360 Part Avenue South, New York, New York 10010-1710. Tel. 212-633-3874, Fax: 212-633-3820, E-mail: reprints@elsevier.com.

Gastroenterology Clinics of North America is also published in Italian by Il Pensiero Scientifico Editore, Rome, Italy; and in Portuguese by Interlivros Edicoes Ltda., Rua Commandante Coelho 1085, 21250 Cordovil, Rio de Janeiro, Brazil.

Gastroenterology Clinics of North America is covered in *MEDLINE/PubMed (Index Medicus)*, *Excerpta Medica*, *Current Contents/Clinical Medicine*, *Science Citation Index*, *ISI/BIOMED*, and *BIOSIS*.

Contributors

CONSULTING EDITOR

GARY W. FALK, MD, MS
Professor of Medicine, Division of Gastroenterology, University of Pennsylvania Perelman School of Medicine, Philadelphia, Pennsylvania

EDITORS

PRASAD G. IYER, MD, MSc, FACG, FASGE, AGAF
Associate Professor; Consultant, Barrett's Esophagus Unit, Division of Gastroenterology and Hepatology, Mayo Clinic, Rochester, Minnesota

NAVTEJ S. BUTTAR, MD
Associate Professor; Consultant, Division of Gastroenterology and Hepatology, Mayo Clinic, Rochester, Minnesota

AUTHORS

JULIAN A. ABRAMS, MD, MS
Assistant Professor of Medicine and Epidemiology, Division of Digestive and Liver Diseases, Columbia University Medical Center, New York, New York

AJAY BANSAL, MD
Associate Professor of Medicine, Division of Gastroenterology and Hepatology, Department of Veterans Affairs Medical Center, Kansas City, Missouri; University of Kansas Medical Center, The Kansas Cancer Institute, Kansas City, Kansas

ANUSHKA BARUAH, MD
Department of Internal Medicine, John H. Stroger, Jr. Hospital of Cook County, Chicago, Illinois

ADAM J. BASS, MD
Department of Medical Oncology, Dana-Farber Cancer Institute, Boston, Massachusetts

NAVTEJ S. BUTTAR, MD
Associate Professor; Consultant, Division of Gastroenterology and Hepatology, Mayo Clinic, Rochester, Minnesota

APOORVA KRISHNA CHANDAR, MBBS, MPH
Research Associate, Division of Gastroenterology and Liver Diseases, Digestive Health Institute, University Hospitals Case Medical Center, Case Western Reserve University, Cleveland, Ohio

KERRY B. DUNBAR, MD, PhD
Assistant Professor, Division of Gastroenterology and Hepatology, Department of Medicine, Dallas VA Medical Center, University of Texas Southwestern Medical Center, Dallas, Texas

GARY W. FALK, MD, MS
Professor of Medicine, Division of Gastroenterology, University of Pennsylvania Perelman School of Medicine, Philadelphia, Pennsylvania

REBECCA C. FITZGERALD, MD
MRC Cancer Unit, Hutchison-MRC Research Centre, University of Cambridge, Cambridge, United Kingdom

LAUREN B. GERSON, MD, MSc
Director of Clinical Research, Gastroenterology Fellowship Program, California Pacific Medical Center, Associate Clinical Professor of Medicine, University of California, San Francisco, San Francisco, California

WILLIAM M. GRADY, MD
Clinical Research Division, Fred Hutchinson Cancer Research Center; Department of Internal Medicine, University of Washington School of Medicine, Seattle, Washington

MILLI GUPTA, MD, FRCP(C)
Clinical Assistant Professor, Division of Gastroenterology and Hepatology, University of Calgary, Calgary, Alberta, Canada

PRASAD G. IYER, MD, MSc, FACG, FASGE, AGAF
Associate Professor; Consultant, Barrett's Esophagus Unit, Division of Gastroenterology and Hepatology, Mayo Clinic, Rochester, Minnesota

VIVEK KAUL, MD, FACG
Segal-Watson Professor of Medicine, Chief, Division of Gastroenterology and Hepatology, Center for Advanced Therapeutic Endoscopy, Strong Memorial Hospital, University of Rochester Medical Center, Rochester, New York

ANDREW M. KAZ, MD
R&D Department, VA Puget Sound Health Care System; Clinical Research Division, Fred Hutchinson Cancer Research Center; Department of Internal Medicine, University of Washington School of Medicine, Seattle, Washington

STEPHEN KIM, MD
Clinical Instructor of Medicine, Division of Digestive Diseases, David Geffen School of Medicine at UCLA, Los Angeles, California

SARAH K. KOSSAK, BS
Division of Gastroenterology and Hepatology, Mayo Clinic, Rochester, Minnesota

SHIVANGI KOTHARI, MD
Assistant Professor of Medicine, Associate Director of Endoscopy, Division of Gastroenterology and Hepatology, Center for Advanced Therapeutic Endoscopy, Strong Memorial Hospital, University of Rochester Medical Center, Rochester, New York

KAUSILIA K. KRISHNADATH, MD, PhD
Professor of Translational Gastroenterology, Department of Gastroenterology and Hepatology, Academic Medical Center, Amsterdam, The Netherlands

KLAUS MÖNKEMÜLLER, MD, PhD, FASGE
Professor, Department of Gastroenterology, Basil I. Hirschowitz Endoscopic
Centre of Endoscopic Excellence, University of Alabama at Birmingham, Birmingham,
Alabama

V. RAMAN MUTHUSAMY, MD
Clinical Professor of Medicine, Division of Digestive Diseases, David Geffen School of
Medicine at UCLA, Los Angeles, California

SHAJAN PETER, MD
Associate Professor, Department of Gastroenterology, Basil I. Hirschowitz Endoscopic
Centre of Endoscopic Excellence, University of Alabama at Birmingham, Birmingham,
Alabama

CHRISTIAN G. PEYRE, MD
Assistant Professor, Division of Thoracic and Foregut Surgery, Department of Surgery,
University of Rochester School of Medicine and Dentistry, Rochester, New York

JOEL H. RUBENSTEIN, MD, MSc
Veterans Affairs Center for Clinical Management Research; Barrett's Esophagus
Program, Division of Gastroenterology, University of Michigan Medical School, Ann Arbor,
Michigan

THOMAS M. RUNGE, MD, MPH
Gastroenterology Research Fellow, Division of Gastroenterology and Hepatology, Center
for Esophageal Diseases and Swallowing, University of North Carolina School of
Medicine, University of North Carolina at Chapel Hill, Chapel Hill, North Carolina

NICHOLAS J. SHAHEEN, MD, MPH
Professor of Medicine and Epidemiology; Chief, Division of Gastroenterology and
Hepatology, Center for Esophageal Diseases and Swallowing, University of North
Carolina School of Medicine, University of North Carolina at Chapel Hill, Chapel Hill,
North Carolina

PRATEEK SHARMA, MD
Division of Gastroenterology and Hepatology, Veterans Affairs Medical Center and
University of Kansas, Kansas City, Missouri

RHONDA F. SOUZA, MD
Professor, Division of Gastroenterology and Hepatology, Department of Medicine, Dallas
VA Medical Center, University of Texas Southwestern Medical Center, Dallas, Texas

STUART J. SPECHLER, MD
Professor, Division of Gastroenterology and Hepatology, Department of Medicine, Dallas
VA Medical Center, University of Texas Southwestern Medical Center, Dallas, Texas

MATTHEW D. STACHLER, MD, PhD
Department of Pathology, Brigham and Women's Hospital, Harvard Medical School,
Boston, Massachusetts

MICHAEL B. WALLACE, MD
Professor of Medicine, Division of Gastroenterology and Hepatology, Mayo School of
Medicine, Jacksonville, Florida

KENNETH K. WANG, MD
Professor, Gastroenterology, Mayo Clinic, Rochester, Minnesota

SACHIN WANI, MD
Assistant Professor of Medicine, Division of Gastroenterology and Hepatology, University of Colorado Anschutz Medical Campus, Aurora, Colorado

THOMAS J. WATSON, MD, FACS
Chief, Division of Thoracic and Foregut Surgery; Professor, Department of Surgery, University of Rochester School of Medicine and Dentistry, University of Rochester Medical Center, Rochester, New York

MATTHEW J. WHITSON, MD
Fellow, Division of Gastroenterology, Hospital of the University of Pennsylvania, University of Pennsylvania Perelman School of Medicine, Philadelphia, Pennsylvania

MUHAMMAD H. ZEB, MD
Division of Gastroenterology and Hepatology, Mayo Clinic, Rochester, Minnesota

Contents

Barrett's esophagus (BE) is the precursor to esophageal adenocarcinoma (EAC), a disease with increasing burden in the Western world, especially in white men. Risk factors for BE include obesity, tobacco smoking, and gastroesophageal reflux disease (GERD). EAC is the most common form of esophageal cancer in the United States. Risk factors include GERD, tobacco smoking, and obesity, whereas nonsteroidal antiinflammatory drugs and statins may be protective. Factors predicting progression from nondysplastic BE to EAC include dysplastic changes on esophageal histology and length of the involved BE segment. Biomarkers have shown promise, but none are approved for clinical use.

This article focuses on recent findings on the molecular mechanisms involved in esophageal columnar metaplasia. Signaling pathways and their downstream targets activate specific transcription factors leading to the expression of columnar and the more specific intestinal-type of genes, which gives rise to Barrett metaplasia. Several animal models have been generated to validate and study these distinct molecular pathways but also to identify the Barrett progenitor cell. Currently, the many aspects involved in the development of esophageal metaplasia that have been elucidated can serve to develop novel molecular therapies to improve treatment or prevent metaplasia. Nevertheless, several key events are still poorly understood and require further investigation.

Central obesity is involved in the pathogenesis and progression of Barrett's esophagus to esophageal adenocarcinoma. Involved are likely both mechanical and nonmechanical effects. Mechanical effects of increased abdominal fat cause disruption of the gastroesophageal reflux barrier leading to increased reflux events. Nonmechanical effects may be mediated by inflammation, via classically activated macrophages, pro-inflammatory cytokines, and adipokines such as Leptin, all of which likely potentiate reflux-mediated inflammation. Insulin resistance, associated with central obesity, is also associated with both Barrett's pathogenesis and progression to adenocarcinoma. Molecular pathways activated in obesity, inflammation and insulin resistance overlap with those involved in Barrett's pathogenesis and progression.

There is substantial interest in identifying patients with premalignant conditions such as Barrett's esophagus (BE), to improve outcomes of subjects with esophageal adenocarcinoma. However, there is limited consensus on the rationale for screening, the appropriate target population, and optimal screening modality. Recent progress in the development and validation of minimally invasive tools for BE screening has reinvigorated interest in BE screening. BE risk scores combining clinical, anthropometric, and laboratory variables are being developed that may allow more precise targeting of screening to high-risk individuals. This article reviews and summarizes data on recent progress and challenges in screening for BE.

Surveillance of Barrett's esophagus for preventing death from esophageal adenocarcinoma is attractive and widely practiced. However, empirical evidence supporting its effectiveness is weak. Longer intervals between surveillance examinations are being recommended, supported by computer simulation analyses. If surveillance is performed, an adequate number of biopsies should be performed or the effect of surveillance would be squandered.

The prevalence of esophageal adenocarcinoma is increasing dramatically. Barrett's esophagus remains the most well-established risk factor for the development of esophageal adenocarcinoma. There are multiple clinical, endoscopic, and pathologic factors that increase the risk of neoplastic progression to high-grade dysplasia or esophageal adenocarcinoma in Barrett's esophagus. This article reviews both risk and protective factors for neoplastic progression in patients with Barrett's esophagus.

A major paradigm shift has occurred in the management of dysplastic Barrett's esophagus (BE) and early esophageal carcinoma. Endoscopic therapy has now emerged as the standard of care for this disease entity. Endoscopic resection techniques like endoscopic mucosal resection and endoscopic submucosal dissection combined with ablation techniques help achieve long-term curative success comparable with surgical outcomes, in this subgroup of patients. This article is an in-depth review of these endoscopic resection techniques, highlighting their role and value in the overall management of BE-related dysplasia and neoplasia.

Barrett's esophagus (BE) is more common in developed countries. Endoscopic therapy is an effective treatment method in management of dysplastic BE. Ablation by thermal energy, freezing, or photochemical injury completely eradicates dysplasia and specialized intestinal metaplasia resulting in neosquamation of esophagus. Among the ablative modalities, radiofrequency ablation (RFA) is the most studied with safe, effective, and durable long-term outcomes. Cryotherapy, argon plasma coagulation, and photodynamic therapy can be offered in select patients when RFA is unavailable, has failed, or is contraindicated. Future research on natural disease progression, biomarkers, advanced imaging, and application of endoscopic techniques will lead to better clinical outcomes for BE-associated neoplasia.

Barrett's esophagus is the only identifiable premalignant condition for esophageal adenocarcinoma. Endoscopic eradication therapy (EET) has revolutionized the management of Barrett's-related dysplasia and intramucosal cancer. The primary goal of EET is to prevent progression to invasive esophageal adenocarcinoma and ultimately improve survival rates. There are several challenges with EET that can be encountered before, during, or after the procedure that are important to understand to optimize the effectiveness and safety of EET and ultimately improve patient outcomes. This article focuses on the challenges with EET and discusses them under the categories of preprocedural, intraprocedural, and postprocedural challenges.

Esophageal adenocarcinoma (EAC) has increased dramatically in the past 3 decades, making its precursor lesion Barrett's esophagus (BE) an important clinical problem. Effective interventions are available, but overall outcomes remain unchanged. Most of the BE population remains undiagnosed; most EACs are diagnosed late, and most BE patients will never progress to cancer. These epidemiologic factors make upper endoscopy an inefficient and ineffective strategy for BE diagnosis and risk stratification. In the current review, biomarkers for diagnosis, risk stratification, and predictors of response to therapy in BE are discussed.

Chemoprevention in Barrett's esophagus is currently applied only in research settings. Identifying pathways that can be targeted by safe, pharmaceutical or natural compounds is key to expanding the scope of chemoprevention. Defining meaningful surrogate markers of cancer progression is critical to test the efficacy of chemopreventive approaches. Combinatorial chemoprevention that targets multiple components of the same pathway or parallel pathways could reduce the risk and improve the efficacy of chemoprevention. Here we discuss the role of chemoprevention as an independent or an adjuvant management option in BE-associated esophageal adenocarcinoma.

Proton pump inhibitors (PPIs) may protect against carcinogenesis in Barrett's esophagus because they eliminate the chronic esophageal inflammation of reflux esophagitis, and because they decrease esophageal exposure to acid, which can cause cancer-promoting DNA damage and increase proliferation in Barrett's metaplasia. Most clinical studies of PPIs and cancer development in Barrett's esophagus have found a cancer-protective effect for these drugs, although there are some contradictory data. Chemoprevention of dysplasia and cancer in Barrett's esophagus with PPIs appears to be cost-effective, and the indirect evidence supporting a cancer-protective role for PPIs is strong enough to warrant PPI treatment of virtually all patients with Barrett's esophagus.

Approximately 10% to 15% of the chronic gastroesophageal reflux disease population is at risk for the development of Barrett's esophagus, particularly in the setting of other risk factors, including male gender, Caucasian race, age more than 50, and central obesity. The risk of cancer progression for patients with nondysplastic BE has been estimated to be approximately 0.2% to 0.5% per year. Given these low progression rates and the high cost of endoscopic surveillance, cost-effectiveness analyses in this area are useful to determine appropriate resource allocation.

Barrett's esophagus (BE) is present in up to 5.6% of the US population and is the precursor lesion for esophageal adenocarcinoma. Surveillance endoscopy is the primary management approach for BE. However, standard protocol biopsies have been associated with significant miss rates of dysplastic lesions in patients with BE. Thus, a variety of methods to optimize the imaging of BE have been developed to improve the efficiency and diagnostic yield of surveillance endoscopy in detecting early neoplasia. These techniques use changes that occur at macroscopic, microscopic, and subcellular levels in early neoplasia and are the focus of this article.

Patients with gastroesophageal reflux disease and Barrett's esophagus can be a management challenge for the treating physician or surgeon.

The goals of therapy include relief of reflux symptoms, induction of histologic regression, and prevention of progression of intestinal metaplasia to dysplasia or invasive carcinoma. Antireflux surgery is effective at achieving these end points, although ongoing follow-up and endoscopic surveillance are essential. In cases of dysplasia or early esophageal neoplasia associated with Barrett's esophagus, endoscopic resection and ablation have supplanted esophagectomy as the standard of care in most cases. Esophageal resection continues to have a role, however, in a minority of appropriately selected candidates.

Esophageal adenocarcinoma (EAC) develops from Barrett's esophagus (BE), wherein normal squamous epithelia is replaced by specialized intestinal metaplasia in response to chronic gastroesophageal acid reflux. BE can progress to low- and high-grade dysplasia, intramucosal, and invasive carcinoma. Both BE and EAC are characterized by loss of heterozygosity, aneuploidy, specific genetic mutations, and clonal diversity. Given the limitations of histopathology, genomic and epigenomic analyses may improve the precision of risk stratification. Assays to detect molecular alterations associated with neoplastic progression could be used to improve the pathologic assessment of BE/EAC and to select high-risk patients for more intensive surveillance.

GASTROENTEROLOGY
CLINICS OF NORTH AMERICA

RELATED INTEREST

Gastrointestinal Endoscopy Clinics of North America
October 2014 (Vol. 24, Issue 4)
Esophageal Function Testing
John Pandolfino, *Editor*

Foreword

Barrett's Esophagus

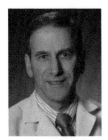

Gary W. Falk, MD, MS
Consulting Editor

The incidence of esophageal adenocarcinoma continues to increase at an alarming rate in the Western world. While the prognosis for early esophageal adenocarcinoma is excellent, the long-term survival of advanced cases remains problematic. Barrett's esophagus is the precursor lesion for esophageal adenocarcinoma, and our approach to both Barrett's esophagus and esophageal adenocarcinoma has changed dramatically in recent years. Key advances in the field, such as high-definition endoscopy, endoscopic mucosal resection, and radiofrequency ablation, have revolutionized the detection and treatment of dysplasia and early neoplasia. However, other areas in Barrett's esophagus remain problematic, including our understanding of the cell or origin, risk factors for the disease and its progression, better population-based screening, and more rational surveillance techniques.

Drs Prasad Iyer and Navtej Buttar have assembled an outstanding group of experts to address many of the challenging issues in the field of Barrett's esophagus today. This issue celebrates some of the advances in our understanding and approach to this disease as well as highlights areas of uncertainty where progress is still needed. These state-of-the-art reviews provide a superb foundation as we try to address the many unresolved issues in the field of Barrett's esophagus.

Gary W. Falk, MD, MS
Division of Gastroenterology
University of Pennsylvania
Perelman School of Medicine
9th Floor, Penn Tower
1 Convention Avenue
Philadelphia, PA 19104-4311, USA

E-mail address:
gary.falk@uphs.upenn.edu

Gastroenterol Clin N Am 44 (2015) xiii
http://dx.doi.org/10.1016/j.gtc.2015.03.003
0889-8553/15/$ – see front matter © 2015 Published by Elsevier Inc.

gastro.theclinics.com

Preface

Barrett's Esophagus: New Insights and Progress

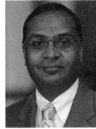 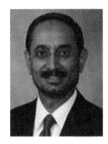

Prasad G. Iyer, MD, MSc, FACG, FASGE, AGAF   Navtej S. Buttar, MD
Editors

Barrett's esophagus (BE) is currently a field in rapid evolution. A number of well established paradigms have been recently challenged with new insights being gained in several areas, such as pathogenesis, screening, and therapy. In this issue of *Gastroenterology Clinics of North America*, we attempt to succinctly summarize and describe challenges being posed to these long-established dogmas by intriguing new data. We also outline new developments that have the potential of greatly expanding our understanding of the pathogenesis, early detection, risk stratification, and treatment of subjects with BE with and without dysplasia/neoplasia.

In this issue, we have brought together established and emerging thought leaders in the field to elucidate this new information. Our topics range from pathogenesis and epidemiology of BE, the strong relationship between obesity and BE, new developments in the early detection of BE to risk stratification with biomarkers, novel advanced imaging techniques and therapy of dysplasia, and neoplasia in BE, including both endoscopy and surgery. Despite impressive advances in the therapeutic armamentarium of BE-related dysplasia, several challenges continue to exist and emerge, which are outlined in a separate article. We also focus on summarizing the current status of chemoprevention, cost effectiveness of current therapeutic approaches in BE, with a final summary of emerging molecular technology (such as genomics), which has the potential of providing insights into hitherto unexplored areas in BE, such as markers to assess cancer risk and progression in BE.

We hope that this issue of *Gastroenterology Clinics of North America* will prove a valuable and indispensable resource to gastroenterologists who have a clinical and research interest in BE. In addition, we also have outlined the research agenda for

Gastroenterol Clin N Am 44 (2015) xv–xvi
http://dx.doi.org/10.1016/j.gtc.2015.03.002
0889-8553/15/$ – see front matter © 2015 Published by Elsevier Inc.

gastro.theclinics.com

the next decade in this exciting field, which we hope will enable reducing the incidence and mortality of esophageal adenocarcinoma.

Prasad G. Iyer, MD, MSc, FACG, FASGE, AGAF
200 1st Street SW
Rochester, MN 55905, USA

Navtej S. Buttar, MD
200 1st Street SW
Rochester, MN 55905, USA

E-mail addresses:
iyer.prasad@mayo.edu (P.G. Iyer)
buttar.navtej@mayo.edu (N.S. Buttar)

Epidemiology of Barrett's Esophagus and Esophageal Adenocarcinoma

Thomas M. Runge, MD, MPH[a], Julian A. Abrams, MD, MS[b],
Nicholas J. Shaheen, MD, MPH[a],*

KEYWORDS

- Barrett's esophagus • Esophageal adenocarcinoma
- Gastroesophageal reflux disease • Epithelium

KEY POINTS

- Barrett's esophagus is a precursor to esophageal adenocarcinoma (EAC).
- The incidence of EAC has increased dramatically and EAC is now the most common form of esophageal cancer in the United States.
- The strongest risk factor for Barrett's esophagus is gastroesophageal reflux (GERD), but central adiposity and tobacco smoking also increase risk.
- Risk factors for EAC include GERD, tobacco smoking, and obesity, whereas *Helicobacter pylori* and nonsteroidal antiinflammatory drugs may be protective.
- Dysplastic changes seen on biopsy predict progression of Barrett's to EAC, but estimates of the incidence of EAC in dysplastic Barrett's epithelium vary.

INTRODUCTION

Barrett's esophagus (BE) is a condition in which the typical squamous epithelium of the esophageal mucosa is replaced with columnar intestinal epithelium.[1,2] BE is a known precursor to the development of esophageal adenocarcinoma (EAC), a

Disclosures: Dr N.J. Shaheen receives research funding from Covidien Medical, CSA Medical, NeoGenomics, Takeda Pharmaceuticals, and Oncoscope. He is a consultant for Oncoscope. Dr J.A. Abrams receives research funding from Covidien Medical, CSA Medical, C2 Therapeutics, and Trio Medicines. He is also a consultant for C2 Therapeutics. Dr T.M. Runge has no conflicts to declare.

This research was funded by T32 DK07634 (Robert Sandler) and K24DK100548 (Nicholas Shaheen).
[a] Division of Gastroenterology and Hepatology, Center for Esophageal Diseases and Swallowing, University of North Carolina School of Medicine, University of North Carolina at Chapel Hill, CB#7080, Chapel Hill, NC 27599-7080, USA; [b] Division of Digestive and Liver Diseases, Columbia University Medical Center, 622 West 168th Street, PH 7W-318D, New York, NY 10032, USA
* Corresponding author.
E-mail address: nshaheen@med.unc.edu

malignancy with a dramatically increasing incidence over the past 40 years.[3–5] The risk of EAC among patients with BE is estimated to be 30-fold to 125-fold greater than that of the general population.[6] Endoscopically, the prevalence of BE has been estimated at 1% to 2% in all patients receiving endoscopy for any indication, and from 5% to 15% in patients with symptoms of gastroesophageal reflux disease (GERD).[7] Although uncommon, EAC has a poor prognosis, and is associated with a 5-year survival rate of less than 20%.[8,9]

The incidence of EAC in patients with BE is considerably higher than that in the general population, but only a minority of patients with BE develop EAC, with annual risk estimated at 0.1% to 0.5%.[10,11] Reasons for the rapid increase in the incidence of EAC are not entirely known. However, risk factors for the development of BE and EAC have been identified. Similarly, risk factors for the progression of BE to EAC have also been identified, and are discussed here.

Epidemiology of Barrett's Esophagus

Prevalence and incidence of Barrett's esophagus

BE primarily affects older adults in the developed world. The prevalence in living adults is difficult to ascertain, because individuals with Barrett's are often asymptomatic and do not seek care. One of the earliest estimates of the prevalence of BE was via an autopsy study.[12] Cameron and colleagues[12] estimated a prevalence of long-segment BE (LSBE) of 376 cases per 100,000, or roughly 0.4% of the population, and suggested that only a small minority of cases were detected clinically. Population-based studies have provided estimates of the prevalence of BE in the general public. A Swedish study by Ronkainen and colleagues[13] estimated the prevalence of BE by performing upper endoscopy on 1000 randomly selected adults. These investigators found BE in 16 (1.6%) of the individuals, with 5 subjects (0.5%) in their study showing long-segment disease.[13]

Tertiary care center endoscopy studies have also attempted to estimate the prevalence of BE. Rex and colleagues[14] performed upper endoscopy in 961 individuals presenting for routine screening colonoscopy. These investigators found an overall prevalence of BE of 6.8%, or 65 of 961 individuals, of whom 12 (1.2%) had LSBE. In patients who reported heartburn, the prevalence was slightly higher at 8.3%, but most of the patients (54%) who were found to have BE reported no reflux symptoms. These estimates may be higher than the prevalence in the general population, because this tertiary center population of volunteers may have had more GERD than a random sample of the adult population. Zagari and colleagues[15] analyzed 1033 patients originally identified as part of a large multicenter cross-sectional study on gallstone disease. Of these patients, 1.3% (13) had histologically confirmed BE, whereas 0.2% (2) had LSBE. These estimates suggest that the prevalence of BE is between 0.5% and 2% of unselected individuals. In individuals with reflux symptoms, prevalence estimates are more variable (**Table 1**), ranging from 5% to 15%.[16]

Given that the use of endoscopy depends on the patient's socioeconomic status, access to care, and other nonmedical factors, the incidence of BE has historically been difficult to ascertain. However, the incidence of endoscopically detected BE seems to have increased dramatically over the past 30 years, a finding that is partially attributable to the increasing frequency of endoscopy during the same period.[17] However, data from the United Kingdom[18] and the Netherlands[19] suggest that incidence rates of BE have increased even after controlling for increasing endoscopy rates. These estimates place the increase in BE incidence at near 65% between 1997 and 2002[19] and 159% between 1993 and 2005. Alarmingly, the greatest proportional

Table 1
Studies examining the prevalence of BE

Authors, Year	Country	Setting, Design	Study Sample	Sample Size	% Male	Average Age (y)	Histologic Confirmation	No. with BE (%)	No. with LSBE (%)	No. with SSBE (%)
Gerson et al,[157] 2002	United States	Single VA center, not population based	Individuals without GERD sx receiving sigmoidoscopy for CRC screening	110	92.0	61.0	Yes	27 (24.5)	19 (17.3)	8 (7.3)
Rex et al,[14] 2003	United States	Multicenter, not population based	Individuals receiving colonoscopy, no GI sx other than reflux or regurgitation	961	59.5	59.0	Yes	65 (6.8)[a]	12 (1.2)	53 (5.5)
Ronkainen et al,[13] 2005	United States	Population-based sample from 2 Swedish communities	Random sample of census-based registry	1000	49.0	53.6	Yes	16 (1.6)[b]	5 (0.5)	11 (1.1)
Ward et al,[158] 2006	United States	Single tertiary care center, not population based	Individuals referred for screening colonoscopy	300	53.7	61.0	Yes	50 (16.7)[c]	4 (1.3)	46 (15.3)
Zagari et al,[15] 2008	Italy	Population-based sample from 2 Italian communities	Individuals remaining from original sample who elected to participate	1033	51.1	59.7	Yes	13 (1.3)[d]	2 (0.2)	11 (1.1)
Zou et al,[159] 2011	China	Population-based sample from 2 Chinese areas	Individuals remaining from random sample who elected to participate	1030	42.3	NR	No	19 (1.8)[e]	NR	NR

Abbreviations: CRC, colorectal cancer; GI, gastrointestinal; NR, not reported; SSBE, short-segment BE; sx, symptoms; VA, Veterans' Affairs.
[a] Prevalence among those with GERD symptoms was 8.3%.
[b] Prevalence among those with GERD symptoms was 2.3%.
[c] Prevalence among those with GERD symptoms was 19.8%.
[d] Prevalence among those with GERD symptoms was 1.5%.
[e] Prevalence among those with GERD symptoms was 2.1%.
Data from Refs.[13–15,157–159]

increase in BE diagnosis was in individuals less than 60 years of age, which is in agreement with other work from Europe.[18]

Age, sex, and ethnic variations in Barrett's esophagus

Men, especially white men, have a strong predilection for the development of BE, with a male/female ratio of 2:1 to 3:1 in most studies (**Table 2**).[1,20] Age at diagnosis can vary widely, because many individuals are asymptomatic and undergo diagnostic endoscopy for other reasons.[21] BE on average is diagnosed in the sixth to seventh decade of life, but may develop earlier.[22] In addition to the greater overall prevalence of BE in men, there is evidence that men develop the disease earlier than women. From a British endoscopy center, Van Blankenstein and colleagues[22] reviewed endoscopy records and histology reports of individuals who received upper endoscopy at a single center. Men on average developed BE about 20 years earlier than women in that study. The overall ratio of BE cases was 2:1 favoring men, but in younger adults the ratio of men to women approached 4:1.[22] A similar trend to early development of BE in men was seen in follow-up studies from Europe.[18,19] White people in general are disproportionately affected compared with other races.[23] In a large cross-sectional study, Ford and colleagues,[24] in a sample from the United Kingdom, found that white people had significantly higher prevalence of BE compared with Asians or Afro-Caribbean people. In that population, LSBE was found in 2.9% of white people, compared with 0.31% of Asians and 0.2% of Afro-Caribbean people.

Studies assessing BE prevalence in Latin Americans also show that BE is considerably less prevalent in Latin Americans compared with white people. In a large study by Abrams and colleagues,[25] the prevalence of BE was significantly lower among those of Latin American background than among white people (1.7% vs 6.1%). Other studies have corroborated variations in BE prevalence among ethnic groups living in the same country, possibly suggesting an effect of as-yet unrecognized polygenetic factors across different ethnicities.

Multiple environmental factors are strongly associated with BE. These factors, such as obesity, GERD, and hiatal hernias, are more common in developed countries. However, genetic factors are likely also at play. Work from twin studies suggests that symptoms of GERD, even when adjusted for obesity and other clinical factors, are more concordant in monozygotic twins than in dizygotic twins.[26]

Selected risk factors for Barrett's esophagus development

Gastroesophageal reflux disease GERD is a central risk factor for BE development. Numerous case-control studies have shown that individuals with GERD are 6 to 8 times more likely to have BE, and the propensity to develop BE increases with more severe symptoms (see **Table 1**).[27–29] Longer duration of GERD may create an environment conducive to the development of BE.[30] However, the presence of reflux symptoms is neither sensitive nor specific for pathologic acid reflux,[31,32] and symptom severity does not correlate well with BE risk.[33,34] Some work has suggested that patients with more significant symptoms may be less likely to have BE,[35] perhaps because of impaired acid sensitivity of the columnar metaplasia compared with normal squamous epithelium. However, longer duration of GERD symptoms predicts increased likelihood of BE.[27] A systematic review on the association between symptoms and BE found no association between reflux symptoms and short-segment BE (SSBE) (odds ratio [OR], 1.15; 95% confidence interval [CI], 0.8–1.7) but found increased odds of LSBE in those with reflux symptoms (OR, 4.92; 95% CI, 2.0, 12.0).[36] Because screening programs target both SSBE and LSBE, significant limitations in using symptom severity remain. When patients with Barrett's are compared

Table 2
Reported risk factors for BE, with magnitudes of association represented as odds ratios (ORs)

Risk Factor	Study, Year	Total (n)	Study Type	Comparison Groups	OR (95% CI)
Symptomatic GERD	Anderson et al,[29] 2007	711	Case control	Population controls, asymptomatic	12.0 (7.6, 18.8)
	Johansson et al,[28] 2007	764	Cross sectional	Population controls, asymptomatic	10.7 (3.5, 33.4)
	Conio et al,[27] 2002	457	Case control	Healthy controls	5.8 (4.0, 8.4)
White race	Ford et al,[24] 2005	20,310	Cross sectional	Afro-Caribbean race	12.2[a]
	Ford et al,[24] 2005	20,310	Cross sectional	South Asian race	6.0 (3.6, 10.2)
	Abrams et al,[25] 2008	2100	Cross sectional	Black people	2.9[a]
	Abrams et al,[25] 2008	2100	Cross sectional	Hispanic people	2.6[a]
Male gender	Ford et al,[24] 2005	20,310	Cross sectional	Female gender	2.7 (2.2, 3.4)
	Van Blankenstein et al,[22] 2005	21,899	Cross sectional	Female gender	2.1 (1.8, 2.6)
	Cook et al,[160] 2005	18,765	Meta-analysis	Female gender	2.0 (1.8, 2.2)
	Abrams et al,[25] 2008	2100	Cross sectional	Female gender	1.9 (1.2, 2.9)
Central adiposity[b]	Edelstein et al,[44] 2007	404	Case control	Low WHR	2.4 (1.4, 3.9)
	Corley et al,[161] 2007	636	Nested case control	Abdominal circumference <80 cm	2.2 (1.1, 3.7)
	Kubo et al,[46] 2013	2502	Pooled analysis	Lowest quartile waist circumference, men	2.2 (1.1–4.7)
				Lowest quartile waist circumference, women	3.8 (1.5, 9.6)
Cigarette smoking	Cook et al,[53] 2012	3534	Pooled analysis	Population controls, nonsmokers	1.7 (1.0, 2.7)
	Steevens et al,[49] 2011	120,852	Prospective cohort	Population controls, nonsmokers	1.3 (1.0, 1.8)
	Thrift et al,[51] 2014	1856	Case control	Primary care controls, nonsmokers	0.8 (0.5, 1.3)
				Elective EGD controls, nonsmokers	1.1 (0.8–1.5)
Helicobacter pylori	Corley et al,[56] 2008	617	Case control	Population controls	0.4 (0.3, 0.7)
	Wang et al,[59] 2009	3529	Meta-analysis	Endoscopically normal controls	0.7 (0.4–1.4)
				Healthy blood donors	2.2 (1.1, 4.6)
Low birth weight	Forssell et al,[62] 2013	1183	Case control	Matched controls	8.2 (2.8, 23.9)
Obstructive sleep apnea	Leggett et al,[64] 2014	188	Case control	Randomly matched controls	1.8 (1.1, 3.2)

Abbreviations: CI, confidence interval; EGD, esophagogastroduodenoscopy; WHR, waist/hip ratio.
[a] CI not available.
[b] Reported magnitude of risk of higher group category (high WHR, high abdominal circumference).
Data from Refs.[22,24,25,27–29,44,46,49,51,53,56,59,62,64,160,161]

with those without, the patients with BE have abundant evidence of aberrant acid exposure: longer episodes of acid exposure, lower pH, and also weak peristaltic contractions and decreased baseline lower esophageal sphincter (LES) tone.[37,38]

Although epidemiologic data suggest that gastric acid suppression with proton pump inhibitors (PPIs) may reduce the chance of developing dysplasia and cancer,[39] the impact PPI use has on development of BE is unknown. Among the many adults who have GERD, only a minority develop BE. The prevalence of BE among those with reflux symptoms is higher than that of the general population, but the relationship is not fully explained by GERD. Obesity may be a common mediator of both GERD and BE. Central adiposity is known to predispose to hiatal hernia development[7] and increased GERD symptoms,[40] and even to directly cause LES relaxations.[41]

In summary, reflux is associated with GERD. However, symptoms of reflux cannot reliably distinguish patients with increased acid reflux from those without. It is likely that a genetic milieu predisposing to the development of BE combined with prolonged acid exposure and mutagenic events, including oxidative stress, may act synergistically in patients who develop EAC.

Obesity Obesity, measured by body mass index (BMI) and central adiposity, has been studied extensively as a risk factor for BE. The incidence of BE and EAC have increased dramatically in the past 40 to 50 years in Western societies, concurrent with rapid increases in the rate of obesity. From 1976 to 1991, the prevalence of obesity at all ages increased from 25% to 33%, and it now approaches 35% in adults.[42] Obesity can be assessed in several ways. High BMIs, and especially central adiposity, have been shown to have a significant association with BE. A 2009 meta-analysis that included 11 observational studies showed an increase in the risk of BE (OR, 1.4) in patients with a BMI greater than 30 kg/m^2 compared with those with BMI less than 30 kg/m^2.[43] Patients with BE have been shown to have higher BMIs than either general controls or individuals with GERD but not BE.[44,45]

Because BMI does not take into account the distribution of body fat, the estimated risk increase in the obese may be poorly estimated by BMI measurements. More recent work has shown that central adiposity, rather than BMI, may be the driver of increased BE risk. Edelstein and colleagues,[44] in a case-control study in 2007, found that the overall risk of BE was significantly greater in those with high waist/hip ratios (WHRs) (OR, 2.4); the risk of LSBE in these patients was even higher (OR, 4.3). A pooled analysis by Kubo and colleagues[46] found that waist circumference, as a proxy measure for central adiposity, increased risk for BE for men (OR, 2.24) and women (OR, 3.75). The impact of obesity on BE risk may vary by race as well. In a US case-control study, Kramer and colleagues[23] studied the effect of BMI and WHR on BE prevalence, and the relationship between WHR and BE was strongest and most significant in white people (OR, 2.5), whereas in African Americans and Latin Americans the associations were not significant. Because the strength of the relationship between WHR and BE was strongest in white people, it was suggested that other ethnic groups could potentially carry as-yet unrecognized genes that protect against BE development.[23] It is possible that the overwhelming male predominance among EAC cases could be explained in part by overweight men distributing fat preferentially to their trunks, and this central adiposity drives the risk increase.[47]

Alcohol Alcohol use has been studied extensively as a possible risk factor for BE.[13,27,48-50] Multiple studies have shown no association between the two, but results have been variable.[48,49,51] Some work has suggested an inverse correlation between wine intake and BE risk.[48] The most robust evidence comes from the Barrett's and

Esophageal Adenocarcinoma Consortium (BEACON) consortium, in which the data from 5 studies were pooled to assess risk of alcohol use.[50] Among 1028 cases and 1282 controls, alcohol use was stratified by gender and by number of drinks per day. There was a borderline significant inverse correlation between BE and any degree of alcohol intake (OR, 0.77, 0.60–1.00). Drinking 3 to less than 5 drinks per day was associated with a statistically significant reduction in BE risk (OR, 0.57, 0.38–0.86), but with more or less alcohol consumed no statistically significant results were found (although there was a trend toward an inverse relationship). When assessing beverage-specific data, wine consumption was associated with an inverse risk of BE (OR, 0.71).[46,48]

At this point the preponderance of evidence supports no association between alcohol intake and BE risk. What was once thought to be a minor risk factor for BE now seems to confer no additional risk. Alcohol might be protective, but in order to fully answer this question, more data are needed.

Cigarette smoking Most studies have found an association between cigarette smoking and an increased risk of developing BE.[52,53] A pooled analysis of 5 case-control studies found a consistent increase in risk of BE over several pack-year cut points, with ORs ranging from 1.44 to 1.99 (**Fig. 1**).[53] However, there was significant heterogeneity between studies, and exclusion of a single study yielded pooled ORs with a higher magnitude across all exposure groups, ranging from 1.75 to 2.89, with an average OR of 2.09.[53] To explore a possible synergistic effect between GERD and tobacco use in the genesis of BE, these investigators conducted additional modeling to assess the concurrent effects of smoking and GERD.[53] The OR of Barrett's increased significantly when both GERD and smoking were present, compared with when smokers did not have GERD.

However, not all studies have identified smoking as a risk factor for BE. Thrift and colleagues[51] studied 258 patients with BE in a case-control study from Houston, Texas. These patients were compared with 2 control groups: one group was composed of patients receiving elective esophagogastroduodenoscopy for any indication, and the other was composed of primary care patients undergoing screening colonoscopy. These researchers found no association between smoking and BE in either group, even when stratified by pack-year exposures, length of time smoking, or number of cigarettes per day. In a prospective study design, Steevens and colleagues[49] found ORs of 1.33 in former smokers and 0.93 in current smokers compared with controls. In conclusion, smoking seems to increase risk of BE, but there is wide variability in risk estimates. Further study may clarify the precise role of tobacco in BE pathogenesis.

Helicobacter pylori Helicobacter pylori (H pylori) infection causes chronic gastritis, peptic ulcer disease, and gastric adenocarcinoma. H pylori is known to have a strong association with intestinal metaplasia in the body and antrum of the stomach.[54] Temporal associations have been made between the decreasing prevalence of H pylori infection in developed countries and the increasing prevalence of EAC.[55] Corley and colleagues[56] showed that H pylori was inversely associated with BE (OR, 0.42) in a case-control study design. Although the mechanisms underlying this inverse association are not fully understood, they may relate to decreased acid production in the setting of H pylori infection (especially with associated atrophic gastritis) or via alterations in the microbiome.

Different strains of H pylori may have different abilities to induce risk. The presence of the cytotoxin-associated gene (CagA) identifies H pylori strains more likely to induce gastritis, more extensive gastric inflammation, and gastric cancer.[57] Vaezi and colleagues[58] addressed the role of H pylori in a case-control study, and found that

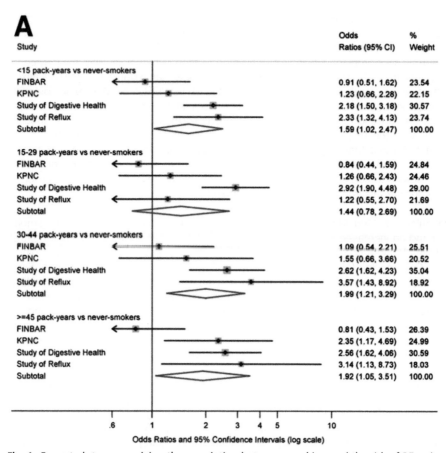

Fig. 1. Forrest plots summarizing the association between smoking and the risk of BE, using population controls. Smoking exposure is grouped by categories. Large unfilled diamonds represent the pooled estimates across all studies within that category. The width of the diamonds represents the 95% CIs. Black squares indicate the point estimate for each individual study. FINBAR, Factors Influencing the Barrett's/Adenocarcinoma Relationship; KPNC, Kaiser Permanente Northern California; UNC, University of North Carolina. (*Adapted from* Cook MB, Shaheen NJ, Anderson LA, et al. Cigarette smoking increases risk of Barrett's esophagus: an analysis of the Barrett's and Esophageal Adenocarcinoma Consortium. Gastroenterology 2012;142:749; with permission.)

patients with BE identified at endoscopy were about 3-fold less likely to be colonized by CagA-positive strains than were controls who did not have BE. However, contradictory findings were noted in a 2009 meta-analysis by Wang and colleagues.[59] Among included studies using endoscopically normal controls, the prevalence of *H pylori* in controls was greater than that in BE, but among those that use healthy blood donors as controls, patients with BE more frequently had *H pylori* infection. The result was a nonsignificant slight trend toward less *H pylori* infection in patients with BE.[59] The investigators cited a need for further study with well-matched cases and controls to make robust conclusions about an association between *H pylori* and BE.

Other possible risk factors Recently, several other possible risk factors for BE have been studied. Low birth weight has been posited as a possible risk factor for BE given the apparent association between preterm birth and systemic inflammation.[60] Forssell and colleagues[61] showed in a Swedish birth cohort that prematurity is associated with the risk of developing esophagitis; a relationship that is most pronounced among those who are small for gestational age (OR, 2.5) or who are born at less than or equal to 32 weeks' gestation (OR, 6.7).[61] Follow-up research by this group suggested that the risk of BE was significantly increased in patients with the lowest birth weights (OR, 8.2).[62] The risk of EAC seems to be increased with reduced gestational time, but the magnitude of effect is smaller (OR, 1.1).[63]

Other factors associated with a proinflammatory state, such as obstructive sleep apnea (OSA) and the metabolic syndrome, seem to increase the risk of BE as well. In a case-control study, Leggett and colleagues[64] found that OSA was associated with an increased risk of BE (OR, 1.8), after controlling for GERD and obesity. Increased levels of adipokines and cytokines have also been found in patients with BE compared with controls.[65] These inflammatory markers may be the intermediaries partially responsible for the increased BE risk seen in individuals with central obesity, OSA, or GERD.

Epidemiology of Esophageal Adenocarcinoma

Prevalence and incidence of esophageal adenocarcinoma

EAC was once a rare form of esophageal malignancy. Surgical series in the early twentieth century showed that EAC made up only 0.8% to 3.7% of all esophageal malignancies.[66] However, by 1990, EAC overtook squamous cell carcinoma of the esophagus, and is now the more common of the two in developed nations.[67] EAC continues to increase in incidence (**Figs. 2** and **3**). In 2014, there are expected to be 18,170 new esophageal cancers diagnosed in the United States.[68] About 15,000 individuals will die from esophageal cancer in 2014, and more than half of these will be from EAC.[68,69]

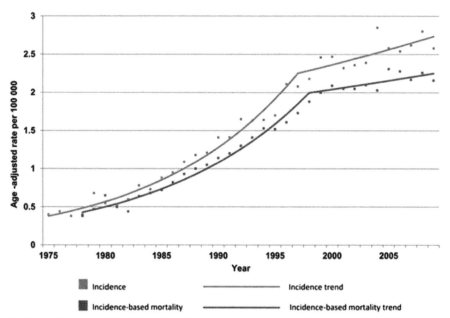

Fig. 2. Incidence and incidence-based mortality from EAC, 1975 to 2009. Produced from SEER 9 data. (*From* Hur C, Miller M, Kong CY, et al. Trends in esophageal adenocarcinoma incidence and mortality. Cancer 2013;119(6):1152; with permission.)

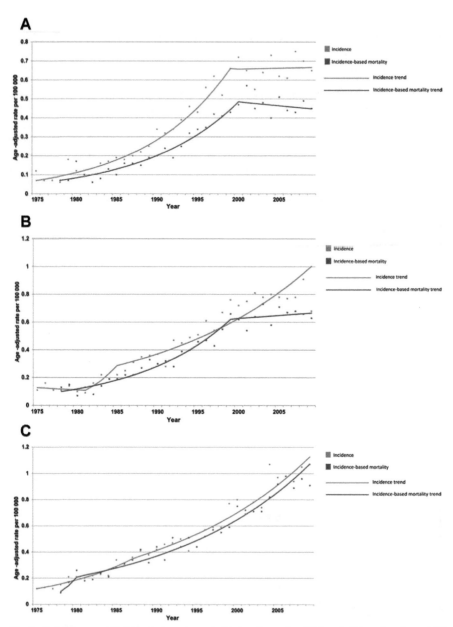

Fig. 3. Incidence and incidence-based mortality by stage, for (*A*) local, (*B*) regional, and (*C*) distant spread of disease. Produced from SEER 9 data. (*From* Hur C, Miller M, Kong CY, et al. Trends in esophageal adenocarcinoma incidence and mortality. Cancer 2013;119(6):1154; with permission.)

Age, sex, and ethnic variations

Esophageal cancer in general affects men in a 4:1 ratio compared with women.[68] With EAC, incidence is highest in white men, with a male/female ratio in white people that approaches 8:1 (See **Table 3**).[70–72] The reported incidence of EAC has risen

Table 3
Reported risk factors for EAC, with magnitudes of association represented as ORs

Risk Factor	Study, Year	Total (n)	Study Type	Comparison Groups	OR (95% CI)
Symptomatic GERD	Lagergren et al,[82] 1999	1271	Case control	Population controls, asymptomatic	43.5[a] (18.3, 103.5)
	Lagergren et al,[82] 1999	1271	Case control	Population controls, asymptomatic	7.7 (5.3, 11.4)
	Whiteman et al,[83] 2008	2373	Case control	Population controls, GERD<once weekly	6.4 (4.5, 9.0)
	Cook et al,[84] 2014	6414	Pooled analysis	Population controls without recurrent heartburn	4.6 (3.3, 6.6)
Male gender	Nordenstedt et al,[70] 2011	9052	Prospective cohort	Women within 13 SEER registries	8.6[b]
	Cook et al,[71] 2009	8783	Prospective cohort	Women within 13 SEER registries	7.7[b]
	Hur et al,[72] 2013	NA	Prospective cohort	Women within SEER registries	7.2[b]
White race	Cook et al,[71] 2009	8783	Prospective cohort	African Americans	4.6[c]
	Nordenstedt et al,[70] 2011	9052	Prospective cohort	African Americans	5.4[c]
	Nordenstedt et al,[70] 2011	9052	Prospective cohort	Hispanics	2.2[c]
Obesity (BMI)	Chow et al,[87] 1998	1284	Case control	Lowest quartile of BMI	3.0[d] (1.7, 5.0)
	Hoyo et al,[90] 2012	12,378	Pooled analysis	Lowest category of BMI	2.8 (1.9, 4.1)
	Steffen et al,[92] 2009	346, 354	Prospective cohort	Lowest quintile of BMI	2.8 (1.3, 5.9)
Obesity (central adiposity)	Steffen et al,[92] 2009	346, 354	Prospective cohort	Lowest quintile of waist circumference	3.4 (1.5, 7.7)
	Singh et al,[93] 2013	841	Meta-analysis	Lowest category of waist circumference	2.0 (1.5, 2.6)
Tobacco use	Cook et al,[94] 2010	10,993	Pooled analysis	Never smokers	2.0 (1.6, 2.3)
	Lagergren et al,[95] 2000	1009	Case control	Never smokers	1.6 (0.9, 2.7)
H pylori	Chow et al,[57] 1998	353	Case control	Population controls	0.4 (0.2, 0.8)
	De Martel et al,[101] 2005	200	Nested case control	Ambulatory patients	0.4 (0.2, 0.9)
NSAIDs	Corley et al,[104] 2003	442	Meta-analysis	Varied[e]	0.7 (0.5, 0.9)
	Abnet et al,[162] 2009	NA	Meta-analysis	Nonusers of NSAIDs[f]	0.65 (0.5, 0.9)

Abbreviations: BMI, body mass index; NA, not available; NSAID, nonsteroidal antiinflammatory drug; SEER, Surveillance, Epidemiology, and End Results.
[a] Severe GERD symptoms.
[b] White women; incidence rate ratios (IRR); no CIs available.
[c] IRRs; no CIs available.
[d] Men only.
[e] Included studies compared with no NSAID use, no acetylsalicylic acid (ASA) use, no ASA use for 1 month, or no daily ASA use for greater than 1 month.
[f] Precise comparison groups not available.
Data from Refs.[57,70–72,82–84,87,90,92–95,101,104,162]

dramatically over the past 30 to 40 years.[3] By some estimates the incidence has increased from 300% to 500% over this time,[2] or by a 10% annual increase in men, and between 5% and 7% annually in women.[73] In the United States from 1975 to 2006, the incidence of EAC increased 7-fold, an increase greater than that of any other major malignancy.[74] Among women, rates of EAC increased from 0.17 per 100,000 in 1975 to 1979 to 0.74 per 100,000 from 2000 to 2004.[73] With EAC similar increases have been seen in the Latin American population of the United States[73] Fewer analyses have been done on African American men or women, often because of significantly lower numbers of reported cases of disease, yielding unstable estimates of risk.[75] In the last quarter of the twentieth century, men more than 65 years of age saw the greatest increase in incidence of EAC (about 600%).[76] Similar increases have been seen in European and some Asian populations as well.[75,77] More recent data suggest that, when separated by stage of disease at diagnosis, incidences of localized EAC have slowed, whereas distant and regional cases have continued a rapid increase (see **Fig. 3**).[72,76]

Multiple studies assessing Surveillance, Epidemiology, and End Results (SEER) data have suggested a ratio of EAC cases in white people to African Americans of approximately 5:1.[71] These results parallel data on the prevalence of both erosive esophagitis and BE in white people versus African Americans, in which rates are significantly higher in white people.[25,78] The increased incidence in EAC among white people is counterintuitive, in that African Americans, white people, and Asians report a similar prevalence of heartburn.[71,78] Similarly, across multiple races, women in general often have fewer complications of GERD, whereas men are more likely to have erosive disease, BE, or EAC.[70]

The greatest gender disparity in EAC cases is seen in white people, with an 8:1 ratio. In African Americans, a 3:1 ratio is seen, and, in Latin Americans, there is a 7:1 predominance of men compared with women.[71] Other work has placed male/female ratios for Latin Americans even higher than those of white people in some age groups.[70]

Recent research suggests that age-related incidence rates show similar patterns in different ethnic groups, and that older individuals are disproportionately affected. Nordenstedt and colleagues,[70] in an analysis of SEER data, showed that incidence of EAC peaks in the 70-year-old and older category in white people, African Americans, and Latin Americans. The reasons for the great gender disparity in EAC incidence are not known. A greater proportion of abdominal fat, or possibly unknown influences of estrogen or testosterone on disease activity and severity, are possible explanations.[70,79]

In the immediate future, the incidence of EAC is expected to continue its increase. Kong and colleagues[80] conducted an analysis of 3 models assessing projections of EAC incidence, progression, and mortality. According to recent predictions, the incidence of EAC is expected to increase until at least 2030 in men. At that point, the estimates place the incidence of EAC at 8.4 to 10.1 per 100,000 person-years.[81]

Selected risk factors for esophageal adenocarcinoma

Gastroesophageal reflux disease The association between GERD symptoms and EAC risk has been shown to be strong, with risk estimates in individuals with frequent GERD symptoms ranging from 3-fold to 5-fold higher or more compared with asymptomatic controls (See **Table 3**).[40,82–84] In a pivotal case-control study in Sweden in 1999, Lagergren and colleagues[82] found that, compared with individuals without GERD symptoms, those with recurrent symptoms had a risk of EAC more than 7 times higher. Among those with severe and long-standing symptoms, the risk was increased dramatically, by a factor of 43, compared with controls (OR, 43.5). This association was also seen in several other studies,[40,83] with estimates of the risk of EAC ranging from 3-fold to 5-fold higher in individuals with GERD. ORs increased with more severe or more frequent symptoms.[40,83] Pooled data from the BEACON consortium, analyzed by Cook and colleagues,[84] found similar effects. Individuals with longer duration of GERD symptoms had an approximately 5-fold increase in risk, and this increased to a 6-fold increase with symptoms longer than 20 years.[84]

What can be concluded from this information? The relationship between GERD symptoms and risk of EAC is predictable and robust. Data supporting this relationship are more robust than those supporting the relationship between GERD and BE, in which an inconsistent relationship between symptom severity and risk of disease is seen.[21] The association between GERD and EAC has been less rigorously studied in minority populations and in women, and estimates of risk may differ when these patient populations are considered.

Obesity Obesity is a risk factor for development of EAC, and some authorities have suggested that obesity is the central driver of BE and EAC rates in the developed world.[30,85] However, the initial increase in EAC incidence predated the obesity epidemic, and thus obesity does not fully explain observed EAC incidence trends.[86] The risk of EAC in patients in the highest categories of BMI has consistently been shown to be 3-fold to 7-fold higher than in those with normal body weight.[74,87,88] This relationship has been reliably shown in other population-based studies as well, and, remarkably, occurs whether or not reflux is present. Other studies have suggested a linear risk increase with increasing BMI (**Fig. 4**).[40,89] A pooled analysis of 10 case-control studies assessed the relationship between BMI and EAC. Compared with the referent group (BMI<25), increasing BMI was associated with increased risk at cut points of 30 to 34.9 (OR, 2.39), 35.0 to 39.9 (OR, 2.79), and greater than 40.0 (OR, 4.76).[90] Prospective studies have shown similar trends. In a prospective cohort study design, Abnet and colleagues[91] compared individuals with BMIs of 18.5 to 25 (normal body weight) with those with obesity (BMI >30.0) and found that the risk of EAC was increased by more than a factor of 2 (hazard ratio [HR], 2.1). The risk of EAC increased further in those with BMIs greater than 35 (HR, 2.64).

As in BE, the obesity risk in EAC may lie primarily in patients with truncal obesity. In a prospective cohort study, Steffen and colleagues[92] found a rate ratio (RR) for EAC of 2.6 compared with those in the highest quartile of waist circumference versus those in the lower quartile. This finding has been corroborated in other recent studies.[93]

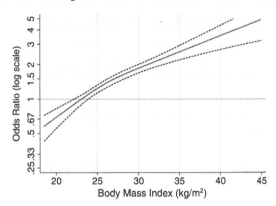

Fig. 4. Restricted cubic regression splines depicting the relationship between BMI and adenocarcinomas of the esophagus and esophageal junction. (*From* Hoyo C, Cook MB, Kamangar F, et al. Body mass index in relation to esophageal and oesophagogastric junction adenocarcinomas: a pooled analysis from the international BEACON consortium. Int J Epidemiol 2012;41:1706–18; with permission.)

Tobacco use Smokers are reported to have at least twice the risk of EAC as non-smokers.[52,94] However, evidence of a possible dose-response relationship has been inconsistent.[94,95] In 2000, Lagergren and colleagues[95] performed a case-control study of possible dose-dependent effects among nearly 200 patients with EAC and 820 controls. In their study, no dose-response trend was seen for either cigarette smokers or pipe smokers, despite such a relationship being seen with esophagogastric junction (EGJ) adenocarcinomas. More recently, in 2010, Cook and colleagues[94] pooled data on tobacco use and EAC risk in both EAC and EGJ adenocarcinoma from the BEACON consortium. An association between smoking and cancer was observed for both EAC (OR, 1.96) and EGJ adenocarcinoma (OR, 2.18). Risks for EAC by gender differed slightly but were not statistically significantly different; there was a trend toward higher risk in men (OR, 2.10 vs 1.74 in women) and a dose-response relationship was seen. Heavy smokers had the highest risk, with ORs of 2.7 (male) and 3.6 (female).[94] These data provide compelling evidence that EAC risk increases with increasing levels of exposure to tobacco. The investigators did not find any modulating effects of GERD or BMI on the effect of smoking and EAC risk.

In summary, smoking for any duration seems to increase risk, and smoking most likely leads to more risk. After quitting, risk likely decreases, but this effect is not immediate.[94] Much of these observed associations may be caused in part by the effects of smoking on both GERD and BE risk. Whether smoking increases the risk of EAC in patients with BE is less clear.

Alcohol Alcohol is strongly associated with squamous cell carcinoma of the esophagus. However, as is seen with BE, alcohol has been shown to have little correlation with development of EAC. In an analysis comparing 260 controls with 227 EAC cases, Anderson and colleagues[96] found no association between any beverage type or amount of alcohol with development of EAC. In a pooled analysis across 11 studies, Freedman and colleagues[97] found no increased risk of EAC in individuals who use alcohol, irrespective of duration or intensity of use. The summary ORs indicated slightly reduced risk in low-alcohol-use and moderate-alcohol-use groups (ORs, 0.78 and 0.77) but there was no association between alcohol and EAC in very-low or high-alcohol-use groups.[97]

Helicobacter pylori *H pylori* causes gastric cancer,[98] but the predominance of data suggest that *H pylori* infection is associated with a decreased risk of EAC.[99] In a case-control study, Chow and colleagues[57] observed an inverse correlation between *H pylori* infection and esophageal or gastric cardia adenocarcinoma (OR, 0.4, 0.2–0.8). Similar inverse relationships have been shown in other studies.[100,101] The mechanism by which *H pylori* could reduce risk for EAC is not known. It has been suggested that the bacteria could reduce the secretion of acid from the stomach, either through direct action on parietal cells or through chronic inflammation.[101,102] It is also not known what effect, if any, eradication of *H pylori* might have on EAC risk.

Nonsteroidal antiinflammatory drugs Some reports have indicated a decreased risk of EAC with nonsteroidal antiinflammatory drug (NSAID) use, both with aspirin and with other nonaspirin drugs.[103,104] Observational studies have had conflicting results.[105,106] A prospective cohort study of 713 patients by Sikkema and colleagues[105] found no association between NSAIDs and cancer risk, whereas Nguyen and colleagues[106] found a reduced risk of EAC (OR, 0.64) in a nested case-control study in 2010. However, systematic reviews have shown a decreased risk of EAC in patients taking NSAIDs. Corley and colleagues[104] found a decreased risk among those using

NSAIDs or aspirin (OR, 0.57; 95% CI, 0.47–0.71). A more recent meta-analysis by Abnet and colleagues in 2009 also found an inverse correlation between NSAID use and EAC (OR, 0.64; 95% CI, 0.52–0.79). In summary, EAC risk may be slightly reduced by taking NSAIDs, but the magnitude of risk reduction is small. A clearer pattern in individual studies would make this conclusion more robust.

Progression of Barrett's Esophagus to Esophageal Adenocarcinoma

Earlier estimates placed the annual rate of progression from BE to EAC at 0.5%.[2,107] However, more recent large cohort studies have reported lower rates of progression, ranging from 0.1% to 0.3%.[10,11,108] Clinical guidelines have recommended periodic endoscopic surveillance for the detection of dysplasia and early cancer in patients with BE. However, surveillance becomes less cost-effective at lower EAC risks, and therefore understanding factors associated with progression are key to guiding management.

Dysplasia in Barrett's esophagus

Dysplasia in BE is a histologic diagnosis suggesting that epithelial cells have acquired genetic or epigenetic alterations that predispose them to the development of malignancy.[1] When identified in a patient with BE, dysplasia predicts a higher risk of EAC, but several issues have limited its utility. For example, sampling error during surveillance endoscopy is an obstacle that has hindered the effectiveness of dysplasia as an accurate marker of cancer risk. Because dysplasia is not readily distinguished endoscopically from typical BE, an area of dysplastic epithelium can easily be missed.[109] Thus, even with extensive sampling, by the time histology shows dysplasia, cancer may be present.[110] Surgical series have shown that cancer was often present at referral for esophagectomy when the referral was for endoscopically diagnosed high-grade dysplasia (HGD).[11,109] Because of sampling error, guidelines recommend use of the Seattle biopsy protocol, an aggressive biopsy technique that seeks to minimize sampling error and improve reliability of cancer and dysplasia detection.[111] Studies have shown that strict adherence to the Seattle protocol improves detection of HGD and cancer.[45] After implementing the strict guidelines, a hospital system in the United Kingdom improved detection of HGD or cancer by more than 4-fold.[112] Despite the benefits of aggressive biopsy protocol, in practice adherence is suboptimal. In a 2009 study by Abrams and colleagues[113] of a national pathology database, these biopsy guidelines were followed in slightly more than half (51.2%) of more than 2200 BE surveillance cases. Furthermore, nonadherence was associated with a significant reduction in dysplasia detection (summary OR, 0.53).

Another issue is the rate of progression. Rates of EAC development in low-grade dysplasia (LGD) were once thought to be as high as 7% to 8% or more per year, or higher.[110,114–117] More recent estimates place the annual risk of progression in BE with LGD closer to 0.5% to 3%, with some newer estimates even lower.[118] However, these estimates are heterogeneous (**Table 4**). Numerous issues confound the accurate interpretation of the presence and severity of dysplasia in BE. Even among experienced pathologists, the extent of interobserver agreement when diagnosing LGD can be less than 50%.[117,119] Other work has shown difficulty in reproducing the diagnosis of BE,[120] in part because inflammation can cause cytologic atypia in the bases of crypts that mimics dysplasia. Regression of LGD, or the failure to detect dysplastic changes on subsequent endoscopies, also occurs in half or more of patients with LGD.[121,122] Because of uncertainties regarding LGD-associated cancer risk, there remains debate over the optimal management strategy in these patients. Incidence of EAC or HGD is estimated at 1.1% to 6% annually but some estimates are as high as 13.4% per year.[10,11,108,123,124] With HGD, interobserver agreement is better but is still less than

Table 4
Prospective and registry-based cohort studies reporting progression risk in LGD, because 2000

Authors, Year	Setting	Study Design	Patients With BE Followed	Male	Incidence of EAC in NDBE (% per y)	Incidence of EAC or HGD in NDBE (% per y)	Incidence of EAC in LGD (% per y)	Incidence of EAC or HGD in LGD (% per y)
Thota et al,[142] 2015	United States	Prospective cohort	299	79.0	NR	NR	0.80	3.10
Picardo et al,[133] 2014	United Kingdom	Prospective cohort	1093	67.1	0.13	0.72	1.98	6.49
Duits et al,[141] 2014	Netherlands	Retrospective cohort	293	76.0	NR	0.60	NR	9.10
Rugge et al,[132] 2012	Italy	Prospective cohort	841	77.0	NR	0.53	NR	3.17
Hvid-Jensen et al,[10] 2011	Netherlands	Prospective cohort	11,028	66.8	0.09	0.25	0.55	1.67
Bhat et al,[11] 2011	United Kingdom	Retrospective cohort	8522	57.9	0.10	0.15	0.92	1.31
Wani et al,[108] 2011	United States	Prospective cohort	1755	85.0	NR	NR	0.44	1.83
Schouten et al,[140] 2011	Netherlands	Retrospective cohort	605	54.0	0.30	NR	0.41	NR
den Hoed et al,[131] 2011	Netherlands	Prospective cohort	133	54.9	NR	0.35	NR	1.62
Jung et al,[139] 2011	United States	Retrospective cohort	355	72.0	0.25$	0.66	0.23	0.71
De Jonge et al,[123] 2010	Netherlands	Retrospective cohort	42,207	62.5	0.39	0.51	0.77	1.06

Study	Country	Study design	N					
Curvers et al,[138] 2010	Netherlands	Retrospective cohort	1198	67.0	NR	0.49	0.34	13.40
Wong et al,[137] 2010	United States	Retrospective cohort	248	NR	0.51	0.61	1.51	1.51
Gatenby et al,[122] 2009	United Kingdom	Retrospective cohort	146	NR	NR	NR	2.70	4.60
Alcedo et al,[136] 2009	Spain	Retrospective cohort	386	79.0	0.52	0.95	0.00	0.00
Swizer-Taylor et al,[130] 2008	United Kingdom	Retrospective cohort	212	69.0	0.68	0.85	0.75	3.16
Lim et al,[129] 2007	United Kingdom	Retrospective cohort	357	57.7	NR	0.62	NR	3.30
Vieth et al,[135] 2006	Germany	Retrospective cohort	748	67.8	0.23	0.23	4.67	4.67
Dulai et al,[128] 2005	United States	Retrospective cohort	575	99.0	0.09	0.36	36.00	1.28
Conio et al,[127] 2003	Italy	Prospective cohort	166	81.3	0.36	0.61	2.27	3.44
Schnell et al,[134] 2001	United States	Retrospective cohort	1099	NR	NR	NR	0.19	NR
Weston et al,[115] 2001	United States	Prospective cohort	48	100.0	NR	NR	0.61	2.43
Reid et al,[109] 2000	United States	Prospective cohort	327	NR	1.05	NR	1.50	NR
Skacel et al,[114] 2000	United States	Retrospective cohort	25	84.0	NR	NR	0.15	0.52

Abbreviation: NDBE, nondysplastic BE.
Data from Refs.[10,11,108,109,114,115,122,123,127–142]

90%.[109] Given the high cumulative incidence of progression from HGD to EAC, current guidelines recommend endoscopic intervention for such patients.[125,126]

Factors that increase risk for dysplasia progression

The strongest predictor of progression to HGD or EAC is baseline LGD. Sikkema and colleagues[105] followed 713 patients with BE with or without LGD for a mean of 4 years, and found that the strongest predictor of incident EAC was the presence of LGD (with OR, 9.6). In longitudinal studies, progression rates are significantly higher in those with LGD, but estimates of increased risk vary widely (see **Table 2**). Most studies following both patients with nondysplastic BE (NDBE) and patients with LGD have found increased risk in the 4-fold to 9-fold range if LGD is present[11,127–133] but estimates have ranged from 2-fold to 27-fold increases in progression rates.[10,11,108,109,114,115,122,123,127,128,130–142]

When patients' slides are reviewed by an expert panel of pathologists, the risk of cancer progression increases because of many patients with LGD being downstaged to NDBE.[138,141] Curvers and colleagues[138] found an annual progression rate of 9.4% in those with LGD confirmed by expert review, compared with an annual risk of 0.53% in those who were downstaged to NDBE after review. This finding was corroborated by Duits and colleagues[141] in 2014. These investigators found that approximately 75% of patients deemed to have LGD by community pathologists were subsequently downgraded to nondysplastic reads by expert pathologists. Among the quarter of patients who had their LGD readings confirmed, progression rates were extremely high: 9.1% of these patients progressed to either HGD or EAC on an annual basis.

Duration of BE is also a risk factor for disease progression. Sikkema and colleagues[105] found that the cumulative incidence of HGD or EAC was 9.6% over 4 years in patients with BE duration greater than 10 years. In those with BE duration less than 10 years, the cumulative incidence was 3.1%. Incidence was 13.3% in those with esophagitis compared with 3.0% in those without.

Among patients with HGD, the risk of cancer is substantially higher. Reid and colleagues[109] reported a cancer risk of 59% over 5 years (or 11.8% annually) in patients with HGD at index endoscopy, compared with 1.5% annual cancer risk in patients with LGD. A meta-analysis published in 2008 yielded a crude incidence rate of 5.6% across 4 studies, with point estimates of annual incidence rates ranging from 2.3% per year to 10.3% per year.[143] Endoscopic therapy is highly effective for the eradication of BE and associated dysplasia, and is now considered the preferred management strategy for patients with HGD.[125]

In summary, LGD represents a marker of increased risk of progression to cancer in patients with BE. However, the magnitude of risk increase is unclear, because reported progression rates to EAC in LGD have been widely variable. This variability is caused in part by the poor reproducibility of this diagnosis. Patients with HGD are at very high risk of progression to cancer, prompting recommendations for therapeutic intervention when it is found. More robust data on progression risk may help better tailor surveillance strategies to each patient in the future.

Barrett's esophagus segment length

Other risk factors have been identified that increase the risk of developing EAC in the setting of BE. Several studies have found that the risk of EAC is greater in longer segments of BE compared with shorter segments.[113,144,145] A study by Weston and colleagues[145] found that the risk increased by a factor of 6 in longer segments. Sikkema and colleagues,[105] in a prospective study design, found that for every additional centimeter of BE the cumulative risk of HGD or EAC increased by 11% over 4 years. The relationship between segment length and increased risk of EAC is not always linear,[146] but the preponderance of evidence suggests that greater surface area of columnar-lined mucosa correlates with increased cancer risk.

Extent of dysplasia

Studies have attempted to determine whether greater extent of dysplasia within a Barrett's segment confers increased risk of neoplastic progression. Studies have had conflicting results as to whether or not more extensive LGD or HGD increases the risk of subsequent EAC.[108,140,147–149] A study by Srivastava and colleagues[147] suggested that, when looking at crypts showing dysplasia (as a criteria for LGD diagnosis), increased fractions of dysplastic crypts correlated with increased EAC risk. Buttar and colleagues[148] also found a 4-fold higher risk of cancer progression in patients with extensive HGD compared with those with unifocal HGD. However, this result could not be duplicated in a follow-up study.[149] Intuitively, it seems that the presence of greater numbers of dysplastic crypts would confer an increased risk of future cancer. However, in part because of sampling error limitations of endoscopic surveillance, the utility of focal versus multifocal dysplasia as a risk stratification tool is unclear.

Molecular/biological markers for progression from Barrett's esophagus to dysplasia/cancer

Numerous studies have attempted to assess the utility of molecular biomarkers to predict progression and assist with risk stratification. If low-risk patients can be accurately identified, then little or no follow-up may be warranted. Alternatively, chemopreventive or endoscopic interventions could be targeted to high-risk patients. However, to date none of the candidate biomarkers has been prospectively validated.

P53 may have the most promise of any of the biomarkers for predicting neoplastic progression in patients with Barrett's. Kastelein and colleagues[150] studied the effect of aberrant p53 expression in a nested case-control study and found striking results. P53 overexpression assessed by immunohistochemistry was associated with significantly increased risk of progression to either HGD or EAC (RR, 5.6; 95% CI, 3.1, 10.3). Among patients with loss of p53 expression, the risk of progression was even higher (RR, 14.0; 95% CI, 5.3, 37.2). LGD alone was far less predictive of progression (RR, 2.4; 95% CI, 0.9, 6.0), and the positive predictive value of progression was 15% with LGD alone compared with 33% in patients with both LGD and aberrant p53 expression.[150] P53 has been found to increase the risk of progression in other studies as well. In a prospective cohort study, Reid and colleagues[151] found that loss of heterozygosity of the chromosome harboring p53 was associated with a 7-fold increase in progression risk.[152]

In a prospective study design, Reid and colleagues[109] analyzed abnormalities in genetic content by flow cytometry and found that, among patients with HGD, incidence of esophageal cancer varied from 58% over 3 years in patients with baseline cytologic abnormalities, to 7.7% in those without baseline cytometric changes. In such lower risk patients, a less invasive management strategy might be warranted. Bird-Lieberman and colleagues[153] performed a retrospective, nested case-control study from a large cohort of patients in Northern Ireland. In that study, LGD, abnormal DNA ploidy, and *Aspergillus oryzae* lectin (AOL) were all risk factors for progression. Expert LGD contributed significantly, but AOL (OR, 3.7) and ploidy (OR, 2.8) were also independent predictors of advancement to EAC.[153]

Another retrospective study found that, among 322 patients with BE, aneuploidy and/or tetraploidy, when assessed by flow cytometry, was associated with an RR of 11.7 for neoplastic progression to cancer.[154]

Fluorescence in situ hybridization (FISH) is a method by which a tissue sample can be tested for a panel of genetic abnormalities.[155] A prospective study by Davelaar and colleagues[156] tested a protocol comparing p53 staining by immunohistochemistry and FISH on brush cytology specimens. They found that p53 abnormalities detected by immunohistochemistry (OR, 17; 95% CI, 3.2, 96) and FISH (OR, 7.3; 95% CI, 1.3, 41) were both independent predictors of progression. In addition, when both p53 and FISH were used, detection of LGD, HGD, and EAC was 100% accurate, both p53 and FISH improved the risk stratification capability of p53 alone, and because flow cytometry requires frozen sections of tissue (something rarely done in clinical practice)[45] the potential for clinical use of FISH may be greater.

Despite the significant advances in biomarker development, significant barriers remain. Of all the biomarkers currently identified, the greatest potential for clinical application may lie with assays using p53. P53 can easily be tested, and in multiple studies has been documented to improve the reproducibility of the diagnosis of dysplasia and to predict neoplastic progression.[155] Because of the imperfect nature of dysplasia alone as a predictor of neoplastic progression, work on molecular biomarkers continues at a rapid pace. However, to date, no biomarkers are approved for diagnosis or risk stratification, and the most recent guidelines from the American Gastroenterological Association recommend against use of molecular biomarkers for risk stratification.[45] Recent British Society of Gastroenterology guidelines propose that p53 immunostaining should be considered, in addition to routine clinical diagnosis, for BE diagnosis.[126] However, pathology societies have yet to develop guidelines for the interpretation and reporting of p53 staining by immunohistochemistry in BE.

SUMMARY

There has been a remarkable increase in the incidence of EAC. In addition, the spectrum of BE and EAC presents multiple challenges to the medical system. Rapidly increasing incidence, high mortality from EAC, and difficulties with risk stratification are all issues to be overcome for effective intervention in this disease state. Some risk factors for BE and EAC are modifiable, such as tobacco use and obesity. In addition to these clinical factors, continued rigorous study of appropriate methods for risk stratification continues. Molecular and genetic biomarkers have considerable promise in risk prediction models, and may in the future be used as part of a prognostic panel, designed to help clinicians focus attention on the patients most at risk.

REFERENCES

1. Spechler SJ. Barrett's esophagus and esophageal adenocarcinoma: pathogenesis, diagnosis, and therapy. Med Clin North Am 2002;86(6):1423–45, vii.
2. Shaheen N, Ransohoff DF. Gastroesophageal reflux, Barrett esophagus, and esophageal cancer: scientific review. JAMA 2002;287(15):1972–81.
3. Blot WJ. Esophageal cancer trends and risk factors. Semin Oncol 1994;21(4): 403–10.
4. Daly JM, Karnell LH, Menck HR. National Cancer Data Base report on esophageal carcinoma. Cancer 1996;78(8):1820–8.
5. Hesketh PJ, Clapp RW, Doos WG, et al. The increasing frequency of adenocarcinoma of the esophagus. Cancer 1989;64(2):526–30.
6. Cameron AJ, Ott BJ, Payne WS. The incidence of adenocarcinoma in columnar-lined (Barrett's) esophagus. N Engl J Med 1985;313(14):857–9.
7. Shaheen NJ, Richter JE. Barrett's oesophagus. Lancet 2009;373(9666):850–61.

8. Lund O, Kimose HH, Aagaard MT, et al. Risk stratification and long-term results after surgical treatment of carcinomas of the thoracic esophagus and cardia. A 25-year retrospective study. J Thorac Cardiovasc Surg 1990;99(2):200–9.
9. Siegel R, Naishadham D, Jemal A. Cancer statistics, 2013. CA Cancer J Clin 2013;63(1):11–30.
10. Hvid-Jensen F, Pedersen L, Drewes AM, et al. Incidence of adenocarcinoma among patients with Barrett's esophagus. N Engl J Med 2011;365(15):1375–83.
11. Bhat S, Coleman HG, Yousef F, et al. Risk of malignant progression in Barrett's esophagus patients: results from a large population-based study. J Natl Cancer Inst 2011;103(13):1049–57.
12. Cameron AJ, Zinsmeister AR, Ballard DJ, et al. Prevalence of columnar-lined (Barrett's) esophagus. Gastroenterology 1990;99(4):918–22.
13. Ronkainen J, Aro P, Storskrubb T, et al. Prevalence of Barrett's esophagus in the general population: an endoscopic study. Gastroenterology 2005;129(6): 1825–31.
14. Rex DK, Cummings OW, Shaw M, et al. Screening for Barrett's esophagus in colonoscopy patients with and without heartburn. Gastroenterology 2003; 125(6):1670–7.
15. Zagari RM, Fuccio L, Wallander MA, et al. Gastro-oesophageal reflux symptoms, oesophagitis and Barrett's oesophagus in the general population: the Loiano–Monghidoro study. Gut 2008;57(10):1354–9.
16. Westhoff B, Brotze S, Weston A, et al. The frequency of Barrett's esophagus in high-risk patients with chronic GERD. Gastrointest Endosc 2005;61(2): 226–31.
17. Conio M, Cameron AJ, Romero Y, et al. Secular trends in the epidemiology and outcome of Barrett's oesophagus in Olmsted County, Minnesota. Gut 2001; 48(3):304–9.
18. Coleman HG, Bhat S, Murray LJ, et al. Increasing incidence of Barrett's oesophagus: a population-based study. Eur J Epidemiol 2011;26(9):739–45.
19. van Soest EM, Dieleman JP, Siersema PD, et al. Increasing incidence of Barrett's oesophagus in the general population. Gut 2005;54(8):1062–6.
20. Cameron AJ, Lomboy CT. Barrett's esophagus: age, prevalence, and extent of columnar epithelium. Gastroenterology 1992;103:1241–5.
21. Wong A, Fitzgerald RC. Epidemiologic risk factors for Barrett's esophagus and associated adenocarcinoma. Clin Gastroenterol Hepatol 2005;3(1):1–10.
22. van Blankenstein M, Looman CW, Johnston BJ, et al. Age and sex distribution of the prevalence of Barrett's esophagus found in a primary referral endoscopy center. Am J Gastroenterol 2005;100(3):568–76.
23. Kramer JR, Fischbach LA, Richardson P, et al. Waist-to-hip ratio, but not body mass index, is associated with an increased risk of Barrett's esophagus in white men. Clin Gastroenterol Hepatol 2013;11(4):373–81.e1.
24. Ford AC, Forman D, Reynolds PD, et al. Ethnicity, gender, and socioeconomic status as risk factors for esophagitis and Barrett's esophagus. Am J Epidemiol 2005;162(5):454–60.
25. Abrams JA, Fields S, Lightdale CJ, et al. Racial and ethnic disparities in the prevalence of Barrett's esophagus among patients who undergo upper endoscopy. Clin Gastroenterol Hepatol 2008;6(1):30–4.
26. Cameron AJ, Lagergren J, Henriksson C, et al. Gastroesophageal reflux disease in monozygotic and dizygotic twins. Gastroenterology 2002;122(1):55–9.
27. Conio M, Filiberti R, Blanchi S, et al. Risk factors for Barrett's esophagus: a case-control study. Int J Cancer 2002;97(2):225–9.

28. Johansson J, Håkansson HO, Mellblom L, et al. Risk factors for Barrett's oesophagus: a population-based approach. Scand J Gastroenterol 2007; 42(2):148–56.
29. Anderson LA, Watson RG, Murphy SJ, et al. Risk factors for Barrett's oesophagus and oesophageal adenocarcinoma: results from the FINBAR study. World J Gastroenterol 2007;13(10):1585.
30. de Jonge PJ, van Blankenstein M, Grady WM, et al. Barrett's oesophagus: epidemiology, cancer risk and implications for management. Gut 2013;63(1): 191–202.
31. Bansal A, Wani S, Rastogi A, et al. Impact of measurement of esophageal acid exposure close to the gastroesophageal junction on diagnostic accuracy and event-symptom correlation: a prospective study using wireless dual pH monitoring. Am J Gastroenterol 2009;104(12):2918–25.
32. Lacy BE, Chehade R, Crowell MD. A prospective study to compare a symptom-based reflux disease questionnaire to 48-h wireless pH monitoring for the identification of gastroesophageal reflux (revised 2-26-11). Am J Gastroenterol 2011; 106(9):1604–11.
33. Avidan B, Sonnenberg A, Schnell TG, et al. Hiatal hernia size, Barrett's length, and severity of acid reflux are all risk factors for esophageal adenocarcinoma. Am J Gastroenterol 2002;97(8):1930–6.
34. Cameron AJ. Barrett's esophagus: prevalence and size of hiatal hernia. Am J Gastroenterol 1999;94(8):2054–9.
35. Eloubeidi MA, Provenzale D. Clinical and demographic predictors of Barrett's esophagus among patients with gastroesophageal reflux disease: a multivariable analysis in veterans. J Clin Gastroenterol 2001;33(4):306–9.
36. Taylor JB, Rubenstein JH. Meta-analyses of the effect of symptoms of gastroesophageal reflux on the risk of Barrett's esophagus. Am J Gastroenterol 2010;105(8):1730–7.
37. Brandt MG, Darling GE, Miller L. Symptoms, acid exposure and motility in patients with Barrett's esophagus. Can J Surg 2004;47(1):47.
38. Singh P, Taylor RH, Colin-Jones DG. Esophageal motor dysfunction and acid exposure in reflux esophagitis are more severe if Barrett's metaplasia is present. Am J Gastroenterol 1994;89(3):349–56.
39. El-Serag HB, Aguirre TV, Davis S, et al. Proton pump inhibitors are associated with reduced incidence of dysplasia in Barrett's esophagus. Am J Gastroenterol 2004;99(10):1877–83.
40. Wu AH, Tseng CC, Bernstein L. Hiatal hernia, reflux symptoms, body size, and risk of esophageal and gastric adenocarcinoma. Cancer 2003;98(5): 940–8.
41. Lagergren J. Influence of obesity on the risk of esophageal disorders. Nat Rev Gastroenterol Hepatol 2011;8(6):340–7.
42. Ogden CL, Carroll MD, Kit BK, et al. Prevalence of childhood and adult obesity in the United States, 2011-2012. JAMA 2014;311(8):806–14.
43. Kamat P, Wen S, Morris J, et al. Exploring the association between elevated body mass index and Barrett's esophagus: a systematic review and meta-analysis. Ann Thorac Surg 2009;87(2):655–62.
44. Edelstein ZR, Farrow DC, Bronner MP, et al. Central adiposity and risk of Barrett's esophagus. Gastroenterology 2007;133(2):403–11.
45. Spechler SJ, Sharma P, Souza RF, et al. American Gastroenterological Association technical review on the management of Barrett's esophagus. Gastroenterology 2011;140(3):e18.

46. Kubo A, Cook MB, Shaheen NJ, et al. Sex-specific associations between body mass index, waist circumference and the risk of Barrett's oesophagus: a pooled analysis from the international BEACON consortium. Gut 2013; 62(12):1684–91.
47. Berger NA, Dannenberg AJ, editors. Obesity, inflammation and cancer. New York (NY): Springer; 2013.
48. Kubo A, Levin TR, Block G, et al. Alcohol types and sociodemographic characteristics as risk factors for Barrett's esophagus. Gastroenterology 2009;136(3): 806–15.
49. Steevens J, Schouten LJ, Driessen AL, et al. A prospective cohort study on overweight, smoking, alcohol consumption, and risk of Barrett's esophagus. Cancer Epidemiol Biomarkers Prev 2011;20(2):345–58.
50. Thrift AP, Cook MB, Vaughan TL, et al. Alcohol and the risk of Barrett's esophagus: a pooled analysis from the International BEACON Consortium. Am J Gastroenterol 2014;109(10):1586–94.
51. Thrift AP, Kramer JR, Richardson PA, et al. No significant effects of smoking or alcohol consumption on risk of Barrett's esophagus. Dig Dis Sci 2014;59(1): 108–16.
52. Lepage C, Drouillard A, Jouve JL, et al. Epidemiology and risk factors for oesophageal adenocarcinoma. Dig Liver Dis 2013;45(8):625–9.
53. Cook MB, Shaheen NJ, Anderson LA, et al. Cigarette smoking increases risk of Barrett's esophagus: an analysis of the Barrett's and Esophageal Adenocarcinoma Consortium. Gastroenterology 2012;142(4):744–53.
54. Stemmermann GN. Intestinal metaplasia of the stomach. A status report. Cancer 1994;74(2):556–64.
55. El-Serag HB, Sonnenberg A. Opposing time trends of peptic ulcer and reflux disease. Gut 1998;43(3):327–33.
56. Corley DA, Kubo A, Levin TR, et al. Helicobacter pylori infection and the risk of Barrett's oesophagus: a community-based study. Gut 2008;57(6):727–33.
57. Chow WH, Blaser MJ, Blot WJ, et al. An inverse relation between cagA+ strains of Helicobacter pylori infection and risk of esophageal and gastric cardia adenocarcinoma. Cancer Res 1998;58(4):588–90.
58. Vaezi MF, Falk GW, Peek RM, et al. CagA-positive strains of Helicobacter pylori may protect against Barrett's esophagus. Am J Gastroenterol 2000;95(9):2206–11.
59. Wang C, Yuan Y, Hunt RH. Helicobacter pylori infection and Barrett's esophagus: a systematic review and meta-analysis. Am J Gastroenterol 2009; 104(2):492–500.
60. Goldenberg RL, Culhane JF, Iams JD, et al. Epidemiology and causes of preterm birth. Lancet 2008;371(9606):75–84.
61. Forssell L, Cnattingius S, Bottai M, et al. Risk of esophagitis among individuals born preterm or small for gestational age. Clin Gastroenterol Hepatol 2012; 10(12):1369–75.
62. Forssell L, Cnattingius S, Bottai M, et al. Increased risk of Barrett's esophagus among individuals born preterm or small for gestational age. Clin Gastroenterol Hepatol 2013;11(7):790–4.
63. Forssell L, Cnattingius S, Bottai M, et al. Risk of oesophageal adenocarcinoma among individuals born preterm or small for gestational age. Eur J Cancer 2013; 49(9):2207–13.
64. Leggett CL, Gorospe EC, Calvin AD, et al. Obstructive sleep apnea is a risk factor for Barrett's esophagus. Clin Gastroenterol Hepatol 2014;12(4): 583–8.e1.

65. Garcia JM, Splenser AE, Kramer J, et al. Circulating inflammatory cytokines and adipokines are associated with increased risk of Barrett's esophagus: a case-control study. Clin Gastroenterol Hepatol 2014;12(2):229–38.e3.
66. Bosch A, Frias Z, Caldwell WL. Adenocarcinoma of the esophagus. Cancer 1979;43(4):1557–61.
67. Devesa SS, Blot WJ, Fraumeni JF. Changing patterns in the incidence of esophageal and gastric carcinoma in the United States. Cancer 1998;83(10):2049–53.
68. American Cancer Society. Cancer facts and figures. Atlanta (GA): American Cancer Society; 2014.
69. Eloubeidi MA, Mason AC, Desmond RA, et al. Temporal trends (1973–1997) in survival of patients with esophageal adenocarcinoma in the United States: a glimmer of hope? Am J Gastroenterol 2003;98(7):1627–33.
70. Nordenstedt H, El-Serag H. The influence of age, sex, and race on the incidence of esophageal cancer in the United States (1992-2006). Scand J Gastroenterol 2011;46(5):597–602.
71. Cook M, Chow W, Devesa S. Oesophageal cancer incidence in the United States by race, sex, and histologic type, 1977–2005. Br J Cancer 2009; 101(5):855–9.
72. Hur C, Miller M, Kong CY, et al. Trends in esophageal adenocarcinoma incidence and mortality. Cancer 2013;119(6):1149–58.
73. Younes M, Henson DE, Ertan A, et al. Incidence and survival trends of esophageal carcinoma in the United States: racial and gender differences by histological type. Scand J Gastroenterol 2002;37(12):1359–65.
74. Pera M, Manterola C, Vidal O, et al. Epidemiology of esophageal adenocarcinoma. J Surg Oncol 2005;92(3):151–9.
75. Reid BJ, Li X, Galipeau PC, et al. Barrett's oesophagus and oesophageal adenocarcinoma: time for a new synthesis. Nat Rev Cancer 2010;10(2):87–101.
76. Brown LM, Devesa SS, Chow WH. Incidence of adenocarcinoma of the esophagus among white Americans by sex, stage, and age. J Natl Cancer Inst 2008; 100(16):1184–7.
77. Vizcaino AP, Moreno V, Lambert R, et al. Time trends incidence of both major histologic types of esophageal carcinomas in selected countries, 1973–1995. Int J Cancer 2002;99(6):860–8.
78. El-Serag HB, Petersen NJ, Carter J, et al. Gastroesophageal reflux among different racial groups in the United States. Gastroenterology 2004;126(7): 1692–9.
79. Lagergren J, Nyrén O. Do sex hormones play a role in the etiology of esophageal adenocarcinoma? A new hypothesis tested in a population-based cohort of prostate cancer patients. Cancer Epidemiol Biomarkers Prev 1998;7(10):913–5.
80. Kong CY, Kroep S, Curtius K, et al. Exploring the recent trend in esophageal adenocarcinoma incidence and mortality using comparative simulation modeling. Cancer Epidemiol Biomarkers Prev 2013;23:997–1006.
81. Thrift AP, Whiteman D. The incidence of esophageal adenocarcinoma continues to rise: analysis of period and birth cohort effects on recent trends. Ann Oncol 2012;23(12):3155–62.
82. Lagergren J, Bergström R, Lindgren A, et al. Symptomatic gastroesophageal reflux as a risk factor for esophageal adenocarcinoma. N Engl J Med 1999; 340(11):825–31.
83. Whiteman DC, Sadeghi S, Pandeya N, et al. Combined effects of obesity, acid reflux and smoking on the risk of adenocarcinomas of the oesophagus. Gut 2008;57(2):173–80.

84. Cook MB, Corley DA, Murray LJ, et al. Gastroesophageal reflux in relation to adenocarcinomas of the esophagus: a pooled analysis from the Barrett's and Esophageal Adenocarcinoma Consortium (BEACON). PLoS one 2014;9(7): e103508.

85. Ryan AM, Duong M, Healy L, et al. Obesity, metabolic syndrome and esophageal adenocarcinoma: epidemiology, etiology and new targets. Cancer Epidemiol 2011;35(4):309–19.

86. Abrams JA, Sharaiha RZ, Gonsalves L, et al. Dating the rise of esophageal adenocarcinoma: analysis of Connecticut Tumor Registry data, 1940–2007. Cancer Epidemiol Biomarkers Prev 2011;20(1):183–6.

87. Chow WH, Blot WJ, Vaughan TL, et al. Body mass index and risk of adenocarcinomas of the esophagus and gastric cardia. J Natl Cancer Inst 1998;90(2):150–5.

88. Lagergren J. Adenocarcinoma of oesophagus: what exactly is the size of the problem and who is at risk? Gut 2005;54(suppl 1):i1–5.

89. Lagergren J, Bergström R, Nyrén O. Association between body mass and adenocarcinoma of the esophagus and gastric cardia. Ann Intern Med 1999; 130(11):883–90.

90. Hoyo C, Cook MB, Kamangar F, et al. Body mass index in relation to oesophageal and oesophagogastric junction adenocarcinomas: a pooled analysis from the International BEACON Consortium. Int J Epidemiol 2012;41(6):1706–18.

91. Abnet CC, Freedman ND, Hollenbeck AR, et al. A prospective study of BMI and risk of oesophageal and gastric adenocarcinoma. Eur J Cancer 2008;44(3): 465–71.

92. Steffen A, Schulze MB, Pischon T, et al. Anthropometry and esophageal cancer risk in the European prospective investigation into cancer and nutrition. Cancer Epidemiol Biomarkers Prev 2009;18(7):2079–89.

93. Singh S, Sharma AN, Murad MH, et al. Central adiposity is associated with increased risk of esophageal inflammation, metaplasia, and adenocarcinoma: a systematic review and meta-analysis. Clin Gastroenterol Hepatol 2013; 11(11):1399–412.e7.

94. Cook MB, Kamangar F, Whiteman DC, et al. Cigarette smoking and adenocarcinomas of the esophagus and esophagogastric junction: a pooled analysis from the international BEACON consortium. J Natl Cancer Inst 2010;102(17):1344–53.

95. Lagergren J, Bergström R, Lindgren A, et al. The role of tobacco, snuff and alcohol use in the aetiology of cancer of the oesophagus and gastric cardia. Int J Cancer 2000;85(3):340–6.

96. Anderson LA, Cantwell MM, Watson RG, et al. The association between alcohol and reflux esophagitis, Barrett's esophagus, and esophageal adenocarcinoma. Gastroenterology 2009;136(3):799–805.

97. Freedman ND, Murray LJ, Kamangar F, et al. Alcohol intake and risk of oesophageal adenocarcinoma: a pooled analysis from the BEACON Consortium. Gut 2011;60(8):1029–37.

98. Parsonnet J, Friedman GD, Vandersteen DP, et al. *Helicobacter pylori* infection and the risk of gastric carcinoma. N Engl J Med 1991;325(16):1127–31.

99. Islami F, Kamangar F. *Helicobacter pylori* and esophageal cancer risk: a meta-analysis. Cancer Prev Res 2008;1(5):329–38.

100. Wu AH, Crabtree JE, Bernstein L, et al. Role of *Helicobacter pylori* CagA+ strains and risk of adenocarcinoma of the stomach and esophagus. Int J Cancer 2003;103(6):815–21.

101. de Martel C, Llosa AE, Farr SM, et al. *Helicobacter pylori* infection and the risk of development of esophageal adenocarcinoma. J Infect Dis 2005;191(5):761–7.

102. Engel LS, Chow WH, Vaughan TL, et al. Population attributable risks of esophageal and gastric cancers. J Natl Cancer Inst 2003;95(18):1404–13.
103. Farrow DC, Vaughan TL, Hansten PD, et al. Use of aspirin and other nonsteroidal anti-inflammatory drugs and risk of esophageal and gastric cancer. Cancer Epidemiol Biomarkers Prev 1998;7(2):97–102.
104. Corley DA, Kerlikowske K, Verma R, et al. Protective association of aspirin/NSAIDs and esophageal cancer: a systematic review and meta-analysis. Gastroenterology 2003;124(1):47–56.
105. Sikkema M, Looman CW, Steyerberg EW, et al. Predictors for neoplastic progression in patients with Barrett's esophagus: a prospective cohort study. Am J Gastroenterol 2011;106(7):1231–8.
106. Nguyen DM, Richardson P, El-Serag HB. Medications (NSAIDs, statins, proton pump inhibitors) and the risk of esophageal adenocarcinoma in patients with Barrett's esophagus. Gastroenterology 2010;138(7):2260–6.
107. Shaheen NJ, Crosby MA, Bozymski EM, et al. Is there publication bias in the reporting of cancer risk in Barrett's esophagus? Gastroenterology 2000;119(2):333–8.
108. Wani S, Falk GW, Post J, et al. Risk factors for progression of low-grade dysplasia in patients with Barrett's esophagus. Gastroenterology 2011;141(4):1179–86.e1.
109. Reid BJ, Levine DS, Longton G, et al. Predictors of progression to cancer in Barrett's esophagus: baseline histology and flow cytometry identify low-and high-risk patient subsets. Am J Gastroenterol 2000;95(7):1669–76.
110. Levine DS, Haggitt RC, Blount PL, et al. An endoscopic biopsy protocol can differentiate high-grade dysplasia from early adenocarcinoma in Barrett's esophagus. Gastroenterology 1993;105:40–50.
111. Wang KK, Sampliner RE, Practice Parameters Committee of the American College of Gastroenterology. Updated guidelines 2008 for the diagnosis, surveillance and therapy of Barrett's esophagus. Am J Gastroenterol 2008;103(3):788–97.
112. Fitzgerald RC, Saeed IT, Khoo D, et al. Rigorous surveillance protocol increases detection of curable cancers associated with Barrett's esophagus. Dig Dis Sci 2001;46(9):1892–8.
113. Abrams JA, Kapel RC, Lindberg GM, et al. Adherence to biopsy guidelines for Barrett's esophagus surveillance in the community setting in the United States. Clin Gastroenterol Hepatol 2009;7(7):736.
114. Skacel M, Petras RE, Gramlich TL, et al. The diagnosis of low-grade dysplasia in Barrett's esophagus and its implications for disease progression. Am J Gastroenterol 2000;95(12):3383–7.
115. Weston AP, Banerjee SK, Sharma P, et al. p53 protein overexpression in low grade dysplasia (LGD) in Barrett's esophagus: immunohistochemical marker predictive of progression. Am J Gastroenterol 2001;96(5):1355–62.
116. Hameeteman W, Tytgat GN, Houthoff HJ, et al. Barrett's esophagus: development of dysplasia and adenocarcinoma. Gastroenterology 1989;96(5 Pt 1):1249–56.
117. Montgomery E, Goldblum JR, Greenson JK, et al. Dysplasia as a predictive marker for invasive carcinoma in Barrett esophagus: a follow-up study based on 138 cases from a diagnostic variability study. Hum Pathol 2001;32(4):379–88.
118. Singh S, Manickam P, Amin AV, et al. Incidence of esophageal adenocarcinoma in Barrett's esophagus with low-grade dysplasia: a systematic review and meta-analysis. Gastrointest Endosc 2014;79(6):897–909.e4.
119. Reid B, Haggitt RC, Rubin CE, et al. Observer variation in the diagnosis of dysplasia in Barrett's esophagus. Hum Pathol 1988;19(2):166–78.

120. Meining A, Ott R, Becker I, et al. The Munich Barrett follow up study: suspicion of Barrett's oesophagus based on either endoscopy or histology only—what is the clinical significance? Gut 2004;53(10):1402–7.

121. Sharma P, Falk GW, Weston A, et al. Dysplasia and cancer in a large multicenter cohort of patients with Barrett's esophagus. Clin Gastroenterol Hepatol 2006; 4(5):566–72.

122. Gatenby P, Ramus J, Caygill C, et al. Routinely diagnosed low-grade dysplasia in Barrett's oesophagus: a population-based study of natural history. Histopathology 2009;54(7):814–9.

123. de Jonge PJ, van Blankenstein M, Looman CW, et al. Risk of malignant progression in patients with Barrett's oesophagus: a Dutch nationwide cohort study. Gut 2010;59(8):1030–6.

124. Gaddam S, Singh M, Balasubramanian G, et al. Persistence of nondysplastic Barrett's esophagus identifies patients at lower risk for esophageal adenocarcinoma: results from a large multicenter cohort. Gastroenterology 2013;145(3): 548–53.e1.

125. Spechler SJ, Sharma P, Souza RF, et al. American Gastroenterological Association medical position statement on the management of Barrett's esophagus. Gastroenterology 2011;140(3):1084–91.

126. Fitzgerald RC, di Pietro M, Ragunath K, et al. British Society of Gastroenterology guidelines on the diagnosis and management of Barrett's oesophagus. Gut 2014;63(1):7–42.

127. Conio M, Blanchi S, Lapertosa G, et al. Long-term endoscopic surveillance of patients with Barrett's esophagus. Incidence of dysplasia and adenocarcinoma: a prospective study. Am J Gastroenterol 2003;98(9):1931–9.

128. Dulai GS, Shekelle PG, Jensen DM, et al. Dysplasia and risk of further neoplastic progression in a regional Veterans Administration Barrett's cohort. Am J Gastroenterol 2005;100(4):775–83.

129. Lim C, Treanor D, Dixon MF, et al. Low-grade dysplasia in Barrett's esophagus has a high risk of progression. Endoscopy 2007;39(07):581–7.

130. Switzer-Taylor V, Schlup M, Lübcke R, et al. Barrett's esophagus: a retrospective analysis of 13 years surveillance. J Gastroenterol Hepatol 2008;23(9):1362–7.

131. den Hoed C, van Blankenstein M, Dees J, et al. The minimal incubation period from the onset of Barrett's oesophagus to symptomatic adenocarcinoma. Br J Cancer 2011;105(2):200–5.

132. Rugge M, Zaninotto G, Parente P, et al. Barrett's esophagus and adenocarcinoma risk: the experience of the North-Eastern Italian Registry (EBRA). Ann Surg 2012;256(5):788–95.

133. Picardo S, O'Brien MP, Feighery R, et al. A Barrett's esophagus registry of over 1000 patients from a specialist center highlights greater risk of progression than population-based registries and high risk of low grade dysplasia. Dis Esophagus 2014;28(2):121–6.

134. Schnell TG, Sontag SJ, Chejfec G, et al. Long-term nonsurgical management of Barrett's esophagus with high-grade dysplasia. Gastroenterology 2001;120(7): 1607–19.

135. Vieth M, Schubert B, Lang-Schwarz K, et al. Frequency of Barrett's neoplasia after initial negative endoscopy with biopsy: a long-term histopathological follow-up study. Endoscopy 2006;38(12):1201–5.

136. Alcedo J, Ferrández A, Arenas J, et al. Trends in Barrett's esophagus diagnosis in Southern Europe: implications for surveillance. Dis Esophagus 2009;22(3): 239–48.

137. Wong T, Tian J, Nagar AB. Barrett's surveillance identifies patients with early esophageal adenocarcinoma. Am J Med 2010;123(5):462–7.
138. Curvers WL, ten Kate FJ, Krishnadath KK, et al. Low-grade dysplasia in Barrett's esophagus: overdiagnosed and underestimated. Am J Gastroenterol 2010; 105(7):1523–30.
139. Jung KW, Talley NJ, Romero Y, et al. Epidemiology and natural history of intestinal metaplasia of the gastroesophageal junction and Barrett's esophagus: a population-based study. Am J Gastroenterol 2011;106(8):1447–55.
140. Schouten LJ, Steevens J, Huysentruyt CJ, et al. Total cancer incidence and overall mortality are not increased among patients with Barrett's esophagus. Clin Gastroenterol Hepatol 2011;9(9):754–61.
141. Duits LC, Phoa KN, Curvers WL, et al. Barrett's oesophagus patients with low-grade dysplasia can be accurately risk-stratified after histological review by an expert pathology panel. Gut 2014. [Epub ahead of print].
142. Thota PN, Lee HJ, Goldblum JR, et al. Risk stratification of patients with Barrett's esophagus and low-grade dysplasia or indefinite for dysplasia. Clin Gastroenterol Hepatol 2015;13(3):459–65.e1.
143. Rastogi A, Puli S, El-Serag HB, et al. Incidence of esophageal adenocarcinoma in patients with Barrett's esophagus and high-grade dysplasia: a meta-analysis. Gastrointest Endosc 2008;67(3):394–8.
144. Wani S, Falk G, Hall M, et al. Patients with nondysplastic Barrett's esophagus have low risks for developing dysplasia or esophageal adenocarcinoma. Clin Gastroenterol Hepatol 2011;9(3):220–7.e1.
145. Weston AP, Badr AS, Hassanein RS. Prospective multivariate analysis of clinical, endoscopic, and histological factors predictive of the development of Barrett's multifocal high-grade dysplasia or adenocarcinoma. Am J Gastroenterol 1999; 94(12):3413–9.
146. Gatenby PA, Caygill CP, Ramus JR, et al. Short segment columnar-lined oesophagus: an underestimated cancer risk? A large cohort study of the relationship between Barrett's columnar-lined oesophagus segment length and adenocarcinoma risk. Eur J Gastroenterol Hepatol 2007;19(11):969–75.
147. Srivastava A, Hornick JL, Li X, et al. Extent of low-grade dysplasia is a risk factor for the development of esophageal adenocarcinoma in Barrett's esophagus. Am J Gastroenterol 2007;102(3):483–93.
148. Buttar NS, Wang KK, Sebo TJ, et al. Extent of high-grade dysplasia in Barrett's esophagus correlates with risk of adenocarcinoma. Gastroenterology 2001; 120(7):1630–9.
149. Dar M, Goldblum JR, Rice TW, et al. Can extent of high grade dysplasia in Barrett's oesophagus predict the presence of adenocarcinoma at oesophagectomy? Gut 2003;52(4):486–9.
150. Kastelein F, Biermann K, Steyerberg EW, et al. Aberrant p53 protein expression is associated with an increased risk of neoplastic progression in patients with Barrett's oesophagus. Gut 2013;62(12):1676–83.
151. Reid BJ, Prevo LJ, Galipeau PC, et al. Predictors of progression in Barrett's esophagus II: baseline 17p (p53) loss of heterozygosity identifies a patient subset at increased risk for neoplastic progression. Am J Gastroenterol 2001; 96(10):2839–48.
152. Allison RK, Skipper HE, Reid MR, et al. Studies on the photosynthetic reaction. I. The assimilation of acetate by Nostoc muscorum. J Biol Chem 1953;204(1): 197–205.

153. Bird-Lieberman EL, Dunn JM, Coleman HG, et al. Population-based study reveals new risk-stratification biomarker panel for Barrett's esophagus. Gastroenterology 2012;143(4):927–35.e3.
154. Rabinovitch PS, Longton G, Blount PL, et al. Predictors of progression in Barrett's esophagus III: baseline flow cytometric variables. Am J Gastroenterol 2001;96(11):3071–83.
155. Timmer M, Sun G, Gorospe EC, et al. Predictive biomarkers for Barrett's esophagus: so near and yet so far. Dis Esophagus 2013;26(6):574–81.
156. Davelaar AL, Calpe S, Lau L, et al. Aberrant TP53 detected by combining immunohistochemistry and DNA-FISH improves Barrett's esophagus progression prediction: a prospective follow-up study. Genes Chromosomes Cancer 2015; 54(2):82–90.
157. Gerson LB, Shetler K, Triadafilopoulos G. Prevalence of Barrett's esophagus in asymptomatic individuals. Gastroenterology 2002;123(2):461–7.
158. Ward EM, Wolfsen HC, Achem SR, et al. Barrett's esophagus is common in older men and women undergoing screening colonoscopy regardless of reflux symptoms. Am J Gastroenterol 2006;101(1):12–7.
159. Zou D, He J, Ma X, et al. Epidemiology of symptom-defined gastroesophageal reflux disease and reflux esophagitis: the systematic investigation of gastrointestinal diseases in China (SILC). Scand J Gastroenterol 2011;46(2):133–41.
160. Cook M, Wild C, Forman D. A systematic review and meta-analysis of the sex ratio for Barrett's esophagus, erosive reflux disease, and nonerosive reflux disease. Am J Epidemiol 2005;162(11):1050–61.
161. Corley DA, Kubo A, Levin TR, et al. Abdominal obesity and body mass index as risk factors for Barrett's esophagus. Gastroenterology 2007;133(1):34–41.
162. Abnet C, Freedman ND, Kamangar F, et al. Non-steroidal anti-inflammatory drugs and risk of gastric and oesophageal adenocarcinomas: results from a cohort study and a meta-analysis. Br J Cancer 2009;100(3):551–7.

Molecular Pathogenesis of Barrett Esophagus

Current Evidence

Kausilia K. Krishnadath, MD, PhD[a],*, Kenneth K. Wang, MD[b]

KEYWORDS

- SSH • BMP4 • pSMAD • CDX2 • Lineage tracing • p63 • WNT • Notch

KEY POINTS

- At present, the SHH-BMP4/pSMAD pathway, its antagonists, and downstream targets seem to be the important signaling pathways involved in the development of earliest stages of columnar metaplasia.
- SHH-BMP4/pSMAD signaling is crucial for the induction of columnar genes leading to the nonintestinal-type of columnar metaplasia.
- Expression of the intestine-specific genes as seen in the later stage of the intestinal-type of Barrett metaplasia seems to be mediated by a pSMAD-CDX2 interaction, Wnt, and Notch signaling.
- Current molecular findings provide important insight in the development of the columnar and intestinal-type metaplasia, which can be used for developing novel molecular therapies.
- With respect to the Barrett cell of origin, there is a need to better characterize the human Barrett progenitor cell to develop appropriate lineage tracing models.

INTRODUCTION

Metaplasia or the dedifferentiation of cells may occur in several organs of the gastrointestinal tract, such as pancreas, stomach, and the esophagus, but also in other locations, such as in lungs, bladder, and cervix. Epithelial metaplasia is caused by constant injury by internal or external factors that give rise to chronic inflammation. In general, metaplastic epithelia are mostly incompletely differentiated, and are often considered to be precancerous lesions. Metaplasia of the distal esophagus is the result of longstanding gastroesophageal reflux disease, in which bile and acid reflux cause chronic inflammation of the esophageal mucosa. In the subsequent process of healing, the epithelium attempts to adapt to its new environment, and hereto may undergo profound phenotypic changes leading to a different type of epithelium that

[a] Department of Gastroenterology and Hepatology, Academic Medical Center, Meibergdreef 9, Amsterdam 1105 AZ, The Netherlands; [b] Gastroenterology, Mayo Clinics, Rochester, MN, USA
* Corresponding author.
E-mail address: k.k.krishnadath@amc.uva.nl

Gastroenterol Clin N Am 44 (2015) 233–247
http://dx.doi.org/10.1016/j.gtc.2015.02.002
0889-8553/15/$ – see front matter © 2015 Elsevier Inc. All rights reserved.

is more resistant to its novel environment. In a surgical animal model, reflux of bile and acid induced the development of nonintestinal and later intestinal metaplasia, supporting the earlier observation in humans that indicated a nonintestinal-type of metaplasia may precede the development of the intestinal-type of metaplasia. Based on observations in human subjects and supported by animal studies and molecular data, the development of the intestinal-type of metaplasia is increasingly recognized as a stepwise process.[1–3] Within this process, inflamed esophageal squamous mucosa is replaced by a transitional epithelium also referred to as multilayer epithelium followed by single layered nonintestinal-type columnar epithelium and finally by the specialized intestinal-type of columnar metaplasia.[1,4,5] This novel concept indicates that the previously defined independent metaplastic phenotypes including the nonintestinal phenotypes, such as junctional/cardia or the gastric/fundic type, and specialized intestinal-type of metaplasia as can be observed in patients with Barrett esophagus are rather related than distinct entities (**Fig. 1**).[6]

Important progress recently has been made in understanding the underlying molecular mechanisms in the process of Barrett metaplasia. The current hypothesis is that the stepwise development of intestinal metaplasia is based on the upregulation of diverse signaling pathways involving SHH, WNTs, Notch, retinoic acid (RA), and bone morphogenetic protein (BMP), which normally are involved in development and homeostasis of the gut and other organs. Through renewed or upregulated activation, these signaling pathways drive the development of epithelial metaplasia by activating specific transcription factors leading to the expression of columnar and more specific intestinal target genes. Much of the current research has focused on the role of factors that regulate these pathways and their downstream targets.

MOLECULAR PATHWAYS INVOLVED IN THE DEVELOPMENT OF COLUMNAR AND SQUAMOUS EPITHELIA

SHH and BMPs are highly influential morphogenes in endoderm development. Both proteins are secreted in the notochord of the esophagus during the early embryonic stages. SHH is a secretory protein. Its signaling is mediated by two membrane-bound receptors: patched (PTCH) and smoothened (SMO). Normally, PTCH inhibits the activation of SMO. On binding to SHH, PTCH is internalized and SMO is released. Active SMO mediates intracellular signaling via several molecules that subsequently cause translocation of transcription factors of the GLI family, which in turn regulates the expression of several genes including BMP4.[7,8] BMP proteins are members of the transforming growth factor-β family.[7,9] Once BMP proteins bind to their type II receptors, type I receptors (BMPR1A or BMPR1B) are recruited, and transduction of a signal by phosphorylation of the SMAD proteins is initiated giving rise to phosphorylated SMAD (pSMAD). The SMAD proteins can be classified into three subgroups based on their distinct functions. The receptor-regulated SMADS (RSMAD1, 2, 3, 5, and 8), on ligand stimulation, are directly phosphorylated by type I BMP receptors.[10] Once activated, these SMADS associate with Smad4. The heteromeric complex translocates into the nucleus, where it mediates the response to specific ligands. Together with the RUNX cofactors, the complex induces transcription of target genes.[11] Downstream targets are, for instance, ID1 and ID2. The RSMADS 1, 5, and 8 act in BMP pathways, whereas R-SMADS 2 and 3 respond to activin/transforming growth factor-β signaling. The inhibitory SMADS (ISMAD6 and SMAD7) prevent the activation of receptor-regulated SMADS or their heteromerization with SMAD4.[12,13]

SHH-BMP cell signaling is essential for the development of organs and tissues and their function is highly conserved between species.[9] Development of the esophagus

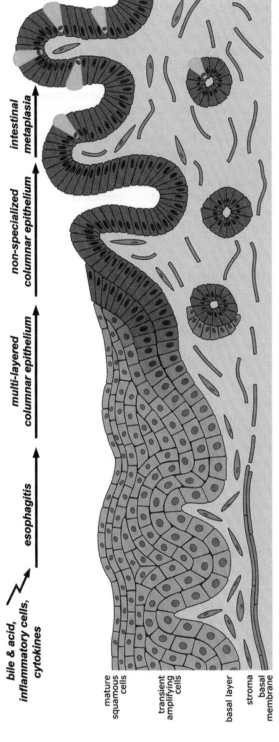

Fig. 1. Stepwise process of development of intestinal-type of metaplasia in the esophagus. Chronic injury and inflammation of the esophageal squamous epithelium is followed by development of multilayered columnar epithelium, which further develops into a single-layered columnar epithelium and finally into the specialized intestinal-type of metaplasia.

has been most extensively studied in mouse, rat, and chicken embryos. The esophagus develops from the anterior foregut. SHH and BMP4 are critical for the development of the foregut and for the separation of trachea from the esophagus.[14] In the foregut the expression of both molecules rapidly decreases at the time that the trachea and esophagus have separated.[15,16] Importantly, the action of BMP4 on the development of the foregut seems to be closely regulated by Noggin, a natural antagonist of BMP proteins. It has been shown that ectopic expression of BMP4 in the esophageal foregut inhibits development of squamous epithelium and promotes columnar differentiation.[17] Likewise knocking out Noggin is associated with esophageal defects and the presence of a columnar epithelial lining in embryos.[18] In other transgenic mouse models it has been demonstrated that differentiation of the foregut epithelium toward stratified squamous epithelium is regulated by SHH and the transcription factors SOX2 and p63.[15] Mice lacking SOX2 and p63 expression develop a columnar-type of epithelium in the esophagus.[19–22] The RA pathway is another pathway that seems to be involved in the development of stratified esophageal epithelium. The effect of RA on cellular differentiation, however, depends on specific receptor activation. This involves the nuclear retinoid acid receptor-alpha and retinoid X receptor-gamma, which are highly expressed in squamous epithelium.[23]

MOLECULAR PATHWAYS INVOLVED IN THE DEVELOPMENT OF COLUMNAR-TYPE OF METAPLASIA

The current concept of esophageal metaplasia is that chronic (inflammatory) injury caused by bile and acid reflux as seen in gastroesophageal reflux disease has led to the upregulation or renewed expression of the SHH-BMP4 signaling pathway, which changes the epithelial environment in favor of columnar cells or drives cells toward a columnar phenotype. In the microenvironment surrounding the epithelial cells these factors are mostly secreted by stromal cells.[7,24,25] The stromal-epithelial interaction of SHH and BMP4 for epithelial remodeling is for instance demonstrated in xenopus.[26] Thus, the cross-talk between epithelium and stroma plays a major role in deciding on cell fate and cell lineage commitment. In adult normal squamous epithelium the expression of SHH and BMP4 is low and confined to the basal layer.[27,28] In Barrett biopsies SHH and its receptor PTCH are increased. Also BMP4 and its downstream target pSMAD are highly expressed, whereas the expression of Noggin, its natural inhibitor, is low.[28,29] Of interest it that increased expression of BMP4 and activation of its pathway is indeed observed in the early stage of esophagitis caused by gastroesophageal reflux disease. In vitro studies showed that BMP4 induced a shift in the gene expression profile of squamous cells toward that of columnar cells, which also included an important shift of the cytokeratin (CK) expression pattern. The cytoskeleton of epithelia, mainly consisting of actin and CKs, highly determines the phenotype of cells. Different types of epithelia have different CK expression patterns. In Barrett esophagus, it is known that CKs specific for columnar cells, such as CK7 and CK8, are highly expressed, whereas normal squamous epithelium show high levels of, for instance, CK10/13 and CK14. In an in vivo transplant culture system using esophageal epithelium expressing SHH, BMP4 and SOX9 were found to be upregulated. SOX9 is a transcription factor of columnar-type of genes.[28] In the organotypic model SOX9 was found to induce the expression of CK8 in squamous cells independent of BMP4.[30] In intestinal cells, however, SOX9 was found to be a WNT target and found to repress CDX2 and MUC2 expression.[31] Both, CDX2 and MUC2 are factors associated with a specific intestinal phenotype. In a transgenic mouse model of chronic inflammation, IL-1β overexpression leads to columnar metaplasia in mice. Columnar metaplasia at the squamocolumnar junction developed after a relatively long period ($\sim$12–15 months) of inflammation. Both, bile acids and carcinogens enhanced the development of metaplasia and dysplasia. Gene expression profiles of the metaplasia in these mice closely resemble gene expression profiles found in human Barrett and the associated cancer.[32] In this model SHH and BMPs were found to be increased in the metaplastic epithelium. Early development of metaplastic columnar glands at the squamocolumnar junction was also demonstrated in a mouse model that overexpressed BMP4 in squamous cells. In these animals the metaplastic glands could be observed at 9 to 12 weeks.[1] In a surgical mouse model in which bile and acid reflux is induced through an esophago-jejunostomy, pSMAD and BMP4 were found to be upregulated in the inflamed esophagus and the metaplastic glands.[1]

MOLECULAR FACTORS INVOLVED IN INTESTINAL DIFFERENTIATION

The intestinal-type of esophageal metaplasia has striking similarities with the specialized intestinal-type of epithelium that can be found in the small and large intestine. Intestinal metaplasia is, for instance, characterized by the presence of periodic acid–Schiff/alcian blue staining goblet cells. SHH and BMP4 are key players in the midgut and hindgut for the early transforming the primordial epithelium of the endoderm into a simple columnar epithelial lining. WNT and Notch signaling subsequently take part in the further differentiation of the intestinal mucosa into crypts and villi, and in the adult small and large intestine these factors are crucial in the homeostasis and crypt renewal.[7,24,25,33] WNT ligands are secreted glycoproteins that bind to cell surface receptors including the transmembrane receptor Frizzled, and the low-density lipoprotein receptor–related proteins 5 and 6 (LRP5/6).[34] WNT signaling may follow the WNT–β-catenin canonical pathway or less defined noncanonical pathways.[35] WNT–β-catenin signaling is essential for growth and differentiation in many tissues, including the intestine.[34–36] A key regulator of canonical WNT signaling is β-catenin. Activation of WNT signaling inhibits degradation of β-catenin, which in turn translocates into the nucleus. β-Catenin through interaction with TCF4/LEF transcription factors promotes transcription of genes involved in growth and proliferation and genes regulating the expression of intestinal-type of genes.[25,37]

Notch signaling is also essential for differentiation, proliferation, and the homeostasis of intestinal epithelium.[38] Activated Notch receptor results in release of the Notch intracellular domain, which can translocate into the nucleus, binds to the transcriptional repressor RBP-J kappa, and recruits coactivators to activate transcription of, for instance, the Hairy enhancer of split1 (HES1) and atonal homolog 1 (ATOH1) genes.[39,40] Notch signaling has a critical role in controlling intestinal cell commitment. The repressor function of the Notch target HES1 and reciprocal function of ATOH1 are critical in the maintenance of stem cell populations and determine the differentiation direction of the intestinal cells.[41–44]

CDX2 is an intestine-specific homeobox gene known to play a critical role in differentiation and maintenance of intestinal epithelial functions. CDX2 is a homologue of the Drosophila Caudal gene and belongs to the family of homeobox genes (HOM cluster in Drosophila). A common feature of these genes is the possession of a "homeobox" DNA binding motif coding for a consensus sequence of 60 to 63 amino acids that acts as a transcriptional regulator of "downstream" genes.[45] Expression of several CDX genes may be regulated through the WNT signaling pathway.[46] In turn CDX2 in cancer has been found to inhibit WNT signaling.[47]

MOLECULAR SIGNALS THAT DRIVE INTESTINAL METAPLASIA

Gene expression profiling of intestinal metaplasia showed that expression of several more specific intestinal-type of genes including CK20, Carbonic Anhydrase 1, VILLIN, Mucins (MUC2), sucrase-isomaltase, human defensin, fatty acid binding protein 6, gap junction protein beta 1, trefoil factors, and others is increased.[48] Transcription of these genes is known to be mediated by the caudal-related homeobox gene CDX2 and CDX1.[49–51] CDX2 is normally not expressed in the normal esophagus or stomach.[52] Several studies demonstrated that nuclear CDX2 and CDX1 expression can be found in the intestinal-type of metaplasia.[53–55] In vitro it was shown that exposure of a human esophageal squamous cell line to acid and bile upregulated CDX2 expression through promoter demethylation.[49] These studies indicate that development of the specialized intestinal phenotype in esophageal metaplasia is mediated by expression of CDX2. To further investigate the role of CDX2 in the development of columnar metaplasia, a transgenic mouse that overexpressed CDX2 in the mouse esophagus under the cytokeratin 14 (K14) promoter was generated. In this model CDX2 overexpression in squamous cells failed to induce a columnar metaplasia.[56] Also, retroviral transduction of human squamous cells with CDX2 did not cause a columnar or intestinal phenotype.[57] Therefore, these results suggest that CDX2 alone is insufficient to induce columnar metaplasia in squamous cells, unlike the metaplasia of the stomach, where overexpression of CDX2 under the H+/K+ATPase promoter clearly leads to intestinal metaplasia of the stomach.[58] In a surgical mouse model it was shown that CDX2 and MUC2 expression are late events in columnar cells, which already have upregulated BMP4-pSMAD pathway. In vitro studies showed that pSMAD and CDX2 form a functional complex that target the Muc2 promoter.[1] This indicates that CDX2 function for transcription of intestinal-type of genes depends on active BMP-pSMAD signaling. This could explain why transgenic overexpression of CDX2 in the stomach but not in the esophagus leads to intestinal metaplasia, because pSMAD is expressed in the stomach.

At the ultrastructural level, primary cultured squamous cells stimulated with an activated BMP4-pSMAD pathway and transfected with CDX2 show morphologic changes toward that of columnar cells. Most remarkable is that the cultured keratinocytes lose their multilayered appearance, reorganize into a monolayer, and develop such features as microvilli (**Fig. 2**).[1]

WNTs and Notch have critical roles in differentiation of the intestinal epithelium. This could mean that these factors may be involved in the development of esophageal metaplasia. So far, canonical WNT–β-catenin signaling has not been observed in the early developmental stage of the nonintestinal-type of metaplasia but the WNT target TCF4 is upregulated in intestinal metaplasia. In vitro analysis also showed that stimulation of keratinocytes with bile and acid upregulates the WNT downstream target TCF4 next to CDX2.[54,59]

Molecules, such as NCID and HES1, which are involved in Notch signaling have been observed in esophageal metaplasia.[60,61] In IL-1ß overexpressing mice, Notch signaling was activated by the binding of the Delta like 1 ligand (DLL1) ligand to Notch. In the intestine ATOH1 drives the differentiation of crypt cells toward goblet cells, a process that is inhibited by HES1.[62] ATOH1 is observed in intestinal metaplasia, where it is mostly confined to the goblet cells. In vitro experiments also showed that bile and acid can upregulate ATOH1 in squamous cells, whereas overexpression of ATOH1 induced expression of intestinal-type of genes including MUC2, alkaline phosphatase, and CK20.[59,63]

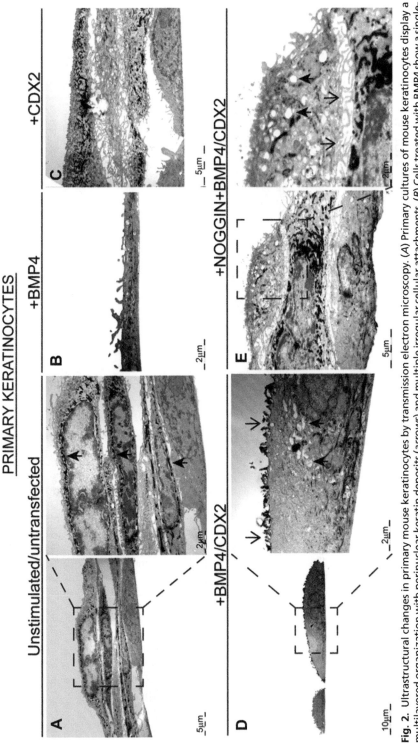

Fig. 2. Ultrastructural changes in primary mouse keratinocytes by transmission electron microscopy. (*A*) Primary cultures of mouse keratinocytes display a multilayered organization with perinuclear keratin deposits (*arrows*) and multiple irregular cellular attachments. (*B*) Cells treated with BMP4 show a single-layered organization, a flat cellular shape, and few vacuoles. (*C*) Cells transfected with CDX2 show a multilayered organization, dense keratin deposits, cytoplasmic vacuoles, and elongated cellular extensions. (*D*) After CDX2 transfection and BMP4 stimulation the cells are organized in single layer and show several secretory-like vacuoles (*thick arrows*) and microvilli-like structures (*thin arrows*) on the cell surface. (*E*) Cells treated with Noggin, before CDX2 transfection and BMP4 stimulation, retain a multilayered organization, showing similar ultrastructural changes of the cells only transfected with CDX2, exhibiting vacuoles (thick *arrows*) and irregular cellular attachments (thin *arrows*).

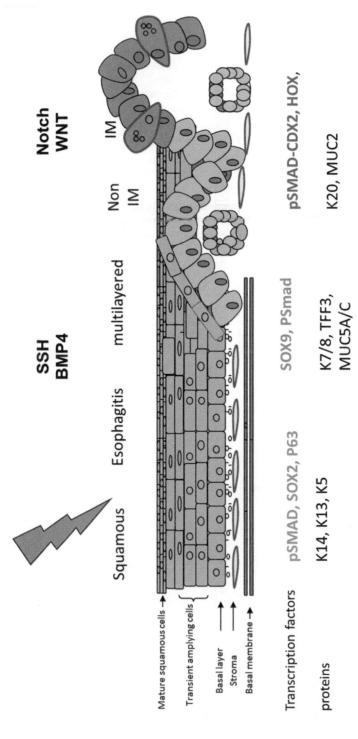

Fig. 3. SHH and BMP4 and downstream targets pSMAD and SOX9 are involved in the earliest stages of development of the nonintestinal-type of columnar metaplasia (non-IM), whereas pSMAD-CDX2, Notch, and WNT signaling are involved in the further development and homeostasis of the intestinal-type of metaplasia (IM). pSMAD, SOX2, and P63 are transcription factors involved in development and homeostasis of normal squamous epithelium.

THE BARRETT CELL OF ORIGIN

A major unanswered question that has been debated for decades is whether the Barrett cell of origin is derived from transdifferentiation of the esophageal squamous epithelium,[64] or originates rather from a progenitor cell in the esophagus,[65] the esophageal submucosal glands,[66] residual embryonic cells located at the squamocolumnar junction,[21] from the gastric cardia,[67] or from circulating cells from the bone marrow (**Fig. 3**).[68] More recent studies using transgenic animal and lineage tracing models point to diverse sites of origin. These studies need to be interpreted with care because the esophagus of rodents and other animals differs in many ways from the human esophagus. For instance, the mouse esophagus is much simpler and devoid of submucosal glands, whereas in humans these submucosal glands may function as a reservoir for different types of progenitors.[3,69] Also in mice the squamocolumnar junction is localized in the stomach and divides the stomach into a fore and distal part. Lgr5-expressing cells have been observed in Barrett metaplasia.[70,71] A Barrett-like metaplasia and neoplasia was found in IL-1ß overexpressing mouse and from lineage tracing experiments it has been suggested that the stem cells that give rise to Barrett esophagus may originate from the neighboring columnar epithelia harboring Lgr5[+] stem cells at the squamocolumnar junction in these mice.[32] In a surgical mouse model lineage tracing of Lgr5[+] cells showed that Lgr5[+] progenitors were not at the basis of the columnar metaplasia that developed at the neosquamocolumnar junction in the tubular esophagus.[32] P63-deficient mice develop columnar epithelium rather than normal squamous epithelium in the forestomach and esophagus. In these mice Carbonic anhydrase 4 (Car4) expressing embryonic progenitors residing at the squamocolumnar junction were able to expand in case squamous cells were injured.[21] It is doubtful if these observations can be translated to humans because metaplasia develops not only in the distal but can also develop in the proximal tubular esophagus (eg, in patients who have undergone esophagocardia resection).[2] In mice it has been recently shown that virtually all basal cells through stochastic divisions serve as squamous progenitors.[72] It is possible that different organ sites involve different progenitors. Therefore, lineage tracing pursuing developmental stem cells in animal models may not clarify the human Barrett progenitor true nature. It is possible that compared with embryonic stem cells the Barrett progenitor cells may present a mixed signature and for instance may also carry cancer (stem) cell features. Indeed, characterizing the Barrett progenitor cell is complex and requires analysis of human metaplastic cell populations to reveal distinct progenitor cell phenotypes. In such analyses, one needs to take into account that Barrett metaplasia is a preneoplastic lesion acquired during adulthood. In humans, the presence of the same mitochondrial mutations in squamous mucosa and Barrett metaplasia may imply a common stem cell for squamous and Barrett cells.[73] Nevertheless, mouse models are crucial to support important molecular observations that occur during the development of metaplasia.

SUMMARY

At present, the SHH-BMP4/pSMAD pathway, its antagonists, and downstream targets seem to be the important signaling pathways involved in the development of earliest stages of columnar metaplasia. SHH-BMP4/pSMAD signaling is crucial for the induction of columnar genes leading to the nonintestinal-type of columnar metaplasia. Expression of the intestine-specific genes as seen in the later stage of the intestinal-type of Barrett metaplasia seems to be mediated by a pSMAD-CDX2 interaction, and in later stage Wnt, and Notch signaling (**Fig. 4**). Several studies have

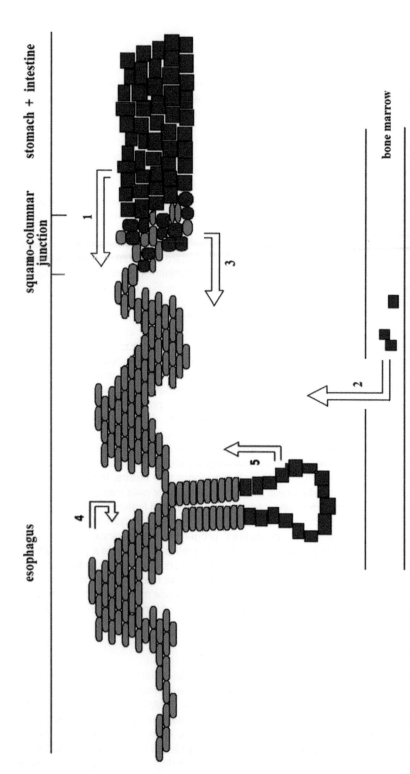

Fig. 4. The proposed origins of the Barrett progenitor cells. (1) Migration of cells from stomach. (2) Migration of cells from bone marrow. (3) "Primitive epithelial cells" (squamocolumnar junction) migrate + replace damaged squamous cells. (4) Transdifferentiation of esophageal cells. (5) Reprogramming of multipotent stem cells in the submucosal glands of the esophagus.

identified several other factors including RA,[23,74,75] FOXA2,[76] KLF4,[77] GATA4[78] and GATA6,[79] and HOX genes[80] that also seem to be involved in the development of metaplasia. It is most likely that the complex process of epithelial metaplasia also involves several of these factors. Therefore, there are still many issues at the molecular level that need to be resolved. Nevertheless, the current molecular findings provide important insight in the development of the columnar- and intestinal-type metaplasia, which can be used for developing novel molecular therapies. With respect to the Barrett cell of origin, there is a need to better characterize the human Barrett progenitor cell to develop appropriate lineage tracing models. This requires human material in which metaplastic cell populations need to be analyzed to distinguish distinct progenitor cell phenotypes. In such analyses one needs to take into account that Barrett metaplasia is a preneoplastic lesion acquired during adulthood and arising from matured tissues. Mouse models are crucial to support important molecular observations that occur during the development of metaplasia, but these models will always fall short in deciphering the origin of the human Barrett progenitor cell, because of the fundamental anatomic differences between the human and mouse esophagus.

REFERENCES

1. Mari L, Milano F, Parikh K, et al. A pSMAD/CDX2 complex is essential for the intestinalization of epithelial metaplasia. Cell Rep 2014;7:1197–210.
2. Castillo D, Puig S, Iglesias M, et al. Activation of the BMP4 pathway and early expression of CDX2 characterize non-specialized columnar metaplasia in a human model of Barrett's esophagus. J Gastrointest Surg 2012;16:227–37.
3. Glickman JN, Chen YY, Wang HH, et al. Phenotypic characteristics of a distinctive multilayered epithelium suggests that it is a precursor in the development of Barrett's esophagus. Am J Surg Pathol 2001;25:569–78.
4. Glickman JN, Spechler SJ, Souza RF, et al. Multilayered epithelium in mucosal biopsy specimens from the gastroesophageal junction region is a histologic marker of gastroesophageal reflux disease. Am J Surg Pathol 2009;33:818–25.
5. Odze RD. Unraveling the mystery of the gastroesophageal junction: a pathologist's perspective. Am J Gastroenterol 2005;100:1853–67.
6. Thompson JJ, Zinsser KR, Enterline HT. Barrett's metaplasia and adenocarcinoma of the esophagus and gastroesophageal junction. Hum Pathol 1983;14: 42–61.
7. Fukuda K, Yasugi S. Versatile roles for sonic hedgehog in gut development. J Gastroenterol 2002;37:239–46.
8. Hammerschmidt M, Brook A, McMahon AP. The world according to hedgehog. Trends Genet 1997;13:14–21.
9. Hogan BL, Blessing M, Winnier GE, et al. Growth factors in development: the role of TGF-beta related polypeptide signalling molecules in embryogenesis. Dev Suppl 1994;53–60.
10. Kretzschmar M, Liu F, Hata A, et al. The TGF-beta family mediator Smad1 is phosphorylated directly and activated functionally by the BMP receptor kinase. Genes Dev 1997;11:984–95.
11. Ito Y, Miyazono K. RUNX transcription factors as key targets of TGF-beta superfamily signaling. Curr Opin Genet Dev 2003;13:43–7.
12. Heldin CH, Miyazono K, Ten DP. TGF-beta signalling from cell membrane to nucleus through SMAD proteins. Nature 1997;390:465–71.
13. Kretzschmar M, Massague J. SMADs: mediators and regulators of TGF-beta signaling. Curr Opin Genet Dev 1998;8:103–11.

14. Jacobs IJ, Ku WY, Que J. Genetic and cellular mechanisms regulating anterior foregut and esophageal development. Dev Biol 2012;369:54–64.
15. Litingtung Y, Lei L, Westphal H, et al. Sonic hedgehog is essential to foregut development. Nat Genet 1998;20:58–61.
16. Narita T, Ishii Y, Nohno T, et al. Sonic hedgehog expression in developing chicken digestive organs is regulated by epithelial-mesenchymal interactions. Dev Growth Differ 1998;40:67–74.
17. Rodriguez P, Da SS, Oxburgh L, et al. BMP signaling in the development of the mouse esophagus and forestomach. Development 2010;137:4171–6.
18. Que J, Choi M, Ziel JW, et al. Morphogenesis of the trachea and esophagus: current players and new roles for noggin and Bmps. Differentiation 2006;74:422–37.
19. Que J, Luo X, Schwartz RJ, et al. Multiple roles for Sox2 in the developing and adult mouse trachea. Development 2009;136:1899–907.
20. Que J, Okubo T, Goldenring JR, et al. Multiple dose-dependent roles for Sox2 in the patterning and differentiation of anterior foregut endoderm. Development 2007;134:2521–31.
21. Wang X, Ouyang H, Yamamoto Y, et al. Residual embryonic cells as precursors of a Barrett's-like metaplasia. Cell 2011;145:1023–35.
22. Daniely Y, Liao G, Dixon D, et al. Critical role of p63 in the development of a normal esophageal and tracheobronchial epithelium. Am J Physiol Cell Physiol 2004;287:C171–81.
23. Chang CL, Lao-Sirieix P, Save V, et al. Retinoic acid-induced glandular differentiation of the oesophagus. Gut 2007;56:906–17.
24. Rubin DC. Intestinal morphogenesis. Curr Opin Gastroenterol 2007;23:111–4.
25. Sancho E, Batlle E, Clevers H. Signaling pathways in intestinal development and cancer. Annu Rev Cell Dev Biol 2004;20:695–723.
26. Ishizuya-Oka A, Hasebe T, Shimizu K, et al. Shh/BMP-4 signaling pathway is essential for intestinal epithelial development during Xenopus larval-to-adult remodeling. Dev Dyn 2006;235:3240–9.
27. van Dop WA, Rosekrans SL, Uhmann A, et al. Hedgehog signalling stimulates precursor cell accumulation and impairs epithelial maturation in the murine oesophagus. Gut 2013;62:348–57.
28. Wang DH, Clemons NJ, Miyashita T, et al. Aberrant epithelial-mesenchymal Hedgehog signaling characterizes Barrett's metaplasia. Gastroenterology 2010; 138:1810–22.
29. Milano F, van Baal JW, Buttar NS, et al. Bone morphogenetic protein 4 expressed in esophagitis induces a columnar phenotype in esophageal squamous cells. Gastroenterology 2007;132:2412–21.
30. Clemons NJ, Wang DH, Croagh D, et al. Sox9 drives columnar differentiation of esophageal squamous epithelium: a possible role in the pathogenesis of Barrett's esophagus. Am J Physiol Gastrointest Liver Physiol 2012;303:G1335–46.
31. Blache P, van de Wetering M, Duluc I, et al. SOX9 is an intestine crypt transcription factor, is regulated by the Wnt pathway, and represses the CDX2 and MUC2 genes. J Cell Biol 2004;166:37–47.
32. Quante M, Bhagat G, Abrams JA, et al. Bile acid and inflammation activate gastric cardia stem cells in a mouse model of Barrett-like metaplasia. Cancer Cell 2012;21:36–51.
33. Batts LE, Polk DB, Dubois RN, et al. Bmp signaling is required for intestinal growth and morphogenesis. Dev Dyn 2006;235:1563–70.
34. Clevers H, Nusse R. Wnt/beta-catenin signaling and disease. Cell 2012;149: 1192–205.

35. Niehrs C. The complex world of WNT receptor signalling. Nat Rev Mol Cell Biol 2012;13:767–79.
36. Habib SJ, Chen BC, Tsai FC, et al. A localized Wnt signal orients asymmetric stem cell division in vitro. Science 2013;339:1445–8.
37. Liu W, Dong X, Mai M, et al. Mutations in AXIN2 cause colorectal cancer with defective mismatch repair by activating beta-catenin/TCF signalling. Nat Genet 2000;26:146–7.
38. Katoh M, Katoh M. Notch signaling in gastrointestinal tract (review). Int J Oncol 2007;30:247–51.
39. Katoh M, Katoh M. Integrative genomic analyses on HES/HEY family: Notch-independent HES1, HES3 transcription in undifferentiated ES cells, and Notch-dependent HES1, HES5, HEY1, HEY2, HEYL transcription in fetal tissues, adult tissues, or cancer. Int J Oncol 2007;31:461–6.
40. Yang Q, Bermingham NA, Finegold MJ, et al. Requirement of Math1 for secretory cell lineage commitment in the mouse intestine. Science 2001;294:2155–8.
41. Katoh M, Katoh M. WNT antagonist, DKK2, is a Notch signaling target in intestinal stem cells: augmentation of a negative regulation system for canonical WNT signaling pathway by the Notch-DKK2 signaling loop in primates. Int J Mol Med 2007;19:197–201.
42. Crosnier C, Vargesson N, Gschmeissner S, et al. Delta-Notch signalling controls commitment to a secretory fate in the zebrafish intestine. Development 2005;132: 1093–104.
43. Kopan R, Ilagan MX. The canonical Notch signaling pathway: unfolding the activation mechanism. Cell 2009;137:216–33.
44. Fre S, Huyghe M, Mourikis P, et al. Notch signals control the fate of immature progenitor cells in the intestine. Nature 2005;435:964–8.
45. Beck F. The role of Cdx genes in the mammalian gut. Gut 2004;53:1394–6.
46. Ikeya M, Takada S. Wnt-3a is required for somite specification along the antero-posterior axis of the mouse embryo and for regulation of cdx-1 expression. Mech Dev 2001;103:27–33.
47. Liu X, Zhang X, Zhan Q, et al. CDX2 serves as a Wnt signaling inhibitor and is frequently methylated in lung cancer. Cancer Biol Ther 2012;13:1152–7.
48. van Baal JW, Milano F, Rygiel AM, et al. A comparative analysis by SAGE of gene expression profiles of Barrett's esophagus, normal squamous esophagus, and gastric cardia. Gastroenterology 2005;129:1274–81.
49. Liu T, Zhang X, So CK, et al. Regulation of Cdx2 expression by promoter methylation, and effects of Cdx2 transfection on morphology and gene expression of human esophageal epithelial cells. Carcinogenesis 2007;28:488–96.
50. Chan CW, Wong NA, Liu Y, et al. Gastrointestinal differentiation marker Cytokeratin 20 is regulated by homeobox gene CDX1. Proc Natl Acad Sci U S A 2009; 106:1936–41.
51. Yamamoto H, Bai YQ, Yuasa Y. Homeodomain protein CDX2 regulates goblet-specific MUC2 gene expression. Biochem Biophys Res Commun 2003;300:813–8.
52. Guo RJ, Suh ER, Lynch JP. The role of Cdx proteins in intestinal development and cancer. Cancer Biol Ther 2004;3:593–601.
53. Huo X, Zhang HY, Zhang XI, et al. Acid and bile salt-induced CDX2 expression differs in esophageal squamous cells from patients with and without Barrett's esophagus. Gastroenterology 2010;139:194–203.
54. Kazumori H, Ishihara S, Rumi MA, et al. Bile acids directly augment caudal related homeobox gene Cdx2 expression in oesophageal keratinocytes in Barrett's epithelium. Gut 2006;55:16–25.

55. Kazumori H, Ishihara S, Kinoshita Y. Roles of caudal-related homeobox gene Cdx1 in oesophageal epithelial cells in Barrett's epithelium development. Gut 2009;58:620–8.
56. Kong J, Crissey MA, Funakoshi S, et al. Ectopic Cdx2 expression in murine esophagus models an intermediate stage in the emergence of Barrett's esophagus. PLoS One 2011;6:e18280.
57. Kong J, Nakagawa H, Isariyawongse BK, et al. Induction of intestinalization in human esophageal keratinocytes is a multistep process. Carcinogenesis 2009; 30:122–30.
58. Mutoh H, Hakamata Y, Sato K, et al. Conversion of gastric mucosa to intestinal metaplasia in Cdx2-expressing transgenic mice. Biochem Biophys Res Commun 2002;294:470–9.
59. Chen X, Jiang K, Fan Z, et al. Aberrant expression of Wnt and Notch signal pathways in Barrett's esophagus. Clin Res Hepatol Gastroenterol 2012;36:473–83.
60. Menke V, van Es JH, de Lau W, et al. Conversion of metaplastic Barrett's epithelium into post-mitotic goblet cells by gamma-secretase inhibition. Dis Model Mech 2010;3:104–10.
61. Mendelson J, Song S, Li Y, et al. Dysfunctional transforming growth factor-beta signaling with constitutively active Notch signaling in Barrett's esophageal adenocarcinoma. Cancer 2011;117:3691–702.
62. van Es JH, van Gijn ME, Riccio O, et al. Notch/gamma-secretase inhibition turns proliferative cells in intestinal crypts and adenomas into goblet cells. Nature 2005;435:959–63.
63. Kong J, Crissey MA, Sepulveda AR, et al. Math1/Atoh1 contributes to intestinalization of esophageal keratinocytes by inducing the expression of Muc2 and Keratin-20. Dig Dis Sci 2012;57:845–57.
64. Yu WY, Slack JM, Tosh D. Conversion of columnar to stratified squamous epithelium in the developing mouse oesophagus. Dev Biol 2005;284:157–70.
65. Kalabis J, Oyama K, Okawa T, et al. A subpopulation of mouse esophageal basal cells has properties of stem cells with the capacity for self-renewal and lineage specification. J Clin Invest 2008;118:3860–9.
66. Leedham SJ, Preston SL, McDonald SA, et al. Individual crypt genetic heterogeneity and the origin of metaplastic glandular epithelium in human Barrett's oesophagus. Gut 2008;57:1041–8.
67. Barbera M, Fitzgerald RC. Cellular origin of Barrett's metaplasia and oesophageal stem cells. Biochem Soc Trans 2010;38:370–3.
68. Sarosi G, Brown G, Jaiswal K, et al. Bone marrow progenitor cells contribute to esophageal regeneration and metaplasia in a rat model of Barrett's esophagus. Dis Esophagus 2008;21:43–50.
69. Glickman JN, Yang A, Shahsafaei A, et al. Expression of p53-related protein p63 in the gastrointestinal tract and in esophageal metaplastic and neoplastic disorders. Hum Pathol 2001;32:1157–65.
70. Becker L, Huang Q, Mashimo H. Lgr5, an intestinal stem cell marker, is abnormally expressed in Barrett's esophagus and esophageal adenocarcinoma. Dis Esophagus 2010;23:168–74.
71. von Rahden BH, Kircher S, Lazariotou M, et al. LgR5 expression and cancer stem cell hypothesis: clue to define the true origin of esophageal adenocarcinomas with and without Barrett's esophagus? J Exp Clin Cancer Res 2011;30:23.
72. Doupe DP, Alcolea MP, Roshan A, et al. A single progenitor population switches behavior to maintain and repair esophageal epithelium. Science 2012;337: 1091–3.

73. Nicholson AM, Graham TA, Simpson A, et al. Barrett's metaplasia glands are clonal, contain multiple stem cells and share a common squamous progenitor. Gut 2012;61:1380–9.
74. Chang CL, Hong E, Lao-Sirieix P, et al. A novel role for the retinoic acid-catabolizing enzyme CYP26A1 in Barrett's associated adenocarcinoma. Oncogene 2008;27:2951–60.
75. Cooke G, Blanco-Fernandez A, Seery JP. The effect of retinoic acid and deoxycholic acid on the differentiation of primary human esophageal keratinocytes. Dig Dis Sci 2008;53:2851–7.
76. Wang DH, Tiwari A, Kim ME, et al. Hedgehog signaling regulates FOXA2 in esophageal embryogenesis and Barrett's metaplasia. J Clin Invest 2014;124: 3767–80.
77. Kazumori H, Ishihara S, Takahashi Y, et al. Roles of Kruppel-like factor 4 in oesophageal epithelial cells in Barrett's epithelium development. Gut 2011;60:608–17.
78. Chen X, Qin R, Liu B, et al. Multilayered epithelium in a rat model and human Barrett's esophagus: similar expression patterns of transcription factors and differentiation markers. BMC Gastroenterol 2008;8:1.
79. Wang J, Qin R, Ma Y, et al. Differential gene expression in normal esophagus and Barrett's esophagus. J Gastroenterol 2009;44:897–911.
80. di Pietro M, Lao-Sirieix P, Boyle S, et al. Evidence for a functional role of epigenetically regulated midcluster HOXB genes in the development of Barrett esophagus. Proc Natl Acad Sci U S A 2012;109:9077–82.

Role of Obesity in the Pathogenesis and Progression of Barrett's Esophagus

Apoorva Krishna Chandar, MBBS, MPH[a],
Prasad G. Iyer, MD, MSc, AGAF[b],*

KEYWORDS

- Barrett's esophagus • Esophageal adenocarcinoma
- Gastroesophageal reflux disease • Obesity • Leptin • Adiponectin
- Insulin resistance • Inflammation

KEY POINTS

- Central obesity is an independent risk factor for Barrett's esophagus (BE) and esophageal adenocarcinoma. Overall body fat content is not a risk factor for BE.
- Central obesity likely mediates its influence on BE via mechanical and metabolic effects.
- Mechanical effects include disruption of the gastroesophageal junction reflux barrier leading to some increase in gastroesophageal reflux.
- Metabolic effects are likely mediated by the visceral abdominal fat compartment, which releases adipokines, and leads to a systemic inflammatory state (mediated via the release of saturated free fatty acids, macrophage activation, and release of pro-inflammatory cytokines), resulting in insulin resistance.
- Several of these inflammatory and proneoplastic pathways can be potentially targeted by novel molecular therapies for chemoprevention.

INTRODUCTION

An exponential increase in the prevalence of obesity has been observed in the United States in recent decades,[1] paralleled by a comparable increase in the incidence of esophageal adenocarcinoma (EAC),[2] a cancer that continues to carry a bleak prognosis.[3] These unprecedented increases in obesity and EAC assume particular

Grant Support: None.
Disclosures: None relevant.
[a] Division of Gastroenterology and Liver Diseases, Digestive Health Institute, University Hospitals Case Medical Center, Case Western Reserve University, 10900 Euclid Avenue, Cleveland, OH 44106, USA; [b] Barrett's Esophagus Unit, Division of Gastroenterology and Hepatology, Mayo Clinic, 200 1st Street South West, Rochester, MN 55905, USA
* Corresponding author.
E-mail address: iyer.prasad@mayo.edu

importance in the context of Barrett's esophagus (BE), the only established premalignant precursor and strongest risk factor of EAC. In BE, the stratified squamous lining of the distal esophagus undergoes a metaplastic change to an intestinal-type columnar epithelium, presumably due to long-standing exposure to gastric refluxate. BE may progress via the development of dysplasia to EAC. The origin of BE and mechanisms of progression to EAC, however, are poorly understood. An obesity and reflux-driven synergism could potentially explain some aspects of the pathogenesis and progression of BE. This review summarizes the current evidence on the role of obesity in the development and progression of BE to EAC.

OBESITY AND BARRETT'S ESOPHAGUS: EVIDENCE FOR ASSOCIATION

Obesity can have wide-ranging consequences on the human body, both metabolic and nonmetabolic, but its association with BE is particularly intriguing. Traditionally, association studies of obesity and BE have used the body mass index (BMI), a convenient, but imprecise tool to measure overall body fat mass. Meta-analyses of observational evidence by Cook et al.[4] and Kamat et al.[5] have shown an association between BMI and BE when using population-based controls without gastroesophageal reflux disease (GERD), but their analyses suffered from the limitation of using unadjusted odds ratios (OR).A GERD-adjusted analysis by Cook showed that the association between BMI and BE was no longer significant when using GERD controls, leading the investigators to speculate that BMI was a risk factor for BE, but with the association mediated through GERD.[4] Given that BMI does not accurately measure body fat content, the findings from studies of association of BMI with BE, or the lack thereof, are not surprising. More recently, researchers have tried to use other measurement tools, such as DEXA (dual-energy X-ray absorptiometry)[6] and bioelectrical impedance analysis (BIA)[7] that can capture body fat mass more precisely. Thrift and colleagues[8] conducted a case-control study in which body fat mass was measured by BIA. They found that BMI was not associated with an increased risk of BE, despite using this more accurate method to measure overall body fat mass.

In contrast to BMI, central obesity has a more robust association with BE. A hospital-based case-control study by Kramer et al.[9] comparing 237 BE cases with 1021 endoscopy controls showed that waist-to-hip ratio (WHR) was associated with a nearly 2-fold increase in BE risk, independent of GERD; this association was further strengthened when the analysis was limited to long-segment Barrett's esophagus (LSBE) and white men. Thrift and colleagues[8] found a similar association between WHR and BE in a case-control study using primary care and endoscopy controls, but the association lost significance when the analysis was adjusted for GERD. Another study found all measures of central obesity (waist circumference [WC], WHR, sagittal abdominal diameter, and waist-to-height ratio) to be strongly associated with increased risk of BE in men, but not in women; this association was reduced slightly after adjusting for GERD symptoms.[10] A recent meta-analysis of 40 observational studies has conclusively shown that central adiposity (measured by either anthropometry or quantitative assessment of intra-abdominal fat: subcutaneous and visceral, by computed tomography [CT]) is associated with an increased risk of BE, even after BMI and GERD are controlled for[11]; the effect estimate was more pronounced in LSBE patients and in men (**Fig. 1**). A dose-response relationship further strengthened this association. This association was seen only with visceral fat and not subcutaneous fat. This association was in addition to strong associations with erosive esophagitis and EAC, phenotypes that are closely linked to BE. An additional meta-analysis using individual patient data from the BEACON consortium has shown

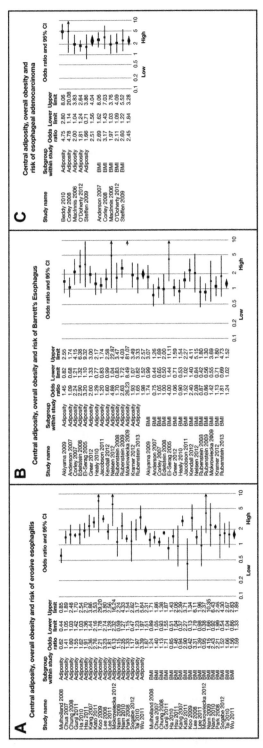

Fig. 1. Central adiposity, overall obesity (BMI), and risk of (A) erosive esophagitis, (B) BE, and (C) EAC. This represents the overall pooled OR by combining categorical OR (for highest category, compared with lowest referent category) with estimated OR from continuous variables. (*From* Singh S, Sharma AN, Murad MH, et al. Central adiposity is associated with increased risk of esophageal inflammation, metaplasia, and adenocarcinoma: a systematic review and meta-analysis. Clin Gastroenterol Hepatol 2013;11(11):1407; with permission.)

that increased WC is associated with a greater than 2-fold higher risk of BE in both men and women, independent of BMI and GERD symptoms.[12]

OBESITY AND BARRETT'S ESOPHAGUS: MECHANISMS OF ASSOCIATION

Ample evidence suggests that abdominal obesity is involved in the pathogenesis of BE. Abdominal obesity is presumably thought to have a dual effect in BE pathogenesis and progression: one that is GERD-dependent (mechanical effect), and another that is GERD-independent (nonmechanical or metabolic effect). Abdominal fat is mainly distributed in 2 compartments: a subcutaneous fat compartment and a visceral fat compartment. Studies that have measured visceral fat using radiographic techniques, such as single-slice abdominal CT (at the level of the L2-L3 interspace), demonstrate that it is indeed the visceral portion of the abdominal fat that is associated with an increased risk of BE, and not subcutaneous fat.[13,14] Although both subcutaneous and visceral fat likely exert mechanical effects, visceral fat is more likely responsible for the metabolic effect. These 2 mechanisms are examined in the following discussion (**Fig. 2**).

Mechanical Effects of Central Obesity

Central obesity, by exerting mechanical effects on the gastroesophageal junction (GEJ), likely results in its anatomic disruption. A prospective study of 285 patients using high-resolution manometry showed that central obesity, measured by WC, had a strong positive correlation with raised intragastric pressure and moderate

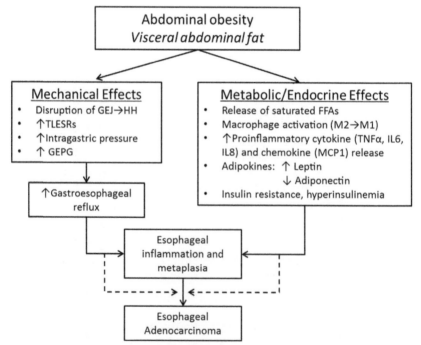

Fig. 2. Potential mechanisms of abdominal obesity–induced esophageal injury, inflammation, and neoplasia. HH, hiatal hernia; M1, classically activated macrophages; M2, alternatively activated macrophages; MCP1, macrophage chemoattractant protein 1; TLESRs, transient lower esophageal sphincter relaxations.

positive correlation with gastroesophageal pressure gradient (GEPG), after controlling for age, sex, and gastroesophageal reflux symptoms.[15] A dose-response relationship between increasing WC and increased intragastric pressure and GEPG was also observed. Furthermore, both BMI and WC were shown to be associated with anatomic disruption of the GEJ (separation of the diaphragmatic hiatus and lower esophageal sphincter), which leads to the formation of a hiatal hernia. These findings have largely been confirmed by Derakhshan et al.[16] in a sample of dyspeptic patients having normal endoscopy (without evidence of a hiatal hernia or erosive esophagitis).

In a Chinese population-based study largely without GERD symptoms, Wu and colleagues[17] found that when compared with controls, a greater proportion of obese patients had an increased frequency of postprandial transient lower esophageal sphincter relaxations (TLESR) with acid reflux, which is another crucial physiologic mechanism of gastroesophageal reflux. The study also demonstrated a significantly increased postprandial GEPG in obese patients. Both BMI and WC were found to correlate well with their findings. Another cross-sectional study involving 206 patients showed a modest association between obesity (BMI $\geq$30 and increased WC) and increased postprandial acid reflux in those who were obese when compared to normal subjects.[18] However, when both BMI and WC (as a measure of central obesity) were examined together, BMI was found to have no association with esophageal acid exposure, indicating that central obesity was likely mediating most of the effects of obesity on GERD. Indeed, meta-analyses have shown that both hiatal hernia and GERD are associated with BE.[19,20]

Despite these reported findings, the mechanical effect alone is insufficient to explain the association of abdominal obesity with BE. For instance, in a prospective cross-sectional study involving 322 patients, there was only a weak positive correlation between intragastric pressure and measures of obesity (both BMI and WC) after adjusting for age, gender, race, and indications for manometry.[21] The absolute increase in reflux episodes with obesity is modest.[18] In addition, other gastrointestinal cancers, which are not influenced by reflux (such as colon[22] and pancreas[23]), are also independently associated with central obesity. Perhaps the most compelling evidence is provided by the meta-analysis by Singh et al.,[11] where, even after adjusting for GERD, the association between abdominal obesity and BE still persisted, indicating that this association might be mediated by GERD independent of nonmechanical effects (see **Fig. 1**). Hence, central obesity, although likely increasing mechanical pressure leading to some increase in gastric reflux, also contributes to BE and EAC risk by nonmechanical means.

Metabolic Effects of Central Obesity

Visceral abdominal fat and obesity

Obesity is widely recognized as a state of chronic low-grade systemic inflammation. Visceral adipose tissue contains an abundance of pro-inflammatory cells, such as classically activated (M1) macrophages, neutrophils, mast cells, Th1 (CD4+, CD8+) T lymphocytes, and B lymphocytes as well as anti-inflammatory cells, such as alternatively activated (M2) macrophages, T regulatory and Th2 lymphocytes, and eosinophils (**Fig. 3**).[24] In normal physiologic states (lean individuals), the overall balance between these cells remains anti-inflammatory, preventing the overexpression of inflammatory mediators. However, in the obese state, adipocyte hypertrophy along with tissue hypoxia leads to a breakdown of this homeostasis.[24] Pro-inflammatory cells, particularly classically activated macrophages (recruited by chemokines such as macrophage chemoattractant protein 1), increase, leading to overexpression and

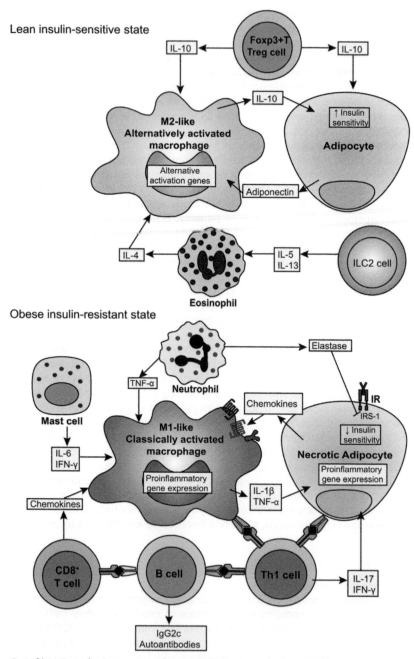

Fig. 3. Infiltration of adipose tissue by pro-inflammatory and anti-inflammatory cells in the lean and obese insulin-resistant state. IFN-γ, interferon-γ; IgG2c, immunoglobulin Gamma 2c; ILC2, innate lymphoid cells type-2; IRS-1, insulin receptor substrate-1. (*From* McNelis JC, Olefsky JM. Macrophages, immunity, and metabolic disease. Immunity 2014;41(1):43; with permission.)

systemic release of pro-inflammatory cytokines (tumor necrosis factor-α [TNF-α], interleukin (IL)-1β, IL-6), lipolysis (which leads to the release of saturated free fatty acids [FFAs]), and a change in the pattern of hormones released by adipocytes (adipokines, such as leptin: increased levels, and adiponectin: decreased levels). Saturated FFA released by lipolysis also promote activation of macrophages to an M1 phenotype. These obesity induced changes cumulatively lead to a systemic inflammatory state and insulin resistance,[25] both of which have been associated with an increased risk of BE and EAC.[26]

In addition to visceral adipose tissue, obesity has been shown to be associated with macrophage-mediated inflammation in other organs, such as the liver, pancreatic islets, hypothalamus, and skeletal muscle (**Fig. 4**).[27,28] Hence, obesity may lead to both

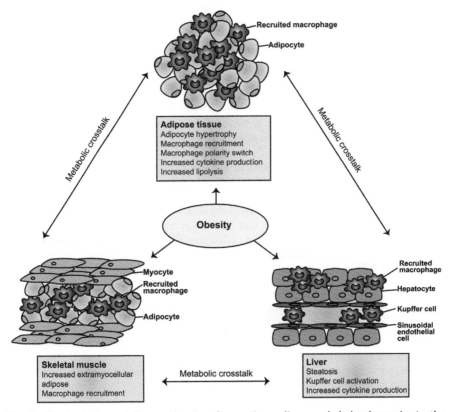

Fig. 4. Obesity induces inflammation in adipose tissue, liver, and skeletal muscle. In the obese state, adipocyte hypertrophy and apoptosis promote the recruitment of monocytes to adipose tissue, where in response to inflammatory stimuli, they differentiate into M1 inflammatory macrophages. In muscle, obesity is associated with increased extramyocellular adipose, which is proposed to recruit macrophages to this site. In the liver, obesity causes increased hepatic lipogenesis and inflammatory gene expression that promotes the activation of resident Kupffer cells and the recruitment of monocytes. M1-like macrophages secrete inflammatory cytokines that can induce insulin resistance locally or enter the peripheral circulation and cause systemic insulin resistance and inflammation. (*Adapted from* Olefsky JM, Glass CK. Macrophages, inflammation, and insulin resistance. Annu Rev Physiol 2010;72:219–46; and *From* McNelis JC, Olefsky JM. Macrophages, immunity, and metabolic disease. Immunity 2014;41(1):41; with permission.)

systemic and localized organ level inflammation in several target organs. Both of these mechanisms may be operative in enhancing esophageal injury and inflammation. Increased peri-esophageal GEJ fat has been demonstrated in subjects with BE and correlates with histologic inflammation and high-grade dysplasia (HGD)[14]; this may enhance esophageal inflammation by paracrine mechanisms. In addition, increased macrophage infiltration has been demonstrated in the BE epithelium of centrally obese BE subjects compared with controls.[29] Most macrophages in the BE epithelium appear to be of a pro-inflammatory (M1) phenotype, which could enhance reflux-mediated inflammation.

Leptin and Barrett's esophagus

Serum leptin, a product of the (ob) gene, is proportional to adipose tissue mass.[30] Leptin levels are substantially higher in women than in men, even after accounting for total body fat.[31] Leptin is angiogenic and mitogenic and regulates neovascularization.[32] It is also anti-apoptotic.[33] Binding of leptin to its receptor results initiates the phosphorylation of JAK2 tyrosine kinase, which in turns starts a cellular signaling cascade that results in further downstream activation of extracellular signal-regulated kinases (ERK), Akt, nuclear factor κB (NFkB), p38, and JNK, all of which are necessary for leptin to exert its anti-apoptotic and proliferative effects.[33,34] It has been shown that the esophageal mucosa is densely packed with leptin receptors.[35] Hence, it is hypothesized that in the obese state, leptin, acting synergistically with stomach acid or alone, induces proliferation in the distal esophagus.

Epidemiologic studies have looked at the association between increased serum leptin and BE. In a GERD-adjusted analysis comparing 306 BE cases and 309 controls, Kendall and colleagues[36] found a 2-fold higher risk of BE when serum leptin levels were high, but only in men. Rubenstein et al.[37] found a similar significant association between high serum leptin and BE risk in men after adjusting for obesity, GERD, and serum insulin. Garcia and colleagues[38] found that high levels of leptin were associated with an 8-fold greater risk of BE in cases than in controls; this association remained significant even after excluding women from the analysis. Thompson et al.,[39] on the contrary, found a greater than 3-fold risk of association between increased serum leptin and BE, but only in women. The reasons for this discrepancy are unclear, but could be related to populations studied, assays used to measure leptin levels, and other unmeasured/unadjusted confounders like insulin, which was adjusted for in only one study.[37] In a recent meta-analysis of 6 studies reporting on the association of serum leptin with BE, Devanna and colleagues[40] found that increased serum leptin was associated with a 2-fold increased risk of BE. This association was strengthened when the analysis was adjusted for GERD, suggesting an independent role of leptin in BE pathogenesis.

Adiponectin and Barrett's esophagus

Adiponectin is a 30-kDa polypeptide secreted predominantly by visceral adipose tissue. Its levels in serum are inversely proportional to the amount of body fat[41] and are lower in men than women.[42] In contrast to leptin, adiponectin exhibits anti-inflammatory[43] and anti-angiogeneic properties.[44] Adiponectin also antagonizes the effect of leptin by inhibiting leptin-induced cellular proliferation.[45] Three adiponectin multimers are recognized in circulating blood, namely, low-molecular-weight (LMW), middle-molecular-weight, and high-molecular-weight (HMW) adiponectin.[46] HMW and LMW adiponectin multimers are known to have contrasting pro-inflammatory and anti-inflammatory actions, respectively.[47]

Two adiponectin receptors are recognized in tissues, namely Adipo-R1 and R2. These receptors have been found to be decreased in BE cell lines.[48] In cell lines, adiponectin inhibits progression of BE into EAC by exerting strong anti-apoptotic effects.[48] BE proliferation is linked to an abnormal activation of the ERK1/2 in the squamous mucosa.[49] Physiologically, high serum adiponectin levels suppress these kinases. In obesity, as a result of low adiponectin, unchecked cellular proliferation takes place.

Mokrowiecka and colleagues[50] found significantly lower serum adiponectin levels in BE cases when compared with control patients. In another study, Rubenstein et al.[51] found an inverse association between low total serum adiponectin and BE after adjusting for GERD, smoking, and WHR. However, the study was limited by its small sample size and only measured total serum adiponectin and not its multi-mers. In a second larger study, the same investigators looked at the differential effects of the 3 multimeric forms of adiponectin.[52] Comparing 112 BE cases and 199 GERD controls, they found high levels of LMW adiponectin to be associated with a significantly lower risk of BE. When stratified by gender, this association became stronger in women, but not in men. The association remained after adjusting for potential confounding by insulin/insulin resistance. Thompson and colleagues[39] also showed an inverse relationship between high levels of total adiponectin and BE after adjusting for age, tobacco use, leptin, and WHR; this association was lost when the analysis was stratified by gender. Two other observational studies found no association between serum adiponectin and BE.[36,38] A systematic review and meta-analysis failed to demonstrate any association between total serum adiponectin and risk of BE.[40] Despite inconclusive results from epidemiologic studies, the study by Rubenstein informs us that the physiologic actions of adiponectin are probably mediated by its LMW multimer. By upregulating anti-inflammatory cytokines and downregulating pro-inflammatory cytokines, LMW adiponectin is thought to prevent inflammatory damage to the squamous epithelium in the setting of GERD and perhaps impedes the development and proliferation of BE.[47] Barrett's epithelium shows greater expression of the pro-inflammatory cytokine IL-6, adding strength to this postulation.[53]

Insulin and insulin resistance
It is now well accepted that obesity is one of the principal contributory factors in the development of insulin resistance (IR). Systemic inflammation associated with obesity has been shown to be a crucial mechanism responsible for IR. Insulin resistance is a condition where peripheral tissues are not sensitive to insulin despite high circulating insulin levels.[54] Insulin stimulates the production of insulin-like growth factor (IGF-1) and downregulates production of IGFBP1, resulting in higher levels of IGF-1 in serum.[55] IGF-1 binds to its receptor (IGF-1R) and this leads to activation of the PI3K/AKT/mTOR pathway, which subsequently promotes mitogenesis and prevents apoptosis.[56] Such an activation of the IGF pathway has been shown to occur in BE.[57] Furthermore, molecular studies have shown that IGF-1 and its binding proteins could influence neoplastic progression in BE.[58] Insulin and insulin-related signaling pathways have been shown to be upregulated in BE and EAC tissue.[57,59] IR is also associated with dysplastic progression in BE,[60] adding further proof that obesity-induced hyperinsulinemia and IR are associated with BE pathogenesis and progression.

Obesity also upregulates several inflammatory pathways, such as NFkB and JNK, which are known to play a role in the development of IR.[61,62] Overexpression of B cells, which occurs in obesity, is also associated with IR.[24] In addition to inflammatory mediators, obesity-induced IR also seems to be mediated by adipokines.[63] Leptin and adiponectin have opposite effects on insulin and IR; elevated serum leptin is strongly associated with IR,[64] whereas high adiponectin increases peripheral tissue sensitivity to insulin. Low adiponectin levels have been implicated in obesity-induced IR.[65]

Several observational studies have looked at the association of insulin, IR, and IGF with BE. Levels of insulin and the pro-inflammatory cytokine, IL-6, were found to be higher in BE cases than controls in a cross-sectional study by Ryan and colleagues.[26] In a large population-based case-control study, type 2 diabetes mellitus was associated with a nearly 50% increase in the risk of BE, independent of other known risk factors such as GERD and BMI; this association was stronger in women than men.[66] Leggett[67] found a 2-fold increase in the risk of BE in those with metabolic syndrome (which is associated with insulin resistance) that was also independent of BMI and GERD. Greer et al.[57] found a strong relationship between increased insulin and IGF-1 levels and risk of BE, but only when compared with healthy controls; this association disappeared when the comparison was GERD controls, indicating that the relationship between insulin and BE could be GERD-dependent. Rubenstein and colleagues,[37] on the other hand, could not find an association between increased insulin levels and higher risk of BE, when controlling for serum leptin. Two other case-control studies similarly failed to show any association between increased insulin and BE.[38,52] There could be several reasons for this nonsignificant result in some studies. Effects on the esophageal mucosa may not be directly mediated by insulin or IR, rather through leptin and/or other adipokines. Insulin could exert its effect through GERD, which has been shown to be increased in hyperinsulinemic and IR states.[68] Hence, adjusting for GERD (which was done in most studies) could have attenuated or removed any significant association between insulin and BE.

THE ROLE OF OBESITY IN BARRETT'S ESOPHAGUS PROGRESSION

Little is known about the role of obesity in the metaplasia-dysplasia-EAC sequence, despite the well-regarded association of obesity with EAC.[11,69] Nevertheless, a few studies have looked at the effect of obesity on BE progression. Thota and colleagues[70] found that a diagnosis of dysplasia or carcinoma was more common than nondysplastic BE in overweight and obese BE patients. In a prospective study of 392 BE patients, increased levels of serum leptin and insulin resistance (measured by the HOMA-IR index) were found to be associated with increased risk for EAC, particularly in men.[60] Although leptin has not been shown to be associated with progression of BE to EAC, despite being increased in the obese state, its effects are tumorigenic. It activates mitogen-activated protein (MAP) kinase, ERK, and phosphatidylinositol 3-kinase/Akt, which are well known to stimulate cellular proliferation and prevent apoptosis.[33] In vitro, leptin also stimulates EAC cell growth. Furthermore, expression of the leptin receptor (ob-R), which is thought to be upregulated with increased visceral adiposity, is predominantly seen in EAC as compared with the normal esophagus.[71]

In a case-control study of 50 BE cases and 50 controls, Nelsen et al.[14] found that both visceral fat and GEJ fat were significantly greater in patients with HGD compared with those without HGD, independent of BMI and GERD. The same study also found these 2 fat stores to be higher in persons with esophageal inflammation than those without, indicating that inflammatory pathways could possibly play a key role in BE progression. Activation of the IL-6/STAT3 pathway in transformed Barrett's epithelial cells inhibits apoptosis, which could be a key mediator of cell survival in the metaplasia-dysplasia-EAC sequence.[72] There is also a progressive increase in

TNF-α expression during metaplasia-dysplasia-EAC sequence in BE.[73] TNF-α, serum levels of which are increased in obesity, also downregulates expression of E-cadherin, which is essential for the maintenance of cellular junctions. Downregulation of E-cadherin expression results in a decrease in the strength of cellular adhesions, which in turn facilitates invasion by cancer cells into surrounding tissues.[74]

THERAPEUTIC IMPLICATIONS

Reversal of obesity and its consequences such as inflammation and IR could potentially inhibit BE pathogenesis and its progression to dysplasia/adenocarcinoma. Regular physical activity can help reduce obesity by leading to a negative energy balance. Although a meta-analysis showed that physical activity was associated with a reduced risk of EAC,[75] studies do not show a consistent effect. A large case-control study (323 BE cases with BE and 1849 controls) conducted in a Veterans' Affairs hospital failed to show a benefit of regular physical activity for BE.[76] It is not clear if physical activity has a direct effect or if it is mediated through a reduction in obesity and likely GERD. Presumably, it could be both. A possible limitation of such studies is the length/duration of intervention. Short-term physical activity interventions may fail to show a benefit and long-term follow-up might be cost-prohibitive.

More radical interventions like bariatric surgery for obesity have shown encouraging results with regards to BE length and dysplasia. In one study, 12 patients (5 patients with LSBE and 7 patients with short-segment Barrett's esophagus [SSBE]) were followed up with repeat endoscopies after their gastric bypass surgery. The authors found that there was regression from intestinal metaplasia to only cardiac mucosa in 4 patients with SSBE, and in one patient with LSBE.[77] In another retrospective chart review study, BE patients who underwent Roux-en-Y gastric bypass showed a decrease in the length of BE and improvement in the degree of dysplasia. In about 50% of these patients, there was complete regression of BE. The beneficial effect of weight loss surgeries on BE could be related to the reduction of visceral fat, which would improve reflux symptoms as well as reduce IR. However, these studies are small and uncontrolled, and larger more definitive studies are needed.

Metformin is a widely used oral hypoglycemic drug, which is known to lower IR.[78] In a randomized controlled trial, researchers studied the effect of metformin on phosphorylated S6 kinase (pS6K1), which is an insulin pathway activation biomarker.[79] Patients were randomly assigned to receive metformin (titrated up to 2000 mg/d) or placebo for 12 weeks. The percentage change in the median level of pS6K1 was not significantly different in the metformin group when compared with the placebo group. Metformin also did not alter epithelial proliferation or apoptosis in esophageal tissues, suggesting that chemoprevention using metformin might not be useful in BE.

Polyunsaturated FFA, particularly omega 3 FFAs, have been shown to modulate the phenotype of macrophages from M1 (pro-inflammatory) to M2 (anti-inflammatory) by acting on the lipid-sensing GPR120 receptor on the macrophage cell surface.[80] In addition, they have anti-inflammatory effects by providing an alternative substrate to the COX-2 enzyme.[81] This anti-inflammatory effect has also been shown to alleviate insulin resistance in some animal studies.[82] A small randomized study showed a potential anti-inflammatory effect of omega 3 FFAs in BE subjects, leading to a decrease in tissue COX-2 but not PGE2 levels.[83] Other compounds such as dietary polyphenols may also possess chemopreventive potential in BE, via inhibiting multiple signaling pathways involved in adipose tissue inflammation and implicated in BE carcinogenesis, such as the NFKB, MAP kinase, and AMPK pathways.[84]

SUMMARY

Central obesity is a reflux independent risk factor for BE and EAC. It likely mediates this effect via mechanical and nonmechanical or systemic effects. Pathways by which nonmechanical effects are mediated are being elucidated, but likely include a combination of systemic/local organ inflammation (inflammatory cell and pro-inflammatory cytokine-mediated), insulin and insulin-like peptides, and adipokines. Signaling cascades involved in these mechanisms likely overlap and may be amenable to therapeutic targeting using novel molecules to impede BE pathogenesis and progression to adenocarcinoma.

REFERENCES

1. Kroep S, Lansdorp-Vogelaar I, Rubenstein JH, et al. Comparing trends in esophageal adenocarcinoma incidence and lifestyle factors between the United States, Spain, and the Netherlands. Am J Gastroenterol 2014;100:330–43 [quiz: 335, 344].
2. Blot WJ, McLaughlin JK. The changing epidemiology of esophageal cancer. Semin Oncol 1999;26:2–8.
3. Siegel R, Ma J, Zou Z, et al. Cancer statistics, 2014. CA Cancer J Clin 2014;64:9–29.
4. Cook MB, Greenwood DC, Hardie LJ, et al. A systematic review and meta-analysis of the risk of increasing adiposity on Barrett's esophagus. Am J Gastro-enterol 2008;103:292–300.
5. Kamat P, Wen S, Morris J, et al. Exploring the association between elevated body mass index and Barrett's esophagus: a systematic review and meta-analysis. Ann Thorac Surg 2009;87:655–62.
6. Kaul S, Rothney MP, Peters DM, et al. Dual-energy X-ray absorptiometry for quan-tification of visceral fat. Obesity (Silver Spring) 2012;20:1313–8.
7. Houtkooper LB, Lohman TG, Going SB, et al. Why bioelectrical impedance analysis should be used for estimating adiposity. Am J Clin Nutr 1996;64:436S–48S.
8. Thrift AP, Kramer JR, Alsarraj A, et al. Fat mass by bioelectrical impedance analysis is not associated with increased risk of Barrett esophagus. J Clin Gastro-enterol 2014;48:218–23.
9. Kramer JR, Fischbach LA, Richardson P, et al. Waist-to-hip ratio, but not body mass index, is associated with an increased risk of Barrett's esophagus in white men. Clin Gastroenterol Hepatol 2013;11:373–81.e1.
10. Kendall BJ, Macdonald GA, Hayward NK, et al, Study of Digestive Health. The risk of Barrett's esophagus associated with abdominal obesity in males and females. Int J Cancer 2013;132:2192–9.
11. Singh S, Sharma AN, Murad MH, et al. Central adiposity is associated with increased risk of esophageal inflammation, metaplasia, and adenocarcinoma: a systematic re-view and meta-analysis. Clin Gastroenterol Hepatol 2013;11:1399–412.e7.
12. Kubo A, Cook MB, Shaheen NJ, et al. Sex-specific associations between body mass index, waist circumference and the risk of Barrett's oesophagus: a pooled analysis from the international BEACON consortium. Gut 2013;62:1684–91.
13. El-Serag HB, Hashmi A, Garcia J, et al. Visceral abdominal obesity measured by CT scan is associated with an increased risk of Barrett's oesophagus: a case-control study. Gut 2014;63:220–9.
14. Nelsen EM, Kirihara Y, Takahashi N, et al. Distribution of body fat and its influence on esophageal inflammation and dysplasia in patients with Barrett's esophagus. Clin Gastroenterol Hepatol 2012;10:728–34 [quiz: e61–2].

15. Pandolfino JE, El-Serag HB, Zhang Q, et al. Obesity: a challenge to esophago-gastric junction integrity. Gastroenterology 2006;130:639–49.
16. Derakhshan MH, Robertson EV, Fletcher J, et al. Mechanism of association between BMI and dysfunction of the gastro-oesophageal barrier in patients with normal endoscopy. Gut 2012;61:337–43.
17. Wu JC, Mui LM, Cheung CM, et al. Obesity is associated with increased transient lower esophageal sphincter relaxation. Gastroenterology 2007;132:883–9.
18. El-Serag HB, Ergun GA, Pandolfino J, et al. Obesity increases oesophageal acid exposure. Gut 2007;56:749–55.
19. Andrici J, Tio M, Cox MR, et al. Hiatal hernia and the risk of Barrett's esophagus. J Gastroenterol Hepatol 2013;28:415–31.
20. Taylor JB, Rubenstein JH. Meta-analyses of the effect of symptoms of gastro-esophageal reflux on the risk of Barrett's esophagus. Am J Gastroenterol 2010; 105:1729–37 [quiz: 1738].
21. El-Serag HB, Tran T, Richardson P, et al. Anthropometric correlates of intragastric pressure. Scand J Gastroenterol 2006;41:887–91.
22. Ma Y, Yang Y, Wang F, et al. Obesity and risk of colorectal cancer: a systematic review of prospective studies. PLoS One 2013;8:e53916.
23. Gukovsky I, Li N, Todoric J, et al. Inflammation, autophagy, and obesity: common features in the pathogenesis of pancreatitis and pancreatic cancer. Gastroenterology 2013;144:1199–209.e4.
24. Lee BC, Lee J. Cellular and molecular players in adipose tissue inflammation in the development of obesity-induced insulin resistance. Biochim Biophys Acta 2014;1842:446–62.
25. McNelis JC, Olefsky JM. Macrophages, immunity, and metabolic disease. Immunity 2014;41:36–48.
26. Ryan AM, Healy LA, Power DG, et al. Barrett esophagus: prevalence of central adiposity, metabolic syndrome, and a proinflammatory state. Ann Surg 2008;247:909–15.
27. Olefsky JM, Glass CK. Macrophages, inflammation, and insulin resistance. Annu Rev Physiol 2010;72:219–46.
28. Osborn O, Olefsky JM. The cellular and signaling networks linking the immune system and metabolism in disease. Nat Med 2012;18:363–74.
29. Malhi H, Gores GJ, Katzka DA, et al. Macrophage related inflammation and phenotype modulation in barrett's esophagus. Gastroenterology 2013;144: S-688.
30. Friedman JM, Halaas JL. Leptin and the regulation of body weight in mammals. Nature 1998;395:763–70.
31. Havel PJ, Kasim-Karakas S, Dubuc GR, et al. Gender differences in plasma leptin concentrations. Nat Med 1996;2:949–50.
32. Sierra-Honigmann MR, Nath AK, Murakami C, et al. Biological action of leptin as an angiogenic factor. Science 1998;281:1683–6.
33. Ogunwobi O, Mutungi G, Beales IL. Leptin stimulates proliferation and inhibits apoptosis in Barrett's esophageal adenocarcinoma cells by cyclooxygenase-2-dependent, prostaglandin-E2-mediated transactivation of the epidermal growth factor receptor and c-Jun NH2-terminal kinase activation. Endocrinology 2006; 147:4505–16.
34. Beales IL, Ogunwobi O, Cameron E, et al. Activation of Akt is increased in the dysplasia-carcinoma sequence in Barrett's oesophagus and contributes to increased proliferation and inhibition of apoptosis: a histopathological and functional study. BMC Cancer 2007;7:97.

35. Francois F, Roper J, Goodman AJ, et al. The association of gastric leptin with oesophageal inflammation and metaplasia. Gut 2008;57:16–24.
36. Kendall BJ, Macdonald GA, Hayward NK, et al, Study of Digestive Health. Leptin and the risk of Barrett's oesophagus. Gut 2008;57:448–54.
37. Rubenstein JH, Morgenstern H, McConell D, et al. Associations of diabetes mellitus, insulin, leptin, and ghrelin with gastroesophageal reflux and Barrett's esophagus. Gastroenterology 2013;145:1237–44.e1–5.
38. Garcia JM, Splenser AE, Kramer J, et al. Circulating inflammatory cytokines and adipokines are associated with increased risk of Barrett's esophagus: a case-control study. Clin Gastroenterol Hepatol 2014;12:229–38.e3.
39. Thompson OM, Beresford SA, Kirk EA, et al. Serum leptin and adiponectin levels and risk of Barrett's esophagus and intestinal metaplasia of the gastroesophageal junction. Obesity (Silver Spring) 2010;18:2204–11.
40. Devanna S, Singh S, Dunagan KT, et al. Association between serum adipokines, insulin and risk of Barrett's esophagus: a systematic review and meta-analysis. Gastroenterology 2014;146:S-310.
41. Scherer PE. Adipose tissue: from lipid storage compartment to endocrine organ. Diabetes 2006;55:1537–45.
42. Coppola A, Marfella R, Coppola L, et al. Effect of weight loss on coronary circulation and adiponectin levels in obese women. Int J Cardiol 2009;134:414–6.
43. Wolf AM, Wolf D, Rumpold H, et al. Adiponectin induces the anti-inflammatory cytokines IL-10 and IL-1RA in human leukocytes. Biochem Biophys Res Commun 2004;323:630–5.
44. Brakenhielm E, Veitonmaki N, Cao R, et al. Adiponectin-induced antiangiogenesis and antitumor activity involve caspase-mediated endothelial cell apoptosis. Proc Natl Acad Sci U S A 2004;101:2476–81.
45. Ogunwobi OO, Beales IL. Globular adiponectin, acting via adiponectin receptor-1, inhibits leptin-stimulated oesophageal adenocarcinoma cell proliferation. Mol Cell Endocrinol 2008;285:43–50.
46. Suzuki S, Wilson-Kubalek EM, Wert D, et al. The oligomeric structure of high molecular weight adiponectin. FEBS Lett 2007;581:809–14.
47. Schober F, Neumeier M, Weigert J, et al. Low molecular weight adiponectin negatively correlates with the waist circumference and monocytic IL-6 release. Biochem Biophys Res Commun 2007;361:968–73.
48. Konturek PC, Burnat G, Rau T, et al. Effect of adiponectin and ghrelin on apoptosis of Barrett adenocarcinoma cell line. Dig Dis Sci 2008;53:597–605.
49. Souza RF, Shewmake KL, Shen Y, et al. Differences in ERK activation in squamous mucosa in patients who have gastroesophageal reflux disease with and without Barrett's esophagus. Am J Gastroenterol 2005;100:551–9.
50. Mokrowiecka A, Daniel P, Jasinska A, et al. Serum adiponectin, resistin, leptin concentration and central adiposity parameters in Barrett's esophagus patients with and without intestinal metaplasia in comparison to healthy controls and patients with GERD. Hepatogastroenterology 2012;59:2395–9.
51. Rubenstein JH, Dahlkemper A, Kao JY, et al. A pilot study of the association of low plasma adiponectin and Barrett's esophagus. Am J Gastroenterol 2008;103:1358–64.
52. Rubenstein JH, Kao JY, Madanick RD, et al. Association of adiponectin multimers with Barrett's oesophagus. Gut 2009;58:1583–9.
53. Dvorakova K, Payne CM, Ramsey L, et al. Increased expression and secretion of interleukin-6 in patients with Barrett's esophagus. Clin Cancer Res 2004;10:2020–8.

54. Schwartz MW, Porte D Jr. Diabetes, obesity, and the brain. Science 2005;307: 375–9.
55. Rubin R, Baserga R. Insulin-like growth factor-I receptor. Its role in cell proliferation, apoptosis, and tumorigenicity. Lab Invest 1995;73:311–31.
56. Kooijman R. Regulation of apoptosis by insulin-like growth factor (IGF)-I. Cytokine Growth Factor Rev 2006;17:305–23.
57. Greer KB, Kresak A, Bednarchik B, et al. Insulin/insulin-like growth factor-1 pathway in Barrett's carcinogenesis. Clin Transl Gastroenterol 2013;4:e31.
58. Siahpush SH, Vaughan TL, Lampe JN, et al. Longitudinal study of insulin-like growth factor, insulin-like growth factor binding protein-3, and their polymorphisms: risk of neoplastic progression in Barrett's esophagus. Cancer Epidemiol Biomarkers Prev 2007;16:2387–95.
59. Clemons NJ, Phillips WA, Lord RV. Signaling pathways in the molecular pathogenesis of adenocarcinomas of the esophagus and gastroesophageal junction. Cancer Biol Ther 2013;14:782–95.
60. Duggan C, Onstad L, Hardikar S, et al. Association between markers of obesity and progression from Barrett's esophagus to esophageal adenocarcinoma. Clin Gastroenterol Hepatol 2013;11:934–43.
61. Yuan M, Konstantopoulos N, Lee J, et al. Reversal of obesity- and diet-induced insulin resistance with salicylates or targeted disruption of Ikkbeta. Science 2001;293:1673–7.
62. Solinas G, Karin M. JNK1 and IKKbeta: molecular links between obesity and metabolic dysfunction. FASEB J 2010;24:2596–611.
63. Silha JV, Krsek M, Skrha JV, et al. Plasma resistin, adiponectin and leptin levels in lean and obese subjects: correlations with insulin resistance. Eur J Endocrinol 2003;149:331–5.
64. Yadav A, Kataria MA, Saini V, et al. Role of leptin and adiponectin in insulin resistance. Clin Chim Acta 2013;417:80–4.
65. Kadowaki T, Yamauchi T, Kubota N, et al. Adiponectin and adiponectin receptors in insulin resistance, diabetes, and the metabolic syndrome. J Clin Invest 2006; 116:1784–92.
66. Iyer PG, Borah BJ, Heien HC, et al. Association of Barrett's esophagus with type II diabetes mellitus: results from a large population-based case-control study. Clin Gastroenterol Hepatol 2013;11:1108–14.e5.
67. Leggett CL, Nelsen EM, Tian J, et al. Metabolic syndrome as a risk factor for Barrett esophagus: a population-based case-control study. Mayo Clin Proc 2013;88(2):157–65.
68. Hsu CS, Wang PC, Chen JH, et al. Increasing insulin resistance is associated with increased severity and prevalence of gastro-oesophageal reflux disease. Aliment Pharmacol Ther 2011;34:994–1004.
69. Kubo A, Corley DA. Body mass index and adenocarcinomas of the esophagus or gastric cardia: a systematic review and meta-analysis. Cancer Epidemiol Biomarkers Prev 2006;15:872–8.
70. Thota PN, Sanaka MR, Singh P, et al. Influence of body mass index (BMI) on the prevalence of dysplasia in barrett's esophagus (BE). Gastroenterology 2014; 146(5):S-302.
71. Howard JM, Beddy P, Ennis D, et al. Associations between leptin and adiponectin receptor upregulation, visceral obesity and tumour stage in oesophageal and junctional adenocarcinoma. Br J Surg 2010;97:1020–7.
72. Zhang HY, Zhang Q, Zhang X, et al. Cancer-related inflammation and Barrett's carcinogenesis: interleukin-6 and STAT3 mediate apoptotic resistance

in transformed Barrett's cells. Am J Physiol Gastrointest Liver Physiol 2011; 300:G454–60.

73. Tselepis C, Perry I, Dawson C, et al. Tumour necrosis factor-alpha in Barrett's oesophagus: a potential novel mechanism of action. Oncogene 2002;21:6071–81.

74. Kavanagh ME, O'Sullivan KE, O'Hanlon C, et al. The esophagitis to adenocarcinoma sequence; the role of inflammation. Cancer Lett 2014;345:182–9.

75. Singh S, Devanna S, Edakkanambeth Varayil J, et al. Physical activity is associated with reduced risk of esophageal cancer, particularly esophageal adenocarcinoma: a systematic review and meta-analysis. BMC Gastroenterol 2014;14:101.

76. Hilal J, Kramer JR, Richardson P, et al. Physical activity and the risk of Barrett's esophagus. Gastroenterol 2014;146:S-307–8.

77. Csendes A, Burgos AM, Smok G, et al. Effect of gastric bypass on Barrett's esophagus and intestinal metaplasia of the cardia in patients with morbid obesity. J Gastrointest Surg 2006;10:259–64.

78. Nagi DK, Yudkin JS. Effects of metformin on insulin resistance, risk factors for cardiovascular disease, and plasminogen activator inhibitor in NIDDM subjects. A study of two ethnic groups. Diabetes Care 1993;16:621–9.

79. Chak A, Buttar NS, Foster NR, et al, Cancer Prevention Network. Metformin does not reduce markers of cell proliferation in esophageal tissues of patients with Barrett's esophagus. Clin Gastroenterol Hepatol 2015;13(4):665–72.

80. Oh da Y, Walenta E, Akiyama TE, et al. A Gpr120-selective agonist improves insulin resistance and chronic inflammation in obese mice. Nat Med 2014;20: 942–7.

81. Cockbain AJ, Toogood GJ, Hull MA. Omega-3 polyunsaturated fatty acids for the treatment and prevention of colorectal cancer. Gut 2012;61:135–49.

82. Kalupahana NS, Claycombe K, Newman SJ, et al. Eicosapentaenoic acid prevents and reverses insulin resistance in high-fat diet-induced obese mice via modulation of adipose tissue inflammation. J Nutr 2010;140:1915–22.

83. Mehta SP, Boddy AP, Cook J, et al. Effect of n-3 polyunsaturated fatty acids on Barrett's epithelium in the human lower esophagus. Am J Clin Nutr 2008;87: 949–56.

84. Siriwardhana N, Kalupahana NS, Cekanova M, et al. Modulation of adipose tissue inflammation by bioactive food compounds. J Nutr Biochem 2013;24: 613–23.

Screening for Barrett's Esophagus

Milli Gupta, MD, FRCP(C)[a], Prasad G. Iyer, MD, MSc, AGAF[b],*

KEYWORDS

- Barrett's esophagus • Screening • Esophageal adenocarcinoma

KEY POINTS

- Although Barrett's esophagus (BE) is the precursor of most esophageal adenocarcinomas, most clinically diagnosed tumors are detected outside of surveillance programs.
- Early stage adenocarcinomas diagnosed in surveillance programs have better outcomes than those diagnosed after the onset of symptoms.
- Epidemiologic studies continue to indicate that most prevalent BE cases in the community remain undetected despite the increasing clinical use of endoscopy.
- Novel minimally invasive tools, such as the cytosponge and unsedated transnasal esophagoscopy, are promising tools for BE screening in the community.
- Need for the development of risk stratification tools for patients with BE is acute, and such tools are necessary for a BE screening program to be successful.

INTRODUCTION

Barrett's esophagus (BE) is a recognized premalignant condition of the esophagus that can progress to esophageal adenocarcinoma (EAC). Despite advances in therapy, the survival of EAC diagnosed after onset of symptoms remains poor, with less than 20% survival at 5 years.[1] The incidence of EAC continues to increase in Western countries, with an estimated 6-fold increase since 1975.[2] Given that BE is the only known precursor of EAC, and a strong risk factor, screening for BE followed by endoscopic surveillance and treatment of dysplasia (or early neoplasia) has been thought to

Disclosures: Advisory Board Member for Forest Clinical Laboratories; Consultant and Educational Grant from Covidien (M. Gupta); Research Funding from Intromedic Inc (Seoul, South Korea) (P.G. Iyer).
Author contributions: Study concept and design, analysis and interpretation of data, drafting of the article, critical revision of the article for important intellectual content (M. Gupta). Study concept and design, analysis and interpretation of data, drafting of the article, critical revision of the article for important intellectual content, study supervision (P.G. Iyer).
[a] Division of Gastroenterology and Hepatology, University of Calgary, 2500 University Dr NW, Calgary, Alberta T2N 1N4, Canada; [b] Division of Gastroenterology and Hepatology, Mayo Clinic, 200 First Street Southwest, Rochester, MN 55905, USA
* Corresponding author.
E-mail address: iyer.prasad@mayo.edu

Gastroenterol Clin N Am 44 (2015) 265–283
http://dx.doi.org/10.1016/j.gtc.2015.02.003
0889-8553/15/$ – see front matter © 2015 Elsevier Inc. All rights reserved.

be an approach that can potentially reduce the incidence of EAC and improve survival. This article reviews and summarizes data on recent progress in screening of BE given the debate in the literature. It outlines the rationale for screening, recent advances in defining the target population, and technologies available for screening, and reviews recent advances in the risk stratification of progression in BE.

RATIONALE FOR SCREENING

The primary purpose of a screening program is to detect premalignant or early stage neoplastic lesions, thereby providing an opportunity to improve outcomes and reduce mortality with early intervention. For BE, screening programs have been recommended by various gastrointestinal (GI) societies.[3–5] However, these guidelines have been qualified as weak recommendations because of the lack of robust evidence.[6] The reasons for discrepancy include lack of randomized, high-quality data showing the lack of reduction in EAC mortality with the implementation of screening[7,8] and inefficient use of resources.[9] The current reference standard technique for screening is the sedated upper endoscopy (sedated esophagogastroduodenoscopy [sEGD]), which is associated with significant costs to the system (eg, use of sedatives, postsedation recovery time, nursing) and to the patient (eg, loss of income for patients and caregivers who take time away from work to complete the procedure). Efforts have been made to find alternative options to sEGD, and these are discussed later.

The second aspect of screening consists of surveillance after the initial identification of BE, so that dysplastic lesions are identified and managed at an earlier stage. There are various grades of dysplasia in BE, with the lowest potential of malignancy being present within nondysplastic BE (NDBE). Although evidence in the past 5 years shows that the incidence of EAC in patients with NDBE is likely to be lower than was previously estimated,[10,11] these numbers often exclude prevalent EAC detected at the time of initial endoscopy. A meta-analysis[12] of 57 studies showed that the annual incidence of EAC in NDBE was 1 in 300 (0.33%). Approximately 7% of patients with BE on initial endoscopy had EAC.[12] By eliminating prevalent EAC from the analysis, the data presented are skewed toward the lower incidence of BE-induced EAC and likely underestimate the true effect of screening on the population. The second concern is that the evidence is retrospective in nature, and associated with lead time bias (time from diagnosis of disease to presentation with symptoms), length time bias (increased survival time related to screening that identifies cases before onset of symptoms), and selection bias (patients willing to receive medical attention). It is uncertain what the true effect of screening is on EAC mortality, and whether it is a cost-effective program. However, a screening or surveillance program in principle can find early stages of disease, identify curable cancers, and still not have a mortality benefit. This possibility is well recognized from large screening studies of lung[13,14] and ovarian[15] cancers. Despite the lack of effect on cancer-specific mortality or all-cause mortality, such results have not reduced the use of transvaginal ultrasounds, cancer antigen 125, or chest radiography.

Screening provides the opportunity to identify tumors at an earlier stage compared with patients without screening.[16–20] Dysplastic BE is a precursor lesion that, if found early and endoscopically treated, can eliminate the need for an esophagectomy. Five-year survival rates of early asymptomatic cancers (T1a and T1b) treated endoscopically are better than those of symptomatic cancers,[21–23] in part because of the availability of endoscopic therapies such as endoscopic mucosal resection and radiofrequency ablation, which are the new definitive therapies for early EAC and dysplastic BE. This development has been positive, because esophagectomy continues to have high morbidity and mortality.[24] The ability to prevent progression of dysplastic/early EAC is a potential incentive to identify patients at risk.

Because of the increasing incidence of EAC, in conjunction with high morbidity/mortality, interest in the population for screening is substantial. Approximately two-thirds of patients, when approached with information on BE and offered the option to be screened, were interested in screening in a population-based survey study. This finding may reflect the raised public profile that BE and EAC have obtained in the last decade. There are also various patient factors to consider following a diagnosis of BE. It has been associated with increased insurance premiums[25] despite patients with BE dying primarily of nonesophageal causes, such as cardiovascular or pulmonary conditions.[7,8] Life expectancy in patients with BE is comparable with that of individuals without BE.[6–8] Moreover, patients with BE have reported reduced quality of life, and increased psychosocial stressors and use of health care resources (compared with patients with gastroesophageal reflux disease [GERD] and the general population).[26] Cost analyses have suggested that 1-time screening endoscopy in patients with GERD is cost-effective[9,27] if surveillance is limited to those who have dysplastic BE. All these factors have increased interest in appropriate screening strategies that are targeted to the correct population, without adding unnecessary anxiety to low-risk patients.

TARGET POPULATION

The high-risk group has the largest potential yield and benefit of screening. However, the target population for BE screening has not been well delineated. Population-based and autopsy studies have shown that only one-third of the prevalent BE cases in the general population are currently identified by clinically indicated endoscopy, despite the sharp increase in the volume of endoscopy in the United States.[28] More than 90% of EAC cases are diagnosed outside of BE surveillance programs, despite the presence of BE histologically.[16]

GERD is the strongest risk factor for BE and EAC. About 10% to 15% of patients with GERD are found to have BE on endoscopy.[29] As obesity increases within North America, the prevalence of GERD has also increased. An update of a 2005 review reflecting on the prevalence of GERD symptoms showed a global increase in weekly symptom scores (10% increase in North America, 15% in Europe, 24% in the Middle East, and 5.5% increase in east Asia).[30] The largest increase in GERD was in North America and east Asia. However, not all patients with BE endorse symptoms of GERD, with some studies reporting that 46% of subjects with BE were asymptomatic for reflux symptoms.[31,32] The prevalence of BE in subjects without, or with infrequent, reflux symptoms has been found to be substantial. In some studies, it is comparable with that of subjects with reflux symptoms. In one study, 8.3% of patients with GERD had BE, compared with 5.6% of patients without GERD.[33] This finding adds to the challenge of finding the right patient population to target for screening. Relying on GERD as the sole risk factor for screening is also impractical because of the millions of subjects with frequent reflux symptoms.[34] A better stratification of patients for screening is sorely needed.

Additional risk factors have been identified over the past few years, to help better delineate patients at risk. Central obesity (in particular visceral abdominal fat, measured by waist/hip ratio or waist circumference, rather than body mass index [BMI]) has been shown to result in increased esophageal injury[35,36] and proinflammatory cytokine[37] release, resulting in systemic inflammation and increased risk of developing BE[38,39] and EAC.[40] These associations have been found to exist independently of GERD.[41] Other risk factors that are associated with BE are (**Table 1**) male

Table 1
Summary of nonmodifiable risk factors for developing BE or progressing to EAC or HGD

Clinical Variable	Reference	Study Design	Sample Size	End Point	Results	Comments
Age	Guardino et al,[50] 2006	Cohort	837	EAC/HGD	OR of 3.5 for age ≥50 y with prevalent EAC compared with age <50 y	Rates of BE progression were similar in both age groups
	Oberg et al,[46] 2005	Cohort	140	EAC/HGD	HR 1.062 (0.98, 1.16)	—
	Eloubeidi and Provenzale,[49] 2001	Case control	211	BE	Age ≥40 y independent predictor (P = .008)	Prospective
	Edelstein et al,[45] 2009	Case control	615	BE	OR per decade for IM 1.3 (95% CI, 1.1–1.5)	—
	Johansson et al,[51] 2007	Case control	764	BE	Prevalence increased 5% by age (95% CI, 1–9)	Prospective study
	Cooper et al,[52] 2014	Case control	3749	EAC	OR, 1.03 (95% CI, 1.01–1.05); P = .005	—
Male gender	Oberg et al,[46] 2005	Cohort	140	EAC/HGD	HR, 1.062 (0.98, 1.16)	—
	Yousef et al,[44] 2008	Meta-analysis	NA	EAC/HGD	Pooled estimate, 10.2 per 1000 person-years in men	Subgroup analysis of 6 studies included
	Edelstein et al,[45] 2009	Case control	615	BE	OR, 1.5 (95% CI, 1.1–2.2)	—
	Menke-Pluymers et al,[47] 1993	Case control	158	EAC	OR, 2.4 (CI not available); P = .06	—
	Gerson et al,[42] 2001	Cohort	517	BE	Logistic regression analysis used to create a prediction model; P = .05	Prospective nature. 7-symptom questionnaire
	Cook et al,[43] 2005	Meta-analysis	NA	BE	Pooled male/female ratio, 1.96:1 (95% CI, 1.77–2.17:1)	32 studies
	Cooper et al,[52] 2014	Case control	3749	EAC	OR, 3.06 (95% CI, 1.50–6.24); P = .002	—

Ethnicity					
Guardino et al,[50] 2006	Cohort	837	EAC/HGD	NA	Mainly white people in the study (76%)
Balasubramaniam et al,[48] 2012	Cohort	1058	BE	OR, 2.40 (95% CI, 1.42–4.03)	Prospective
Length of BE					
Guardino et al,[50] 2006	Cohort	837	EAC/HGD	NA	On multivariate analysis, length ≥ 3 cm resulted in $2.5\times$ risk of developing EAC or HGD
Edelstein et al,[45] 2009	Case control	615	BE	OR for LSBE 1.4 (95% CI, 1.5–11.4)	—
Yousef et al,[44] 2008	Meta-analysis	NA	EAC/HGD	Incidence in LSBE and SSBE was comparable (6.7 and 6.1/1000 patient-y respectively)	Subgroup analysis of 26 studies
Sato et al,[88] 2008	Case control	62	EAC/HGD	Association between LSBE and EAC/HGD reported	Individual HRs not provided
Rudolf et al,[89] 2000	Cohort study	309	EAC	Risk of EAC in SSBE similar to LSBE ($P>.2$). If HGD on index EGD, no association of length and EAC risk	Prospective. Baseline dysplasia is an important factor to consider

Age was modeled as a continuous variable in all studies but Guardino and colleagues[50] (it was dichotomous: either <50 or >50 years old). Gender was modeled as dichotomous variable. Ethnicity was modeled as dichotomous variable. Length of BE segment was modeled as continuous variable in all studies.

Abbreviations: CI, confidence interval; HR, hazard ratio; IM, intestinal metaplasia; LSBE, long-segment BE; NA, not applicable; OR, odds ratio; SSBE, short-segment BE.

Data from Refs. [42–52,88,89]

gender,[42–47] non-Hispanic white ethnicity,[48] older age,[45,46,49–52] family history of BE or EAC,[53,54] obstructive sleep apnea,[55] and smoking.[47,51,52,56–59] A combination of these factors likely increases the risk of BE and EAC in an additive or synergistic manner.

These findings have led to increased interest in creating risk scores for BE. Three such tools have been created, but their utility in clinical practice is unknown at this time. The initial tool, created in 2012, was externally validated and showed age, gender, highest level of education, smoking history, BMI, and use of acid suppressants as predictors of BE.[60] The area under the curve (AUC) was 0.70 on the initial test model, and 0.60 for the independent validation dataset. In contrast, the AUC for using only GERD as a predictor of BE was 0.61 (P<.001).[61] The second tool is the Michigan Barrett's Esophagus Prediction Tool.[61] It is a model that predicts the likelihood of BE based on age, GERD symptoms, waist/hip ratio, and pack years of cigarette smoking. This model was generated after evaluating subjects undergoing screening colonoscopy with a research upper endoscopy for BE. All variables listed are equally weighted, and the AUC was 0.72. The third tool[62] combined clinical (GERD symptom frequency and duration, age, gender, ethnicity, waist/hip ratio, and Helicobacter pylori status) and circulating cytokine markers (serum levels of interleukin [IL] 12p70, IL6, IL8, IL10, and leptin). The AUC for this model was 0.85, which was significantly improved from a GERD-only model, but external validation is still pending. These models give hope. Since the last cost-effective analysis was performed ~12 years ago, there is interest in identifying the patient population that is best served by screening. Other than the broad categories mentioned earlier, there has been an interest in creating predictive tools.

MINIMALLY INVASIVE BARRETT'S ESOPHAGUS SCREENING TECHNIQUES

The most used modality for BE screening is sEGD. It is the current benchmark against which other tools are assessed. As mentioned previously, there are issues with accessibility, cost, and use. Some alternatives to sEGD have been explored, such as esophageal video capsule endoscopy (VCE), transnasal endoscopy (TNE), and noninvasive esophageal capsule cytology (cytosponge).

A population-based study[63] evaluated the acceptability of VCE, TNE, and sEGD in a community population. It found that two-thirds of the population was interested in BE screening using noninvasive means. This finding is in contrast with a Veterans' Affairs (VA) study[64] that showed only 15% acceptability of VCE and TNE. However, in the VA study, patients had limited knowledge of BE and EAC. Nevertheless, in both studies, VCE was the preferred modality, although the difference was not statistically significant. The performance characteristics of VCE are currently suboptimal for BE diagnosis,[65] with a meta-analysis[66] quoting pooled rates of sensitivity and specificity as 77% and 86% respectively. In addition, the technique is not cost-effective, given current costs and need for confirmatory sEGD.[67] Reduction of costs may render this technology cost-effective in the future. With potential advances in VCE technology (ability to zoom, addition of filter to change white light to blue light), it may be possible to improve diagnostic accuracy for BE.

Another option for visualizing the esophagus is to use a transnasal endoscope (TNE). This device uses a thinner caliber scope (diameter, 5.4 mm vs 9.8 mm) and enters the esophagus via the mouth or nares (**Fig. 1**A). It has the benefit of being used without sedation and has accuracy for BE detection that is comparable with sEGD.[68] Endoscopic assessment of BE and detection of intestinal metaplasia (IM) was equivalent between TNE and sEGD in a randomized trial[69] from the United Kingdom. Tolerability was equivalent, with preference of TNE because of the lack of

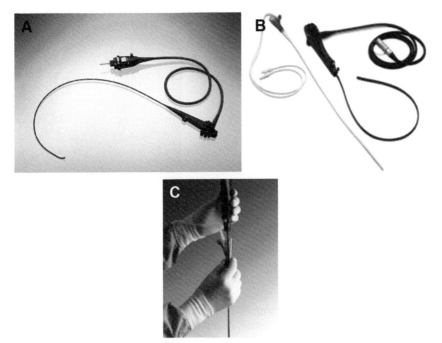

Fig. 1. (*A*) Conventional TNE. (*B*) TNE and (*C*) disposable Endosheath. (*Courtesy of* Vision Sciences, Orangeburg, NY; with permission).

sedation and associated patient costs. Physician extenders can be successfully trained in the use of TNE for BE screening, with comparable accuracy and tolerability rates.[64,70] An esophagoscope with a disposable sheath (Vision Sciences, Orangeburg, NY) with or without a biopsy channel has recently been developed (see **Fig. 1**B, C). The sheath can be disposed of after a single use, with the endoscope ready for use without conventional disinfection. A recent randomized controlled trial found that the acceptability, quality, and yield of TNE performed in a hospital endoscopy unit (huTNE) and in a mobile research van (muTNE) was comparable with sEGD performed in a hospital endoscopy unit.[71] TNE was well tolerated, with comparable yield (BE, esophagitis) and with substantially shorter time to complete esophageal evaluation.

Another transnasal device (EG2 scan, Intromedic Inc, Seoul, Korea) is being investigated (NCT02066233) as a potential minimally invasive, unsedated technique for BE screening (**Fig. 2**). This novel device has a probe capable of 30 frames per second with a 125° field of view. It is maneuverable along a single axis and is single use. The device has no suction or biopsy channel, but does allow insufflation with air. Initial tolerability, safety, and accuracy for the diagnosis of BE seem to be reasonable.

A nonendoscopic option being developed is esophageal capsule cytology, called the cytosponge. This device is the size of a pill and is ingested (**Fig. 3**).[72] It contains a compressed ball-shaped mesh on a string. The patient is asked to swallow the pill with the string attached. The string is held without any tension to allow the capsule to enter the stomach. Once it is inside the patient's stomach, the gelatin layer dissolves to release the sponge (measuring 25 mm in diameter). As it is withdrawn from the patient, it brushes the gastroesophageal junction and esophageal epithelium to capture cells for analysis. The cytology specimen is then sent for histologic and immunohistochemical analysis. The cytology specimen is analyzed for trefoil factor

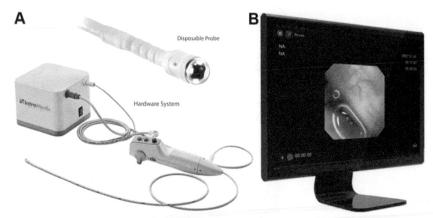

Fig. 2. Components of the E.G. Scan system (second generation) include (*A*) a probe (disposable) containing the camera capsule, bending module, and data connector; (*B*) software that is provided to display the findings of the scope in real time. (*Courtesy of* IntroMedic, Seoul, Korea; with permission).

3 (TFF3), a recently identified marker of columnar epithelium.[72,73] Compared with sEGD, the sensitivity of cytosponge/TFF3 assay is 73% and specificity 93.8% for BE segments greater than 1 cm. Sensitivity increases to 90% and specificity remains at 93.5% for BE segments greater than 2 cm. If validated in other cohorts, the cytosponge has the potential to replace sEGD, because it is noninvasive and easy to perform in the primary care setting. In a recent economic assessment,[74] it was a cost-effective method to screen 50-year-old men with GERD for BE, versus no screening or screening with conventional endoscopy. If dysplastic BE or early EAC is detected by this method, it will be followed by sEGD and endotherapy for definitive management. One of the concerns with this technology was the low acceptability by patients (18%).[72] Validation studies in other countries are currently underway, and

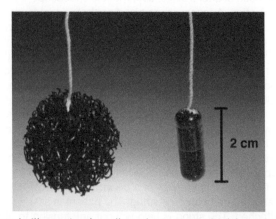

Fig. 3. Gelatin-based pill contains the collapsed cytosponge (*right*). It expands in the stomach after the outer layer has dissolved, to release the mesh sponge (*left*). As the cytosponge is pulled out of the patient's mouth (attached to the string), the mesh captures epithelial cells of the esophagus and gastroesophageal junction. (*From* Kadri SR, Lao-Sirieix P, O'Donovan M, et al. Acceptability and accuracy of a non-endoscopic screening test for Barrett's esophagus in primary care: cohort study. BMJ 2010;341:c4372; with permission).

may shed further light on the feasibility of this technique. The balloon cytology device is another nonendoscopic technique that has been studied. However, it has poor sensitivity (80% for high-grade dysplasia [HGD] but 22% for low-grade dysplasia [LGD]) and tissue sample acquisition (70%).[75] Therefore, there is limited use for it in the current paradigm.

A new noninvasive technique has been developed that provides information not only on esophageal mucosa but also on the architecture and microscopic structures of the esophageal wall. Such cross-sectional imaging has mostly been applied as an adjunct to sEGD (such as optical coherence tomography). Tethered capsule endomicroscopy (TCE) uses a capsule attached to a thin sheath (comprising an optic fiber and drive-shaft) called the tether. The tether transmits light to and from the capsule to capture images on a software program. Once the capsule has been swallowed to its distal-most location (stomach), the driveshaft within the tether allows the operator to control the position of the capsule within the GI tract as it is withdrawn.[76] The capsule is smaller than a penny, spins and mechanically rotates on its axis to provide three-dimensional images, and is reusable (**Fig. 4**). This test has the potential to be per-formed in a primary care setting. This technique is unlike string capsule endoscopy, in which only mucosal images are captured for review. A pilot study of healthy volun-teers and those with BE showed excellent tolerability and image capture/resolution with TCE.[77] However, more data are needed before application in clinical practice.

RISK STRATIFICATION OF BARRETT'S ESOPHAGUS

Given the low rates of progression to HGD and/or EAC in subjects with NDBE[12] and the limitations in surveillance endoscopy, BE screening is likely to be practical only

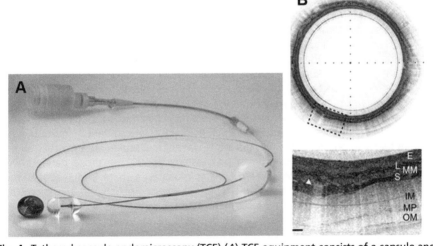

Fig. 4. Tethered capsule endomicroscopy (TCE) (*A*) TCE equipment consists of a capsule and a fiber optic sheath called the tether. The tether is flexible and has a plastic ball attached to facilitate manipulation. (*B*) The normal esophagus in 3 dimensions obtained from a normal volunteer in vivo. The lower image shows a 3× expanded view of the normal esophageal wall architecture, including squamous epithelium (E), muscularis mucosa (MM), lamina propria (L), submucosa (S) containing blood vessels (*arrowhead*), inner and outer muscularis (IM and OM), and myenteric plexus (MP). (*From* Gora MJ, Sauk JS, Carruth RW, et al. Teth-ered capsule endomicroscopy enables less invasive imaging of gastrointestinal tract micro-structure. Nat Med 2013;19(2):238–40; with permission.)

if risk stratification for patients with BE allows the identification of low-risk individuals who can be discharged from surveillance, making the pool of patients with BE in surveillance potentially smaller and more manageable. Patients with NDBE constitute more than 80% of the population with BE in the community. Clinical and demographic characteristics that increase the risk of progression in BE are identified and categorized in **Table 2**. Dysplasia is the only currently used factor for risk stratification, but it is fraught with several limitations, including a patchy distribution and lack of interobserver agreement among pathologists. Moreover, compliance with current recommendations remains poor.

Biomarkers can predict progression to carcinoma, and potentially can define the patient population that should undergo intensive surveillance or therapy. Reducing costs and redirecting limited resources toward patients who are at risk of progressing is desirable, and biomarkers have the potential to alter the current paradigm. Another benefit of biomarkers is the lack of interobserver variability, which is present in pathology and endoscopy.

Presence of multiple unstable genetic markers increases the likelihood of progressing to EAC. Genetic patterns between BE and EAC support the hypothesis that both share a common background of molecular changes, and that BE is an intermediary step to EAC.[78] There are various molecular abnormalities that have been detected. A subgroup of patients with LGD and NDBE have a high risk of progression to EAC if they have abnormalities in DNA content, such as tetraploidy or aneuploidy (relative risk [RR], 11; 95% confidence interval [CI], 5.5–21).[79] Similarly, patients have a 16-fold increase in progression to HGD or EAC if they have loss of heterozygosity (LOH) of p53, resulting in overexpression of p53.[80] Hypermethylation of p16, which inactivates cell cycle control, has also been independently found to increase progression from IM to HGD/EAC (odds ratio [OR], 1.74; 95% CI, 1.33–2.20).[81]

Genetic abnormalities recognized to have an association with dysplastic BE/EAC can be combined to predict the likelihood of developing EAC. For example, in a multicenter study, an 8-gene methylation panel[82] comprising p16, HPP1, RUNX3, NELL1, TAC1, SST, AKAP12, and CDH13 predicted progression of NDBE to HGD/EAC in 50% of patients. Another study evaluated a panel of DNA abnormalities, including LOH of 17p (TP53) and 9p (p16 locus), over a 10-year period, and found a high risk of EAC development (RR, 38.7; 95% CI, 10.8–138.5).[83] However, this was a retrospective study performed on prospectively collected samples, and external validation is lacking. Given that dysplasia in BE is patchy,[84] there has been interest in assessing clonal diversity as a marker of progression. Clonal diversity refers to variety in the genetic markers that can be present within the same patient's samples. Analysis of 239 patients[85] showed a strong likelihood of progression (P<.001) in those patients with clonal diversity within the DNA content, LOH, microsatellite shifts, and sequence mutations in p53 and p16. However, this is a laborious and complicated methodology that is not likely to be commercially available in the near future.[86] It has also not been externally validated, which limits its use. At present, all of these studies have been performed on tissue samples. Alternative methods of testing these genetic abnormalities are needed that can be applied widely and without tissue sampling.

The Northern Ireland Register assessed patients with BE for clinical variables (age, sex, and year of BE diagnosis) and biomarkers [DNA ploidy, p53, cyclin A expression, Lewis(a), Lewis(x), *Aspergillus oryzae* lectin (AOL), and binding of wheat germ agglutinin] that increase the likelihood of progressing to HGD/EAC.[87] Because of the retrospective nature of this study, biomarker assessment was performed on paraffin-embedded tissue. For progression, the presence of LGD and all biomarkers [except Lewis(x)] was associated with EAC or HGD. Independently, LGD (OR, 11),

Table 2
Summary of modifiable risk factors for BE progressing to EAC or HGD

Clinical Variable	Reference	Study Design	Sample Size	End Point	Results	Comments
GERD	Eloubeidi and Provenzale,[49] 2001	Case control	211	BE	Heartburn >1/wk ($P = .007$); heartburn or acid regurgitation ($P = .007$)	Less likely to report severe GERD ($P<.01$) or nocturnal symptoms ($P = .03$)
	Oberg et al,[46] 2005	Cohort	140	EAC/HGD	RR, 1.3 (1.2–1.7)	Longer duration of symptoms was independently associated with developing HGD/EAC
	Smith et al,[56] 2005	Case control	428	BE and dysplasia	Weekly GERD and BE: OR, 29.7 (95% CI, 12.2–72.6). Weekly GERD and dysplasia: OR, 59.7 (95% CI, 18.5–193)	Population
	Johansson,[51] 2007	Case control	764	BE	OR, 10.7 (95% CI, 3.5–33.4)	Interaction noted between reflux and smoking (OR, 51.4; 95% CI, 14.1–188)
	Anderson et al,[58] 2007	Case control	451	BE and EAC	GERD and BE: OR, 12 (95% CI, 7.64–18.7). GERD and EAC: OR, 3.48 (95% CI, 2.25–5.41)	Prospective Population based
	Taylor and Rubenstein,[90] 2010	Meta-analysis	NA	BE	OR, 2.90 (95% CI, 1.86–4.5)	26 studies. OR for LSBE in GERD, 4.92 (95% CI, 2.01–12)
	Balasubramaniam et al,[48] 2012	Cohort	1058	BE	OR, 1.50 (95% CI, 1.07–2.09)	Patients with heartburn for more than 5 y
	Gerson et al,[42] 2001	Cohort	517	BE	Logistic regression analysis used to create a prediction model; $P = .05$	Heartburn, nocturnal pain, odynophagia were positively associated. Dysphagia was negatively associated with BE

(continued on next page)

Table 2
(continued)

Clinical Variable	Reference	Study Design	Sample Size	End Point	Results	Comments
Central Obesity	Corley et al,[91] 2007	Case control	953	BE	Waist circumference >80 cm: OR, 2.24 (95% CI, 1.21–4.15)	—
	Edelstein et al,[92] 2007	Case control	404	BE	Higher waist/hip ratio: OR, 2.4 for all cases (95% CI, 1.4–3.9); OR, 4.3 (95% CI, 1.9–9.9) for LSBE	Prospective study. Results are independent of BMI
	Singh et al,[41] 2013	Meta-analysis	NA	BE and EAC	Risk of BE: OR, 1.93 (95% CI, 1.52–2.57). Risk of EAC: OR, 2.51 (95% CI, 1.54–4.06)	17 studies
	Nelsen et al,[93] 2012	Cohort	100	BE and EAC	Abdominal circumference associated with BE: OR, 9.1 (95% CI, 1.4–57.2); P = .02	Patients with higher visceral fat area (P = .02) were more likely to have HGD
OSA	Leget et al,[55] 2014	262	Case control	BE	OR, 1.8 (95% CI, 1.1–3.2)	Independent of age, sex, BMI, GERD, and smoking
Smoking	Menke-Pluymers et al,[47] 1993	Case control	158	EAC	2.3-fold increased risk for smokers	—
	Johansson et al,[51] 2007	Case control	764	BE	Smokers: 3.3-fold increased risk (95% CI, 1.1–9.9)	Prospective
	Smith et al,[56] 2005	Case control	428	BE	OR, 3.1 for smoking (CI, not available)	Prospective. Interaction noted between reflux and smoking
	Cook et al,[57] 2012	Meta-analysis	NA	BE	Smokers: OR, 1.67 (95% CI, 1.04–2.67) vs controls and OR, 1.61 (95% CI, 1 33–1.96) vs GERD controls	5 case control studies. Association strengthened with increased pack years until 20 pack years, when it started to plateau. Synergistic effects with GERD
	Thrift et al,[59] 2014	Case control	1856	BE	No association	Based on intensity, duration, pack years, cessation
	Anderson et al,[58] 2007	Case control	451	BE and EAC	EAC more likely in smokers (OR, 4.84; 95% CI, 2.72–8.61)	No significant association between BE and smoking
	Cooper et al,[52] 2014	Case control	3749	EAC	OR, 2.36 (95% CI, 1.13–4.93); P = .023	On multivariate analysis, association between smoking and EAC was lost

Alcohol					
Kubo et al,[94] 2009	Case control	953	BE	No association; trend toward wine reducing BE	Wine consumption and education status inversely related
Thrift et al,[59] 2014	Case control	1856	BE	Moderate intake inversely associated with BE (14–28 drinks/wk: OR, 0.39; 95% CI, 0.15–1.00)	—
Anderson et al,[95] 2009	Case control	941	BE and EAC	No association with either BE or EAC	—
Yates et al,[96] 2014	Cohort	24,068	BE and EAC	Inverse association of alcohol (≥7 units/wk) with EAC (HR, 0.49; 95% CI, 0.23–1.04). $P = .06$	No association with developing BE

GERD was treated differently by each study, and description is provided within the comment section of this table. Central obesity consisted of either waist/hip ratio or waist circumference. Both were modeled as dichotomous variables. Obstructive sleep apnea (OSA) was modeled as a dichotomous variable. Smoking was modeled as a dichotomous variable. Alcohol was modeled as a dichotomous variable. BMI, body mass index; GERD, gastroesophageal reflux disease; HGD, high grade dysplasia; OR, odds ratio; RR, relative risk.

Data from Refs.[41,42,46–49,51,52,56–59,90–96]

DNA ploidy (OR, 3.2), AOL (OR, 3), and Lewis(a) (OR, 1.7) were each associated with HGD or EAC. Biomarker p53 was associated with progression to EAC (OR, 1.95) only, but not HGD. For patients with dysplasia and biomarker abnormality, the OR was 2.99 (95% CI, 1.72–5.20) compared with patients with dysplasia alone (OR, 3.74; 95% CI, 2.43–5.79). Despite the retrospective nature of this study, it showed that a combination of clinical and biomarker panels is feasible to implement, with the potential for widespread applicability.

SUMMARY

Progress has been made in several directions in BE screening but primarily in the area of noninvasive/minimally invasive tools, which may be comparable with conventional endoscopy in quality, accuracy, and acceptability. Initial progress has been made in the development of prediction models incorporating several risk factors for BE. Validation of these models in unselected populations is required before they can be widely used for clinical purposes. Risk stratification of patients diagnosed from clinically indicated or population-screening endoscopy is essential to make screening a practical proposition. This requirement may be the rate-limiting factor in the widespread dissemination of screening for BE. However, substantial work is ongoing in this area with progress likely in the near future.

REFERENCES

1. Pohl H, Sirovich B, Welch HG. Esophageal adenocarcinoma incidence: are we reaching the peak? Cancer Epidemiol Biomarkers Prev 2010;19(6):1468–70.
2. Hur C, Miller M, Kong CY, et al. Trends in esophageal adenocarcinoma incidence and mortality. Cancer 2013;119(6):1149–58.
3. Wang KK, Sampliner RE. Updated guidelines 2008 for the diagnosis, surveillance and therapy of Barrett's esophagus. Am J Gastroenterol 2008;103(3):788–97.
4. Spechler SJ, American Gastroenterological Association, Sharma P, et al. American Gastroenterological Association medical position statement on the management of Barrett's esophagus. Gastroenterology 2011;140(3):1084–91.
5. Hirota WK, Zuckerman MJ, Adler DG, et al. ASGE guideline: the role of endoscopy in the surveillance of premalignant conditions of the upper GI tract. Gastrointest Endosc 2006;63(4):570–80.
6. Sharma P, McQuaid K, Dent J, et al. A critical review of the diagnosis and management of Barrett's esophagus: the AGA Chicago Workshop. Gastroenterology 2004;127(1):310–30.
7. Eckardt VF, Kanzler G, Bernhard G. Life expectancy and cancer risk in patients with Barrett's esophagus: a prospective controlled investigation. Am J Med 2001; 111(1):33–7.
8. van der Burgh A, Dees J, Hop WC, et al. Oesophageal cancer is an uncommon cause of death in patients with Barrett's oesophagus. Gut 1996;39(1):5–8.
9. Inadomi JM, Sampliner R, Lagergren J, et al. Screening and surveillance for Barrett esophagus in high-risk groups: a cost-utility analysis. Ann Intern Med 2003; 138(3):176–86.
10. Bhat S, Coleman HG, Yousef F, et al. Risk of malignant progression in Barrett's esophagus patients: results from a large population-based study. J Natl Cancer Inst 2011;103(13):1049–57.
11. Hvid-Jensen F, Pedersen L, Drewes AM, et al. Incidence of adenocarcinoma among patients with Barrett's esophagus. N Engl J Med 2011;365(15):1375–83.

12. Desai TK, Krishnan K, Samala N, et al. The incidence of oesophageal adenocarcinoma in non-dysplastic Barrett's oesophagus: a meta-analysis. Gut 2012;61(7): 970–6.
13. Oken MM, Hocking WG, Kvale PA, et al. Screening by chest radiograph and lung cancer mortality: the Prostate, Lung, Colorectal, and Ovarian (PLCO) randomized trial. JAMA 2011;306(17):1865–73.
14. Infante M, Cavuto S, Lutman FR, et al. A randomized study of lung cancer screening with spiral computed tomography: three-year results from the DANTE trial. Am J Respir Crit Care Med 2009;180(5):445–53.
15. Buys SS, Partridge E, Black A, et al. Effect of screening on ovarian cancer mortality: the Prostate, Lung, Colorectal and Ovarian (PLCO) Cancer Screening Randomized Controlled Trial. JAMA 2011;305(22):2295–303.
16. Corley DA, Levin TR, Habel LA, et al. Surveillance and survival in Barrett's adenocarcinomas: a population-based study. Gastroenterology 2002;122(3): 633–40.
17. Corley DA, Mehtani K, Quesenberry C, et al. Impact of endoscopic surveillance on mortality from Barrett's esophagus-associated esophageal adenocarcinomas. Gastroenterology 2013;145(2):312–9.e1.
18. Rubenstein JH, Sonnenberg A, Davis J, et al. Effect of a prior endoscopy on outcomes of esophageal adenocarcinoma among United States veterans. Gastrointest Endosc 2008;68(5):849–55.
19. van Sandick JW, van Lanschot JJ, Kuiken BW, et al. Impact of endoscopic biopsy surveillance of Barrett's oesophagus on pathological stage and clinical outcome of Barrett's carcinoma. Gut 1998;43(2):216–22.
20. Ferguson MK, Durkin A. Long-term survival after esophagectomy for Barrett's adenocarcinoma in endoscopically surveyed and nonsurveyed patients. J Gastrointest Surg 2002;6(1):29–35 [discussion: 36].
21. Prasad GA, Wu TT, Wigle DA, et al. Endoscopic and surgical treatment of mucosal (T1a) esophageal adenocarcinoma in Barrett's esophagus. Gastroenterology 2009;137(3):815–23.
22. Wani S, Drahos J, Cook MB, et al. Comparison of endoscopic therapies and surgical resection in patients with early esophageal cancer: a population-based study. Gastrointest Endosc 2014;79(2):224–32.e1.
23. Das A, Singh V, Fleischer DE, et al. A comparison of endoscopic treatment and surgery in early esophageal cancer: an analysis of Surveillance Epidemiology and End Results data. Am J Gastroenterol 2008;103(6):1340–5.
24. Smith I, Kahaleh M. Endoscopic versus surgical therapy for Barrett's esophagus neoplasia. Expert Rev Gastroenterol Hepatol 2015;9:31–5.
25. Shaheen NJ, Dulai GS, Ascher B, et al. Effect of a new diagnosis of Barrett's esophagus on insurance status. Am J Gastroenterol 2005;100(3):577–80.
26. Crockett SD, Lippmann QK, Dellon ES, et al. Health-related quality of life in patients with Barrett's esophagus: a systematic review. Clin Gastroenterol Hepatol 2009;7(6):613–23.
27. Gerson LB, Groeneveld PW, Triadafilopoulos G. Cost-effectiveness model of endoscopic screening and surveillance in patients with gastroesophageal reflux disease. Clin Gastroenterol Hepatol 2004;2(10):868–79.
28. Jung KW, Talley NJ, Romero Y, et al. Epidemiology and natural history of intestinal metaplasia of the gastroesophageal junction and Barrett's esophagus: a population-based study. Am J Gastroenterol 2011;106(8):1447–55.
29. Dent J, El-Serag HB, Wallander MA, et al. Epidemiology of gastro-oesophageal reflux disease: a systematic review. Gut 2005;54(5):710–7.

30. El-Serag HB, Sweet S, Winchester CC, et al. Update on the epidemiology of gastro-oesophageal reflux disease: a systematic review. Gut 2014;63(6):871–80.

31. Gerson LB, Shetler K, Triadafilopoulos G. Prevalence of Barrett's esophagus in asymptomatic individuals. Gastroenterology 2002;123(2):461–7.

32. Ward EM, Wolfsen HC, Achem SR, et al. Barrett's esophagus is common in older men and women undergoing screening colonoscopy regardless of reflux symptoms. Am J Gastroenterol 2006;101(1):12–7.

33. Rex DK, Cummings OW, Shaw M, et al. Screening for Barrett's esophagus in colonoscopy patients with and without heartburn. Gastroenterology 2003;125(6):1670–7.

34. Camilleri M, Dubois D, Coulie B, et al. Prevalence and socioeconomic impact of upper gastrointestinal disorders in the United States: results of the US upper gastrointestinal study. Clin Gastroenterol Hepatol 2005;3(6):543–52.

35. Corley DA, Kubo A, Zhao W. Abdominal obesity, ethnicity and gastro-oesophageal reflux symptoms. Gut 2007;56(6):756–62.

36. El-Serag HB, Graham DY, Satia JA, et al. Obesity is an independent risk factor for GERD symptoms and erosive esophagitis. Am J Gastroenterol 2005;100(6):1243–50.

37. Garcia JM, Splenser AE, Kramer J, et al. Circulating inflammatory cytokines and adipokines are associated with increased risk of Barrett's esophagus: a case-control study. Clin Gastroenterol Hepatol 2014;12(2):229–38.e3.

38. Prasad GA, Bansal A, Sharma P, et al. Predictors of progression in Barrett's esophagus: current knowledge and future directions. Am J Gastroenterol 2010;105(7):1490–502.

39. El-Serag HB, Kvapil P, Hacken-Bitar J, et al. Abdominal obesity and the risk of Barrett's esophagus. Am J Gastroenterol 2005;100(10):2151–6.

40. Nocon M, Labenz J, Jaspersen D, et al. Association of body mass index with heartburn, regurgitation and esophagitis: results of the Progression of Gastroesophageal Reflux Disease study. J Gastroenterol Hepatol 2007;22(11):1728–31.

41. Singh S, Sharma AN, Murad MH, et al. Central adiposity is associated with increased risk of esophageal inflammation, metaplasia, and adenocarcinoma: a systematic review and meta-analysis. Clin Gastroenterol Hepatol 2013;11(11):1399–412.e7.

42. Gerson LB, Edson R, Lavori PW, et al. Use of a simple symptom questionnaire to predict Barrett's esophagus in patients with symptoms of gastroesophageal reflux. Am J Gastroenterol 2001;96(7):2005–12.

43. Cook MB, Wild CP, Forman D. A systematic review and meta-analysis of the sex ratio for Barrett's esophagus, erosive reflux disease, and nonerosive reflux disease. Am J Epidemiol 2005;162(11):1050–61.

44. Yousef F, Cardwell C, Cantwell MM, et al. The incidence of esophageal cancer and high-grade dysplasia in Barrett's esophagus: a systematic review and meta-analysis. Am J Epidemiol 2008;168(3):237–49.

45. Edelstein ZR, Bronner MP, Rosen SN, et al. Risk factors for Barrett's esophagus among patients with gastroesophageal reflux disease: a community clinic-based case-control study. Am J Gastroenterol 2009;104(4):834–42.

46. Oberg S, Wenner J, Johansson J, et al. Barrett esophagus: risk factors for progression to dysplasia and adenocarcinoma. Ann Surg 2005;242(1):49–54.

47. Menke-Pluymers MB, Hop WC, Dees J, et al. Risk factors for the development of an adenocarcinoma in columnar-lined (Barrett) esophagus. The Rotterdam Esophageal Tumor Study Group. Cancer 1993;72(4):1155–8.

48. Balasubramanian G, Singh M, Gupta N, et al. Prevalence and predictors of columnar lined esophagus in gastroesophageal reflux disease (GERD) patients undergoing upper endoscopy. Am J Gastroenterol 2012;107(11):1655–61.
49. Eloubeidi MA, Provenzale D. Clinical and demographic predictors of Barrett's esophagus among patients with gastroesophageal reflux disease: a multivariable analysis in veterans. J Clin Gastroenterol 2001;33(4):306–9.
50. Guardino JM, Khandwala F, Lopez R, et al. Barrett's esophagus at a tertiary care center: association of age on incidence and prevalence of dysplasia and adenocarcinoma. Am J Gastroenterol 2006;101(10):2187–93.
51. Johansson J, Håkansson HO, Mellblom L, et al. Risk factors for Barrett's oesophagus: a population-based approach. Scand J Gastroenterol 2007;42(2):148–56.
52. Cooper S, Menon S, Nightingale P, et al. Risk factors for the development of oesophageal adenocarcinoma in Barrett's oesophagus: a UK primary care retrospective nested case-control study. United European Gastroenterol J 2014; 2(2):91–8.
53. Chak A, Lee T, Kinnard MF, et al. Familial aggregation of Barrett's oesophagus, oesophageal adenocarcinoma, and oesophagogastric junctional adenocarcinoma in Caucasian adults. Gut 2002;51(3):323–8.
54. Juhasz A, Mittal SK, Lee TH, et al. Prevalence of Barrett esophagus in first-degree relatives of patients with esophageal adenocarcinoma. J Clin Gastroenterol 2011; 45(10):867–71.
55. Leggett CL, Gorospe EC, Calvin AD, et al. Obstructive sleep apnea is a risk factor for Barrett's esophagus. Clin Gastroenterol Hepatol 2014;12(4):583–8.e1.
56. Smith KJ, O'Brien SM, Smithers BM, et al. Interactions among smoking, obesity, and symptoms of acid reflux in Barrett's esophagus. Cancer Epidemiol Biomarkers Prev 2005;14(11 Pt 1):2481–6.
57. Cook MB, Shaheen NJ, Anderson LA, et al. Cigarette smoking increases risk of Barrett's esophagus: an analysis of the Barrett's and Esophageal Adenocarcinoma Consortium. Gastroenterology 2012;142(4):744–53.
58. Anderson LA, Watson RG, Murphy SJ, et al. Risk factors for Barrett's oesophagus and oesophageal adenocarcinoma: results from the FINBAR study. World J Gastroenterol 2007;13(10):1585–94.
59. Thrift AP, Kramer JR, Richardson PA, et al. No significant effects of smoking or alcohol consumption on risk of Barrett's esophagus. Dig Dis Sci 2014;59(1): 108–16.
60. Thrift AP, Kendall BJ, Pandeya N, et al. A clinical risk prediction model for Barrett esophagus. Cancer Prev Res (Phila) 2012;5(9):1115–23.
61. Rubenstein JH, Morgenstern H, Appelman H, et al. Prediction of Barrett's esophagus among men. Am J Gastroenterol 2013;108(3):353–62.
62. Thrift AP, Garcia JM, El-Serag HB. A multibiomarker risk score helps predict risk for Barrett's esophagus. Clin Gastroenterol Hepatol 2014;12(8):1267–71.
63. Gupta M, Beebe TJ, Dunagan KT, et al. Screening for Barrett's esophagus: results from a population-based survey. Dig Dis Sci 2014;59(8):1831–50.
64. Chak A, Alashkar BM, Isenberg G, et al. Comparative acceptability of transnasal esophagoscopy and esophageal capsule esophagoscopy: a randomized, controlled trial in veterans. Gastrointest Endosc 2014;80(5):774–82.
65. Waterman M, Gralnek IM. Capsule endoscopy of the esophagus. J Clin Gastroenterol 2009;43(7):605–12.
66. Bhardwaj A, Hollenbeak CS, Pooran N, et al. A meta-analysis of the diagnostic accuracy of esophageal capsule endoscopy for Barrett's esophagus in patients with gastroesophageal reflux disease. Am J Gastroenterol 2009;104(6):1533–9.

67. Gerson L, Lin OS. Cost-benefit analysis of capsule endoscopy compared with standard upper endoscopy for the detection of Barrett's esophagus. Clin Gastroenterol Hepatol 2007;5(3):319–25.

68. Atkinson M, Chak A. Unsedated small-caliber endoscopy–a new screening and surveillance tool for Barrett's esophagus? Nat Clin Pract Gastroenterol Hepatol 2007;4(8):426–7.

69. Shariff MK, Bird-Lieberman EL, O'Donovan M, et al. Randomized crossover study comparing efficacy of transnasal endoscopy with that of standard endoscopy to detect Barrett's esophagus. Gastrointest Endosc 2012;75(5):954–61.

70. Alashkar B, Faulx AL, Hepner A, et al. Development of a program to train physician extenders to perform transnasal esophagoscopy and screen for Barrett's esophagus. Clin Gastroenterol Hepatol 2014;12(5):785–92.

71. Sami SS, Dunagan KT, Johnson ML, et al. A randomized comparative effectiveness trial of novel endoscopic techniques and approaches for Barrett's esophagus screening in the community. Am J Gastroenterol 2015;110(1):148–58.

72. Kadri SR, Lao-Sirieix P, O'Donovan M, et al. Acceptability and accuracy of a non-endoscopic screening test for Barrett's oesophagus in primary care: cohort study. BMJ 2010;341:c4372.

73. Lao-Sirieix P, Boussioutas A, Kadri SR, et al. Non-endoscopic screening biomarkers for Barrett's oesophagus: from microarray analysis to the clinic. Gut 2009;58(11):1451–9.

74. Benaglia T, Sharples LD, Fitzgerald RC, et al. Health benefits and cost effectiveness of endoscopic and nonendoscopic cytosponge screening for Barrett's esophagus. Gastroenterology 2013;144(1):62–73.e6.

75. Falk GW, Chittajallu R, Goldblum JR, et al. Surveillance of patients with Barrett's esophagus for dysplasia and cancer with balloon cytology. Gastroenterology 1997;112(6):1787–97.

76. Seibel EJ, Carroll RE, Dominitz JA, et al. Tethered capsule endoscopy, a low-cost and high-performance alternative technology for the screening of esophageal cancer and Barrett's esophagus. IEEE Trans Biomed Eng 2008;55(3):1032–42.

77. Gora MJ, Sauk JS, Carruth RW, et al. Tethered capsule endomicroscopy enables less invasive imaging of gastrointestinal tract microstructure. Nat Med 2013; 19(2):238–40.

78. Selaru FM, Zou T, Xu Y, et al. Global gene expression profiling in Barrett's esophagus and esophageal cancer: a comparative analysis using cDNA microarrays. Oncogene 2002;21(3):475–8.

79. Rabinovitch PS, Longton G, Blount PL, et al. Predictors of progression in Barrett's esophagus III: baseline flow cytometric variables. Am J Gastroenterol 2001; 96(11):3071–83.

80. Reid BJ, Prevo LJ, Galipeau PC, et al. Predictors of progression in Barrett's esophagus II: baseline 17p (p53) loss of heterozygosity identifies a patient subset at increased risk for neoplastic progression. Am J Gastroenterol 2001;96(10): 2839–48.

81. Schulmann K, Sterian A, Berki A, et al. Inactivation of p16, RUNX3, and HPP1 occurs early in Barrett's-associated neoplastic progression and predicts progression risk. Oncogene 2005;24(25):4138–48.

82. Jin Z, Cheng Y, Gu W, et al. A multicenter, double-blinded validation study of methylation biomarkers for progression prediction in Barrett's esophagus. Cancer Res 2009;69(10):4112–5.

83. Galipeau PC, Li X, Blount PL, et al. NSAIDs modulate CDKN2A, TP53, and DNA content risk for progression to esophageal adenocarcinoma. PLoS Med 2007;4(2):e67.

84. Leedham SJ, Preston SL, McDonald SA, et al. Individual crypt genetic heterogeneity and the origin of metaplastic glandular epithelium in human Barrett's oesophagus. Gut 2008;57(8):1041–8.

85. Merlo LM, Shah NA, Li X, et al. A comprehensive survey of clonal diversity measures in Barrett's esophagus as biomarkers of progression to esophageal adenocarcinoma. Cancer Prev Res (Phila) 2010;3(11):1388–97.

86. Timmer MR, Sun G, Gorospe EC, et al. Predictive biomarkers for Barrett's esophagus: so near and yet so far. Dis Esophagus 2013;26(6):574–81.

87. Bird-Lieberman EL, Dunn JM, Coleman HG, et al. Population-based study reveals new risk-stratification biomarker panel for Barrett's esophagus. Gastroenterology 2012;143(4):927–35.e3.

88. Sato F, Jin Z, Schulmann K, et al. Three-tiered risk stratification model to predict progression in Barrett's esophagus using epigenetic and clinical features. PLoS One 2008;3(4):e1890.

89. Rudolph RE, Vaughan TL, Storer BE, et al. Effect of segment length on risk for neoplastic progression in patients with Barrett esophagus. Ann Intern Med 2000;132(8):612–20.

90. Taylor JB, Rubenstein JH. Meta-analyses of the effect of symptoms of gastroesophageal reflux on the risk of Barrett's esophagus. Am J Gastroenterol 2010; 105(8):1729, 1730–7 [quiz: 1738].

91. Corley DA, Kubo A, Levin TR, et al. Abdominal obesity and body mass index as risk factors for Barrett's esophagus. Gastroenterology 2007;133(1):34–41 [quiz: 311].

92. Edelstein ZR, Farrow DC, Bronner MP, et al. Central adiposity and risk of Barrett's esophagus. Gastroenterology 2007;133(2):403–11.

93. Nelsen EM, Kirihara Y, Takahashi N, et al. Distribution of body fat and its influence on esophageal inflammation and dysplasia in patients with Barrett's esophagus. Clin Gastroenterol Hepatol 2012;10(7):728–34 [quiz: e61–2].

94. Kubo A, Levin TR, Block G, et al. Alcohol types and sociodemographic characteristics as risk factors for Barrett's esophagus. Gastroenterology 2009;136(3): 806–15.

95. Anderson LA, Cantwell MM, Watson RG, et al. The association between alcohol and reflux esophagitis, Barrett's esophagus, and esophageal adenocarcinoma. Gastroenterology 2009;136(3):799–805.

96. Yates M, Cheong E, Luben R, et al. Body mass index, smoking, and alcohol and risks of Barrett's esophagus and esophageal adenocarcinoma: a UK prospective cohort study. Dig Dis Sci 2014;59(7):1552–9.

Surveillance in Barrett's Esophagus
Utility and Current Recommendations

 CrossMark

Joel H. Rubenstein, MD, MSc[a,b],*

KEYWORDS

- Esophageal neoplasms • Surveillance • Endoscopy

KEY POINTS

- Empirical evidence supporting the efficacy of surveillance of Barrett's esophagus is limited to observational studies with important limitations.
- Guidelines provide weak recommendations in favor of surveillance of Barrett's esophagus.
- In nondysplastic Barrett's esophagus, it is recommended to not perform surveillance more frequently than every 3 years.
- Adequate biopsies should be performed during surveillance endoscopies (4 quadrant every 2 cm plus of any mucosal irregularities).

INTRODUCTION

The notion of endoscopic surveillance of Barrett's esophagus with the aim of decreasing the burden of esophageal adenocarcinoma (EAC) is very attractive for several reasons. The incidence of EAC has risen dramatically over the past 4 decades in many Western nations. The mortality rate from the cancer is high. There exists a relatively easily identifiable precursor lesion in Barrett's esophagus, and tissue can be acquired from the lesion for histology with relative ease and safety (when compared with sampling, for instance, lesions of the pancreas, kidney, liver, or lung). Although survival from even most early-stage esophageal cancers is still poor,[1] a growing body of evidence has demonstrated the efficacy of endoscopic therapy directed at dysplasia and even adenocarcinoma confined to the mucosa (invading the lamina propria or muscularis mucosae, T1a cancers).[2,3] Therefore, it would seem reasonable that an effort should be made to reduce the burden of EAC by performing periodic

Conflict of Interest: J.H. Rubenstein has been a paid consultant for ORC International.
[a] Veterans Affairs Center for Clinical Management Research, VA Medical Center 111-D, 2215 Fuller Road, Ann Arbor, MI 48105, USA; [b] Barrett's Esophagus Program, Division of Gastroenterology, University of Michigan Medical School, 3912 Taubman Center, SPC 5362, Ann Arbor, MI 48109, USA
* VA Medical Center, 111-D, 2215 Fuller Road, Ann Arbor, MI 48105.
E-mail address: jhr@umich.edu

endoscopic surveillance in patients with Barrett's esophagus in order to identify and intervene on patients who develop dysplasia or intramucosal cancer. Herein, the author reviews the evidence regarding the effectiveness and efficiency of surveillance, caveats in interpreting that evidence, recommendations from published guidelines, details regarding the logistics of how surveillance should be conducted, and potential future directions.

INCIDENCE OF CANCER IN BARRETT'S ESOPHAGUS

Whether surveillance of Barrett's esophagus is rational depends heavily on the incidence of EAC in that setting. Some relatively small cohorts have published estimates of the incidence of EAC in nondysplastic Barrett's esophagus exceeding 2% per year.[4] However, there was likely a bias for disseminating the studies with the greatest observed risk. A recent meta-analysis of cohort studies has estimated the incidence at 0.33% per year.[5] Some large cohort studies have estimated the incidence as low as 0.12% per year.[6,7] When the risk of cancer is as low as 2% per decade, it is not clear that any intervention, even if it is efficacious for preventing cancer mortality, is worth the expected expense and complications. In low-grade dysplasia, the incidence of cancer may be higher, but it still ranges between 0.2% and 0.4% per year.[8–10] The incidence is clearly greater when high-grade dysplasia is present, but in that case, the standard of care has become endoscopic therapy rather than surveillance.[11]

LEAD-TIME AND LENGTH-TIME BIASES

In order to interpret the results of surveillance in Barrett's esophagus, an understanding of lead-time and length-time biases is necessary. Studies of the effects of screening or surveillance on cancer mortality are inherently fraught with the potential for bias by lead-time and length-time effects. Lead-time effects are best understood through a thought experiment (**Fig. 1**). A hypothetical set of twin brothers is imagined who were born on the same day, destined to develop EAC on the same day, and destined to die from EAC on the same day. Twin A does not undergo any screening or surveillance and instead is diagnosed with EAC when he presents with dysphagia, say at the age of 68 years. Assuming he dies at the age of 70 years, his survival time with EAC is 2 years. Twin B decided to undergo screening, was found to have Barrett's esophagus, and underwent surveillance; he was diagnosed with EAC while asymptomatic, say at the age of 63 years. He undergoes esophagectomy but still ends up dying from recurrent metastatic EAC at the age of 70 years. His survival time with EAC is observed to be 7 years. In practice, it is not known when someone is destined to develop cancer or when one is destined to die (even among twins), so this difference of 5 years between the 2 patients would be mistakenly attributed as an extension of the duration of life by 5 years, when in fact all that was accomplished with screening and surveillance was increasing the proportion of life with a known diagnosis of EAC in twin B and not delaying the date of his death at all. Even if there is a true effect of screening and surveillance on survival, it can be expected that lead-time effects will bias the observation of survival toward a stronger effect.

Length-time effects refer to the predilection of screening and surveillance examinations to identify indolent disease. Cancers are heterogeneous, with some progressing quickly and others slowly (**Fig. 2**). Any screening or surveillance examination is more likely to identify a slow-growing tumor than a fast-growing one because there is more time available to detect the cancer between onset and death. A reasonable assumption is that a slow-growing tumor is also less likely to be fatal than a fast-growing tumor; so any screening or surveillance examination is more likely to detect cancers

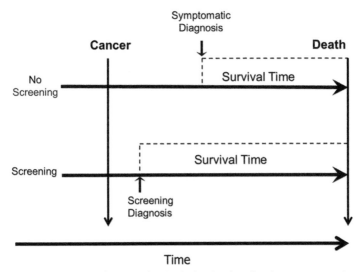

Fig. 1. Lead-time bias. Each of a pair of twins is destined to develop cancer on the same day and die from cancer on the same day. One twin does not undergo screening and is diagnosed with cancer because of symptoms. The other twin is diagnosed with cancer when he undergoes screening. If it is not known that they are destined to live the exact same number of days in their entire life, it would be observed that the second twin survives longer with his cancer than the first twin. But in fact, screening did not extend his life; it only increased the proportion of his life with a diagnosis of cancer.

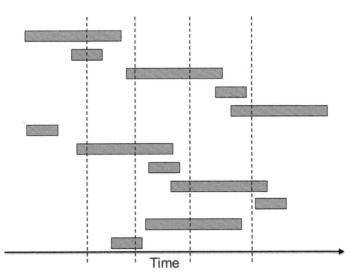

Fig. 2. Length-time bias. Cancers are heterogeneous. Slow-growing (less-fatal) cancers are represented by long bars (duration of time a patient is alive with the cancer). Fast-growing (more fatal) cancers are represented by short bars. In this example, the prevalence of slow-growing and fast-growing cancers is equal (there are 6 of each type). Surveillance is performed at the 4 times represented by the dashed lines. Because the slow-growing cancers are present for a longer period, surveillance is inherently more likely to identify slow-growing tumors (all 6 in this example), but miss fast-growing tumors (only 2 of 6 are detected in this example).

that are less fatal. The observed longer survival in surveillance-detected cases could be entirely because of the differences in the biology of the tumors detected by surveillance versus symptom-detected tumors and not a causal effect of surveillance. The potential for length-time bias can be aggravated by the manner in which cases and controls are classified. For instance, in one analysis of the effect of surveillance of Barrett's esophagus, the cases were defined as cancers detected by surveillance and controls as cancers detected by symptoms in the interval between surveillance. Such a design inherently compares slow-growing to fast-growing cancers; the investigators found a strong inverse association between surveillance (and likely preferential detection of slow-growing cancers) and mortality.[12] Analyzing the data from the same population in a different manner wherein patients with fatal cancer were compared with those with Barrett's esophagus for the presence of a prior endoscopy, the same investigators strikingly found no evidence of a protective effect of endoscopy.[13] The only way to entirely avoid length-time effects in studies of surveillance (even in randomized trials) is to perform surveillance so frequently that all tumors are detected by surveillance and not in the interval between surveillance (for instance, in an absurd scenario, with weekly or even daily endoscopies).

EMPIRICAL STUDIES OF THE EFFECTIVENESS OF SURVEILLANCE ENDOSCOPY

There have not been any published randomized trials of surveillance in Barrett's esophagus. Several retrospective studies have suggested that prior upper endoscopy among patients with EAC is associated with earlier stage of cancer at the time of initial diagnosis and improved survival. One must pay careful attention to the design of those studies in order to interpret the results. For instance, in a retrospective review of 589 patients with adenocarcinoma of either the esophagus or the gastroesophageal junction diagnosed within an integrated health system of Kaiser Permanente Northern California, Corley and colleagues[12] found 23 patients who had been diagnosed with Barrett's esophagus at least 6 months before the diagnosis of cancer. Of these 23 patients, 15 had their cancer detected during a surveillance endoscopy, and 8 patients were detected due to symptoms, none of whom had undergone any surveillance endoscopies. The age at diagnosis of patients in whom cancer was detected by surveillance was similar to that of patients without a prior diagnosis of Barrett's esophagus, but less than that of those with a prior Barrett's esophagus diagnosis who were not undergoing surveillance. The cancers in patients with a prior diagnosis of Barrett's esophagus who were not undergoing surveillance were diagnosed at a later stage than the surveillance-detected cancers ($P = .02$; the latter group with none worse than stage IIA). Adjusting for age, the patients with surveillance-detected cancer survived longer than those with the symptom-detected cancer with prior Barrett's esophagus (hazard ratio [HR], 0.25; 95% confidence interval [CI], 0.06–1.0). However, defining cases and controls based on surveillance detection of cancer inherently aggravates the potential for length-time bias. After 11 years, Corley and colleagues[13] updated the review of their health system's data to assess the role of surveillance in cancer mortality; they identified 38 deaths from adenocarcinoma of the esophagus or gastroesophageal junction in patients with a diagnosis of Barrett's esophagus at least 6 months before their cancer diagnosis and compared these to 101 patients with Barrett's esophagus matched for age, sex, and year of Barrett's esophagus diagnosis. In this analysis, they did not find any association between cancer mortality and receipt of surveillance endoscopy within 3 years prior (odds ratio [OR], 0.99, 95% CI, 0.36–2.75).

In a case-control study within the US Veterans Health Administration, Kearney and colleagues[14] identified 245 cases of death from adenocarcinoma of the esophagus or gastric cardia in patients diagnosed with gastroesophageal reflux disease (GERD) using International Classification of Diseases diagnostic billing codes, and compared them to 980 controls with GERD, matched for age, sex, and race. Receipt of a prior upper endoscopy at least 1 year prior was associated with a decreased odds of death from cancer (OR, 0.66; 95% CI, 0.45–0.96), but the investigators noted that none of the controls had been diagnosed with EAC and none had undergone esophagectomy, raising the likelihood that the results were biased in some way. For instance, those who underwent upper endoscopy may have been more conscious of their health and may have had other health-conscious habits such as avoidance of tobacco, healthy diet, and exercise, which were not measured. The author's group also examined the effect of prior upper endoscopy on patients with EAC with GERD using the same database.[15] Differences in the analysis were that data from 4 additional years were included, all subjects were required to have at least 1 encounter with the Veterans Health Administration in each of the 5 years preceding the diagnosis of cancer, and electronic medical records were reviewed to verify case status, dates of endoscopies, stage at diagnosis, and follow-up. From 311 potential subjects using administrative data, 155 subjects with EAC and a prior diagnosis of GERD were verified. Of the 155 subjects with EAC, 25 cases had undergone upper endoscopy between 1 and 5 years before the diagnosis of cancer. Those undergoing prior upper endoscopy were diagnosed at an earlier stage ($P = .03$), but there was no survival benefit (HR, 0.93; 95% CI, 0.58–1.50, adjusting for age, comorbidities, and year of diagnosis). Adherence with the recommended interval of surveillance (eg, 3 years for nondysplastic Barrett's esophagus), trended toward an association with improved survival (adjusted HR, 0.52; 95% CI, 0.24–1.12), but even among patients who did not undergo cancer resection, there seemed to be an association between adherence and survival (adjusted HR, 0.42; 95% CI, 0.16–1.09). This observation suggests that even if there had been a statistically significant association between surveillance and survival from EAC, it may not be a causal relation, but instead the result of bias such as selection of health-conscious patients for endoscopy and other biases described below.

In an analysis of the US Surveillance, Epidemiology, and End Results (SEER) cancer registry linked to Medicare data, Cooper and colleagues[16] identified 777 patients with EAC who were at least 70 years old at diagnosis. An upper endoscopy was performed at least 1 year before cancer diagnosis in 13%, but Barrett's esophagus was coded in only 7%. The stage of cancer was earlier in those with a prior upper endoscopy (62% vs 35% local cancer or dysplasia; notably, approximately 12% of the patients with a prior upper endoscopy and classified as having cancer by the study actually only had dysplasia). Patients classified with EAC with a prior upper endoscopy had longer median survival time (7 months vs 5 months, P<.01). Adjusting for age, sex, race, and comorbidities, prior upper endoscopy was associated with improved survival (HR, 0.73; 95% CI, 0.57–0.93). Results were similar for patients who not only underwent a prior upper endoscopy but also were diagnosed with Barrett's esophagus.

Cooper and colleagues[17] updated their analysis of the SEER-Medicare linked database 7 years later but limited the newer analysis to the receipt of an upper endoscopy between 6 months and 3 years before the diagnosis of EAC and lowered the minimum age to 68 years. A total of 2754 patients with EAC were identified, 11.5% of whom had undergone upper endoscopy within the defined time, and Barrett's esophagus was coded in 8.1%. Among those who had undergone prior upper endoscopy, the median number of prior endoscopies was 4. A prior diagnosis of Barrett's esophagus was more strongly associated with both earlier stage and improved survival than merely a prior upper endoscopy (for survival: prior Barrett's esophagus HR, 0.45; 95% CI, 0.25–0.80 vs prior endoscopy HR, 0.66; 95% CI, 0.47–0.93).

Verbeek and colleagues[18] analyzed data from the Netherlands National Cancer Registry linked to a nationwide pathology registry. The investigators identified 9780 cases of EAC, 791 (8%) of whom had a diagnosis of Barrett's esophagus at least 1 year before the cancer diagnosis, including 452 undergoing adequate surveillance (defined as at least 1 additional set of biopsies performed within 1.5 times the recommended interval; eg, 4.5 years for nondysplastic Barrett's esophagus). Those classified as undergoing adequate surveillance were more likely to be detected at stage I (47% vs 18% for inadequate surveillance, 17% for no surveillance but prior diagnosis of Barrett's esophagus, and 6% for no known prior Barrett's esophagus). Adequate surveillance was associated with improved 5-year survival compared with those without a prior diagnosis of Barrett's esophagus (OR, 0.74; 95% CI, 0.58–0.94, adjusting for sex, age, year of diagnosis, academic vs community hospital, location of tumor, stage, differentiation, and type of treatment). Although Barrett's esophagus with inadequate surveillance or without surveillance were both associated with improved survival in univariate analysis, there were no associations in the adjusted analyses. The definition for adequate surveillance used in this study aggravates the potential for length-time bias because patients with only 1 endoscopy before the diagnosis of EAC would be classified as no surveillance, even if that procedure had been performed within 4.5 years of the cancer diagnosis. This fact likely explains why patients classified as not undergoing surveillance had a shorter interval between diagnosis of Barrett's esophagus and EAC than those classified as adequate surveillance (median 5.2 years vs 7.5 years). Patients with inadequate surveillance were older at the time of diagnosis than those with adequate surveillance but had longer interval between diagnosis of Barrett's esophagus and EAC (median 12.6 years), suggesting that their age at diagnosis of Barrett's esophagus may have been similar. As the survival analyses were conducted starting at the age of diagnosis of cancer, this suggests that at least some of the observed association between adequate surveillance and survival is likely because of lead-time bias. Strangely, the association of adequate surveillance with survival persisted after adjusting for stage and treatment modality; if the effect of surveillance is mediated through earlier stage at diagnosis and greater likelihood of surgical resection, then it should be expected that association with adequate surveillance should no longer be evident after adjusting for those factors. This suggests that at least some of the observed association between surveillance and survival is biased by length-time effects and/or confounded by other unmeasured factors such as comorbidities or health-conscious behaviors.

Recently, Bhat and colleagues[19] reported results from a population-based study in Northern Ireland. The investigators identified 716 cases of EAC, 52 (7.3%) of whom had a diagnosis of Barrett's esophagus at least 6 months prior. Those with a prior diagnosis of Barrett's esophagus were more likely to be diagnosed at stage I or II (44.2% vs 11.1%) and more likely to undergo surgical resection (50.0% vs 25.5%). Patients with EAC with a prior diagnosis of Barrett's esophagus seemed to survive longer (HR, 0.44; 95% CI, 0.30–0.64; adjusted for age, sex, and tumor grade). However, there was a survival benefit of prior Barrett's esophagus even in patients who did not undergo esophagectomy (HR, 0.50; 95% CI, 0.32–0.79), suggesting that the estimate of the effect was likely biased. The investigators attempted to adjust for the potential of lead-time bias by estimating the duration of asymptomatic, but clinically detectable cancer (the sojourn time) by comparing the average age at cancer diagnosis between those with and without prior Barrett's esophagus diagnosis (67.4 vs 69.9 years, a difference of 2.5 years). In the analysis adjusting for lead-time bias, the effect of a prior diagnosis of Barrett's esophagus on survival was attenuated (HR, 0.65; 95% CI, 0.45–0.95). The investigators also attempted to adjust for the potential of length-time bias by accounting for the relative proportions of low-grade differentiated tumors in both groups, and the expected survival difference between grades of differentiation, finding that it only slightly altered the estimate for the effect of prior diagnosis of Barrett's esophagus on survival.

In summary, several retrospective studies have observed apparent associations between surveillance and improved survival from EAC, but the results have not been consistent and the studies are prone to several important potential biases.

WHAT IS THE TRUE EFFECTIVENESS OF SURVEILLANCE?

Given the inherent predilection of studies of surveillance to be biased by lead-time and length-time effects, and the likely selection effects for health-conscious patients to undergo surveillance in the observational studies, the available empirical data on surveillance almost certainly overestimate the magnitude of the effect of surveillance of Barrett's esophagus on improving survival from EAC. Of the studies described above, there was no evidence of an effect of surveillance in the Kaiser Permanente Northern California system or in the US Veterans Health Administration, but both effect estimates had fairly wide CIs, which could allow for some substantial undetected effect. In the larger SEER-Medicare linked data set and in the much larger Dutch national study, the effect estimates for mortality ranged from 0.45 to 0.74. These effects should be interpreted as the best-case scenario; the true effect is likely weaker, and it is conceivable that there is no true effect. In the Northern Ireland study, which formally attempted to account for the potential for lead-time and length-time effects, a prior diagnosis of Barrett's esophagus was associated with an HR of approximately 0.65.

Notably, all the studies described estimated the effect of surveillance on survival from EAC. In the current era of endoscopic therapy, there is the potential for an additional effect of surveillance on preventing EAC. Endoscopic therapy in dysplastic Barrett's esophagus prevents progression to EAC, at least in the short term.[2,20] However, 60% to 67% of patients with Barrett's esophagus who have been adherent with surveillance and yet progressed to invasive cancer were never found to have high-grade dysplasia on any surveillance endoscopy and 30% to 54% were never found to have low-grade dysplasia either.[18,21] So even if endoscopic therapy could prevent progression to EAC in 100% of patients with dysplastic Barrett's esophagus, a substantial proportion of patients undergoing surveillance would still develop EAC. A randomized controlled trial of surveillance plus endoscopic therapy for dysplasia compared with no surveillance would be needed to better estimate the efficacy and effectiveness of surveillance.

COST-EFFECTIVENESS OF SURVEILLANCE

Several investigators have sought to estimate the cost-effectiveness of surveillance. These estimates depend on the effectiveness of surveillance, which is not known with much precision. For the purposes of their analyses, the investigators have all assumed that surveillance is indeed effective. Before the widespread advent of endoscopic therapy, Inadomi and colleagues[22] published a cost-effectiveness analysis, which found that screening for Barrett's esophagus and surveillance in patients with dysplasia was cost-effective, but that additionally performing surveillance in patients with nondysplastic Barrett's esophagus even as infrequently as every 5 years cost $596,000 per quality-adjusted life-year (QALY) gained; the typically accepted willingness-to-pay thresholds of society ranges from $50,000 to $250,000 per QALY. In a model incorporating endoscopic therapy for high-grade dysplasia and surveillance every 2 years for nondysplastic Barrett's esophagus, Gordon and colleagues[23] estimated that surveillance would prevent 28% of EAC and cost $60,858 per QALY. In a European model of long-segment Barrett's esophagus incorporating endoscopic therapy for high-grade dysplasia, Kastelein and colleagues[24] estimated that surveillance every 5 years cost €5283 per QALY compared with no surveillance. Surveillance every 4 years cost an additional €62,619 per QALY compared with every 5 years and surveillance every 3 years cost an additional €105,755 per QALY compared with every 4 years. Similar to the study by Inadomi and colleagues,[22] they found that a strategy of surveillance every 5 years without endoscopic therapy would cost €413,500 per QALY compared with no surveillance. The investigators concluded that the optimal strategy was surveillance every 5 years with endoscopic therapy for high-grade dysplasia. Although these studies do not prove that surveillance is effective, they demonstrate that if surveillance is indeed effective, then surveillance followed by endoscopic therapy for high-grade dysplasia is likely cost effective. However, surveillance of nondysplastic Barrett's esophagus without endoscopic therapy for high-grade dysplasia (as had been practiced for many years before the advent of endoscopic resection and radiofrequency ablation) was likely a very inefficient practice.

GUIDELINE RECOMMENDATIONS

The published guidelines regarding surveillance of Barrett's esophagus have evolved over time (Table 1). The 1998 guidelines from the American College of Gastroenterology recommended surveillance with biopsies every 2 to 3 years in patients without dysplasia

Table 1
A history of guideline recommendations regarding surveillance of Barrett's esophagus

Year	Society	Recommendation	Grade
1998	ACG[25]	Surveillance every 2–3 y after 2 sets of biopsies without dysplasia	N/A
2002	ACG[23]	Surveillance every 3 y after 2 sets of biopsies without dysplasia	N/A
2005	BSG[41]	Surveillance every 2 y	C (weakest)
2005	AGA[42]	Surveillance at 1 y, then every 5 y	N/A
2006	ASGE[43]	Surveillance at 1 y, then every 3 y	N/A
2007	FSDE[27]	Surveillance every 2 y for >6 cm, 3 y for 3–6 cm, and 5 y for <3 cm	N/A
2008	ACG[30]	Surveillance every 3 y after 2 sets of biopsies without dysplasia	N/A
2011	AGA[11]	Surveillance every 3–5 y	Weak
2012	DSGH[44]	Surveillance every 3 y	IIIB (on scale of IA to IV with IA being best-quality evidence)
2012	ACP[45]	Surveillance every 3–5 y	May be indicated
2012	ASGE[26]	Surveillance every 3–5 y	Low-quality evidence
2014	BSG[28]	Surveillance should be offered: • For ≥3 cm, every 2–3 y • For <3 cm with intestinal metaplasia, every 3–5 y	B C (weakest) C (weakest)

Abbreviations: ACG, American College of Gastroenterology; ACP, American College of Physicians; AGA, American Gastroenterology Association; ASGE, American Society for Gastrointestinal Endoscopy; BSG, British Society of Gastroenterology; DSGH, Danish Society of Gastroenterology and Hepatology; FSDE, French Society of Digestive Endoscopy; N/A, not applicable.
Data from Refs.[11,23,25–28,30,41–45]

on at least 2 prior endoscopies (because of concern of sampling error for missing dysplasia on the first endoscopy).[25] The 2011 guidelines from the American Gastroenterology Association dropped the recommendation for a repeat endoscopy within 1 year after the initial diagnosis of Barrett's esophagus and gave a weak recommendation for surveillance every 3 to 5 years in nondysplastic Barrett's esophagus.[11] Similarly, the 2012 guidelines from the American Society for Gastrointestinal Endoscopy specifically recommended against surveillance at 1 year from the initial diagnosis and recommended surveillance every 3 to 5 years in nondysplastic Barrett's esophagus.[26] In 2007, the French Society of Digestive Endoscopy introduced the recommendation of surveillance interval stratified by the length of Barrett's esophagus.[27] The most recent guidelines from the British Society of Gastroenterology endorsed a similar framework.[28] All these recommendations have been characterized as weak and based on low-quality evidence. The general theme over time has been a prolongation of the recommended interval between surveillance, such that current US guidelines recommend surveillance every 3 to 5 years. The Choosing Wisely campaign of the American Board of Internal Medicine and Consumer Reports is aimed at decreasing overutilization of testing and therapy. In 2012, the American Gastroenterology Association included in its list for Choosing Wisely of Five Things Physicians and Patients Should Question surveillance endoscopy in Barrett's esophagus more frequently than every 3 years.

EMPIRICAL EVIDENCE FOR THE FREQUENCY OF SURVEILLANCE

Despite the trend toward recommendations for less-frequent surveillance intervals, there is very little empirical data to guide the decision about the correct interval. The initial recommendation of surveillance every 2 to 3 years was justified by the expectation that the incidence of EAC in nondysplastic Barrett's esophagus is likely low and more frequent surveillance would not be justified.[25] Some guidelines have cited the earlier case-control study within the US Veterans Health Administration described above, which found that an endoscopy performed between 2 and 4 years prior was the only interval studied that was statistically significantly associated with a decreased odds of death from EAC.[14] However, as described above, the investigators themselves noted that the results of the study were suspect because none of the controls were ever diagnosed with EAC or underwent esophagectomy, suggesting that the association of endoscopy (at any interval) with protection from EAC mortality was likely biased by selection effects. The trend toward recommendations of less-frequent intervals seems to be driven primarily by the emerging data that the true incidence of EAC in nondysplastic Barrett's esophagus is lower than it was believed when the initial guidelines were published. The cost-effectiveness analysis by Kastelein and colleagues[24] found that surveillance more frequently than every 5 years was expensive but did not examine surveillance intervals less frequent than every 5 years. Given the rarity of incident EAC in nondysplastic Barrett's esophagus, a surveillance interval as long as every 10 years might even be reasonable. On the other hand, if the transition from dysplasia to cancer is a rapid event, lengthening the interval of surveillance might substantially reduce the effectiveness of surveillance because most patients would develop their cancer in the interval between surveillances. For instance, in the Seattle Barrett's Esophagus Study cohort of patients with high-grade dysplasia under surveillance every 3 months, those who ultimately progressed to cancer had somatic chromosomal alterations present at the earliest 2 to 4 years before their cancer.[29] So it is unclear what the correct interval of surveillance should be. In light of the uncertainty, the very low incidence of EAC in Barrett's esophagus argues in favor of infrequent surveillance, if surveillance is performed at all.

BIOPSY PROTOCOL IN SURVEILLANCE

Guidelines have recommended biopsies of visible mucosal abnormalities in addition to random biopsies in 4 quadrants every 2 cm in nondysplastic Barrett's esophagus and every 1 cm in dysplastic Barrett's esophagus.[11,26,28,30] Unfortunately, adherence to the protocol has been demonstrated to be inversely associated with the length of Barrett's esophagus; patients with longer Barrett's esophagus and thus at highest risk of progression are the least likely to undergo an adequate biopsy regimen.[31,32] The observation of nonadherence in longer segments of Barrett's esophagus suggests that endoscopist fatigue, time pressures, and financial incentives may be responsible. Adherence to the biopsy protocol has been associated with an increased detection of dysplasia and cancer.[31,33] If one is going to undertake the risks and costs of surveillance, one ought to make certain that the surveillance endoscopy is as effective as possible, even if that requires a few more minutes for the procedure.

FUTURE DIRECTIONS

Although surveillance of Barrett's esophagus has been recommended, it is not clear if it is effective. A randomized trial of surveillance would provide higher-quality evidence regarding whether time is being wasted with surveillance. Such a trial would have to be very large, but the cost would be a very small proportion of the money currently spent on screening and surveillance in Barrett's esophagus. The efficiency of surveillance might be improved by developing and implementing risk-stratified strategies of surveillance. For instance, the French Society of Digestive Endoscopy and the British Society of Gastroenterology have recommended surveillance intervals stratified by the length of Barrett's esophagus.[27,28] Other potential clinical markers that could be leveraged for risk stratification include age, sex, obesity, tobacco use, and family history.[34–36] Aside from clinical markers, the use of molecular biomarkers might improve the efficiency of surveillance. Promising examples include loss of heterozygosity in the p53 gene, abnormally increased tetraploidy, aneuploidy, hypermethylated genes, and specific lectins.[37–39] Use of such markers to guide surveillance decisions could improve the cost-effectiveness of surveillance.[23] In addition, strategies that use adjunctive imaging technologies during endoscopy could improve the accuracy of detection of neoplasia, thereby decreasing the number of biopsies required and potentially lengthening the duration required between surveillance procedures. Finally, nonendoscopic technologies for performing surveillance, such as the cytosponge device, if both accurate and inexpensive could improve the effectiveness of surveillance, possibly at a lower cost than endoscopic surveillance.[40]

SUMMARY

Surveillance of Barrett's esophagus for incident dysplasia or EAC has become an accepted practice, receiving weak recommendations in favor from multiple specialty societies. Although the strategy makes good sense intuitively, the body of evidence supporting the practice is relatively weak and there are legitimate concerns that the practice may not be particularly effective. As such, there has been momentum toward at least decreasing the frequency of surveillance. In addition, if surveillance is undertaken, then evidence does demonstrate that an adequate biopsy protocol should be performed. Otherwise, endoscopists squander much of whatever chance they have for effectively reducing the burden of EAC.

REFERENCES

1. Hur C, Miller M, Kong CY, et al. Trends in esophageal adenocarcinoma incidence and mortality. Cancer 2013;119:1149–58.
2. Shaheen NJ, Sharma P, Overholt BF, et al. Radiofrequency ablation in Barrett's esophagus with dysplasia. N Engl J Med 2009;360:2277–88.
3. Pech O, May A, Manner H, et al. Long-term efficacy and safety of endoscopic resection for patients with mucosal adenocarcinoma of the esophagus. Gastroenterology 2014;146:652–60.e1.
4. Shaheen N, Crosby M, Bozymski E, et al. Is there publication bias in the reporting of cancer risk in Barrett's esophagus? Gastroenterology 2000;119:333–8.
5. Desai TK, Krishnan K, Samala N, et al. The incidence of oesophageal adenocarcinoma in non-dysplastic Barrett's oesophagus: a meta-analysis. Gut 2012;61:970–6.
6. Hvid-Jensen F, Pedersen L, Drewes AM, et al. Incidence of adenocarcinoma among patients with Barrett's esophagus. N Engl J Med 2011;365:1375–83.
7. Wani S, Falk G, Hall M, et al. Patients with nondysplastic Barrett's esophagus have low risks for developing dysplasia or esophageal adenocarcinoma. Clin Gastroenterol Hepatol 2011;9:220–7 [quiz: e26].
8. Wani S, Falk GW, Post J, et al. Risk factors for progression of low-grade dysplasia in patients with Barrett's esophagus. Gastroenterology 2011;141:1179–86.
9. Bhat S, Coleman HG, Yousef F, et al. Risk of malignant progression in Barrett's esophagus patients: results from a large population-based study. J Natl Cancer Inst 2011;103:1049–57.
10. de Jonge PJ, van Blankenstein M, Looman CW, et al. Risk of malignant progression in patients with Barrett's oesophagus: a Dutch nationwide cohort study. Gut 2010;59:1030–6.
11. Spechler SJ, Sharma P, Souza RF, et al. American gastroenterological association medical position statement on the management of Barrett's esophagus. Gastroenterology 2011;140:1084–91.
12. Corley DA, Levin TR, Habel LA, et al. Surveillance and survival in Barrett's adenocarcinomas: a population-based study. Gastroenterology 2002;122:633–40.
13. Corley DA, Mehtani K, Quesenberry C, et al. Impact of endoscopic surveillance on mortality from Barrett's esophagus–associated esophageal adenocarcinomas. Gastroenterology 2013;145:312–9.
14. Kearney DJ, Crump C, Maynard C, et al. A case-control study of endoscopy and mortality from adenocarcinoma of the esophagus or gastric cardia in persons with GERD. Gastrointest Endosc 2003;57:823–9.
15. Rubenstein JH, Sonnenberg A, Davis J, et al. Prior endoscopy does not improve long-term survival from esophageal adenocarcinoma among United States veterans. Am J Gastroenterol 2006;101:S46 [Abstract].
16. Cooper GS, Yuan Z, Chak A, et al. Association of prediagnosis endoscopy with stage and survival in adenocarcinoma of the esophagus and gastric cardia. Cancer 2002;95:32–8.
17. Cooper GS, Kou TD, Chak A. Receipt of previous diagnoses and endoscopy and outcome from esophageal adenocarcinoma: a population-based study with temporal trends. Am J Gastroenterol 2009;104:1356.
18. Verbeek RE, Leenders M, Ten Kate FJ, et al. Surveillance of Barrett's esophagus and mortality from esophageal adenocarcinoma: a population-based cohort study. Am J Gastroenterol 2014;109:1215–22.
19. Bhat SK, McManus DT, Coleman HG, et al. Oesophageal adenocarcinoma and prior diagnosis of Barrett's oesophagus: a population-based study. Gut 2015;64:20–5.

20. Phoa KN, van Vilsteren FG, Weusten BL, et al. Radiofrequency ablation vs endoscopic surveillance for patients with Barrett esophagus and low-grade dysplasia: a randomized clinical trial. JAMA 2014;311:1209–17.

21. Rubenstein JH, Sonnenberg A, Davis J, et al. Effect of a prior endoscopy on outcomes of esophageal adenocarcinoma among United States veterans. Gastrointest Endosc 2008;68:849–55.

22. Inadomi JM, Sampliner R, Lagergren J, et al. Screening and surveillance for Barrett esophagus in high-risk groups: a cost-utility analysis. Ann Intern Med 2003;138:176–86.

23. Gordon LG, Mayne GC, Hirst NG, et al. Cost-effectiveness of endoscopic surveillance of non-dysplastic Barrett's esophagus. Gastrointest Endosc 2014;79: 242–56.e6.

24. Kastelein F, van Olphen S, Steyerberg EW, et al. Surveillance in patients with long-segment Barrett's oesophagus: a cost-effectiveness analysis. Gut 2014. [Epub ahead of print].

25. Sampliner RE. Practice guidelines on the diagnosis, surveillance, and therapy of Barrett's esophagus. The Practice Parameters Committee of the American College of Gastroenterology. Am J Gastroenterol 1998;93:1028–32.

26. Evans JA, Early DS, Fukami N, et al. The role of endoscopy in Barrett's esophagus and other premalignant conditions of the esophagus. Gastrointest Endosc 2012; 76:1087–94.

27. Boyer J, Laugier R, Chemali M, et al. French Society of Digestive Endoscopy SFED guideline: monitoring of patients with Barrett's esophagus. Endoscopy 2007;39:840–2.

28. Fitzgerald RC, di Pietro M, Ragunath K, et al. British Society of Gastroenterology guidelines on the diagnosis and management of Barrett's oesophagus. Gut 2014; 63:7–42.

29. Li X, Galipeau PC, Paulson TG, et al. Temporal and spatial evolution of somatic chromosomal alterations: a case-cohort study of Barrett's esophagus. Cancer Prev Res (Phila) 2014;7:114–27.

30. Wang KK, Sampliner RE. Practice parameters committee of the American college of G. Updated guidelines 2008 for the diagnosis, surveillance and therapy of Barrett's esophagus. Am J Gastroenterol 2008;103:788–97.

31. Abrams JA, Kapel RC, Lindberg GM, et al. Adherence to biopsy guidelines for Barrett's esophagus surveillance in the community setting in the United States. Clin Gastroenterol Hepatol 2009;7:736–42 [quiz: 710].

32. Curvers WL, Peters FP, Elzer B, et al. Quality of Barrett's surveillance in the Netherlands: a standardized review of endoscopy and pathology reports. Eur J Gastroenterol Hepatol 2008;20:601–7.

33. Fitzgerald RC, Saeed IT, Khoo D, et al. Rigorous surveillance protocol increases detection of curable cancers associated with Barrett's esophagus. Dig Dis Sci 2001;46:1892–8.

34. Hardikar S, Onstad L, Blount PL, et al. The role of tobacco, alcohol, and obesity in neoplastic progression to esophageal adenocarcinoma: a prospective study of Barrett's esophagus. PLoS One 2013;8:e52192.

35. Coleman HG, Bhat S, Johnston BT, et al. Tobacco smoking increases the risk of high-grade dysplasia and cancer among patients with Barrett's esophagus. Gastroenterology 2012;142:233–40.

36. Prasad GA, Bansal A, Sharma P, et al. Predictors of progression in Barrett's esophagus: current knowledge and future directions. Am J Gastroenterol 2010; 105:1490–502.

37. Jin Z, Cheng Y, Gu W, et al. A multicenter, double-blinded validation study of methylation biomarkers for progression prediction in Barrett's esophagus. Cancer Res 2009;69:4112–5.
38. Bird-Lieberman E, Dunn J, Coleman H, et al. Population-based study reveals new risk-stratification biomarker panel for Barrett's esophagus. Gastroenterology 2012;143:927–35.e3.
39. Reid BJ, Levine DS, Longton G, et al. Predictors of progression to cancer in Barrett's esophagus: baseline histology and flow cytometry identify low- and high-risk patient subsets. Am J Gastroenterol 2000;95:1669–76.
40. Kadri SR, Lao-Sirieix P, O'Donovan M, et al. Acceptability and accuracy of a non-endoscopic screening test for Barrett's oesophagus in primary care: cohort study. BMJ 2010;341:c4372.
41. Watson A, Heading RC, Shepherd NA. Guidelines for the diagnosis and management of Barrett's columnar-lined oesophagus. 2005. Available at: http://www.bsg.org.uk/bsgdisp1.php?id=3f4a76385e42599499e9&h=1&sh=1&i=1&b=1&m=00023. Accessed January 22, 2007.
42. Wang KK, Wongkeesong M, Buttar NS. American Gastroenterological Association medical position statement: role of the gastroenterologist in the management of esophageal carcinoma. Gastroenterology 2005;128:1468–70.
43. Hirota W, Zuckerman M, Adler D, et al. ASGE guideline: the role of endoscopy in the surveillance of premalignant conditions of the upper GI tract. Gastrointest Endosc 2006;63:570–80.
44. Bremholm L, Funch-Jensen P, Eriksen J, et al. Barrett's esophagus. Diagnosis, follow-up and treatment. Dan Med J 2012;59:C4499.
45. Shaheen NJ, Weinberg DS, Denberg TD, et al. Upper endoscopy for gastro-esophageal reflux disease: best practice advice from the clinical guidelines committee of the American College of Physicians. Ann Intern Med 2012;157:808–16.

Predictors of Progression to High-Grade Dysplasia or Adenocarcinoma in Barrett's Esophagus

Matthew J. Whitson, MD, Gary W. Falk, MD, MS*

KEYWORDS

- Barrett's esophagus • Esophageal adenocarcinoma • Dysplasia • Risk factors
- Neoplastic progression

KEY POINTS

- Barrett's esophagus is the most well-established risk factor for the development of esophageal adenocarcinoma.
- Risk factors for neoplastic progression in patients with Barrett's esophagus include endoscopic findings (ie, erosive esophagitis), pathologic findings (ie, dysplasia), and clinical aspects (ie, male sex, older age, tobacco).
- Protective factors against neoplastic progression include medication use (ie, statins, aspirin) and dietary considerations.

INTRODUCTION

The incidence of esophageal adenocarcinoma, a disease characterized by high mortality and an estimated 5-year survival rate of 20%, has increased dramatically in recent decades.[1,2] Barrett's esophagus is the most well-established risk factor for the development of esophageal adenocarcinoma.[3] The annual risk of progression from Barrett's esophagus to adenocarcinoma is approximately 0.33% per year.[4] When including both esophageal adenocarcinoma and high-grade dysplasia as a combined end point of progression, the incidence rate is approximately 0.9% to 1.0% per year.[5,6] Despite this neoplastic risk, the vast majority of patients with Barrett's esophagus die of causes other than esophageal adenocarcinoma.[7] At present, it remains unclear which patients

This work was supported in part by the NIH/NCI U54-CA163004, NIH/NIDDK P30-DK050306 (and its Molecular Pathology and Imaging and Molecular Biology Cores), NIH/NCI P01-CA098101 and institutional funds.
Division of Gastroenterology, Hospital of the University of Pennsylvania, University of Pennsylvania Perelman School of Medicine, 7th floor, South Pavillion, 3400 Civic Center Boulevard, Philadelphia, PA 19104, USA
* Corresponding author.
E-mail address: gary.falk@uphs.upenn.edu

Gastroenterol Clin N Am 44 (2015) 299–315
http://dx.doi.org/10.1016/j.gtc.2015.02.005
0889-8553/15/$ – see front matter © 2015 Elsevier Inc. All rights reserved.

with Barrett's esophagus progress on to neoplasia, a fact that makes current surveillance programs problematic. This article examines the endoscopic, pathologic, and epidemiologic risk factors for neoplastic progression in Barrett's esophagus (**Table 1**).

ENDOSCOPIC RISK FACTORS
Segment Length

While esophageal adenocarcinoma can develop in both short and long segments of Barrett's esophagus (traditionally defined as >3 cm), the understanding of the relationship between segment length and the risk of progression has evolved in recent years.[8] A 2012 meta-analysis found a lower annual incidence of esophageal adenocarcinoma in patients with short-segment Barrett's esophagus (<3 cm) than in the overall Barrett's esophagus population (0.19% vs 0.33% per year).[4] Work from the Northern Ireland Barrett's Esophagus Registry demonstrated an increased risk for progression to adenocarcinoma or high-grade dysplasia in long-segment Barrett's esophagus (hazard ratio [HR], 7.1; 95% confidence interval [CI], 1.74–29.04).[9] A recent case-control study from Berlin also found an association of segment length with progression to adenocarcinoma or high-grade dysplasia.[10] Patients with long-segment Barrett's esophagus had an increased risk of progression when compared with those with short-segment Barrett's esophagus (odds ratio [OR], 2.69; 95% CI, 1.48–4.88).

Newer studies have examined the relationship of segment length and risk of progression not only as a binary variable of long versus short but also as a continuous variable. In a large multicenter study, increasing segment length was an independent risk factor for neoplastic progression in patients with nondysplastic Barrett's esophagus.[11] Patients who progressed to adenocarcinoma or high-grade dysplasia had a longer Barrett's segment (6.1 cm vs 3.5 cm). Perhaps more importantly, the risk for neoplastic progression increased by 28% for every 1-cm increase in length of the Barrett's segment. Similarly, a Netherlands cohort study of more than 700 patients with nondysplastic Barrett's esophagus or low-grade dysplasia confirmed the concept of increasing risk with increasing segment length.[12] The relative risk of neoplastic progression to adenocarcinoma or high-grade dysplasia was 1.11 (95% CI, 1.01–1.2) per 1-cm increase in segment length. The recently completed SURF (Surveillance vs Radiofrequency Ablation) trial of radiofrequency ablation in patients with Barrett's esophagus with low-grade dysplasia also found segment length to be an independent predictor of neoplastic progression in the surveillance arm of the study (OR, 1.35 per cm; 95% CI, 1.04–1.76).[13]

Table 1	
Risk factors for neoplastic progression to esophageal adenocarcinoma	
Clinical	Older age
	White race
	Male sex
	Family history
	Tobacco
	Obesity
Endoscopic	Long-segment Barrett's esophagus
	Hiatal hernia
	Mucosal abnormalities
	Right hemisphere position
Pathologic	Intestinal metaplasia
	Dysplasia
	p53 Overexpression

However, progression does occur in shorter segments of Barrett's esophagus, and a population-based study of over 8000 patients in Ireland found no relationship between segment length and risk of progression.[14] Taken together, it would seem that longer segments of Barrett's esophagus are associated with an increased risk of progression to adenocarcinoma or high-grade dysplasia.

Hiatal Hernia

Hiatal hernia is a well-documented risk factor for the development of Barrett's esophagus.[15] In addition, some data suggest that a larger hiatal hernia size may increase the risk of neoplastic progression in Barrett's esophagus (OR, 1.20 per cm hiatal hernia; 95% CI, 1.04–1.39).[16] In a cohort study of 550 patients from the Veterans Affairs Medical Center, Kansas City, a large hiatal hernia (>6 cm) was associated with an increased risk of neoplastic progression to adenocarcinoma or high-grade dysplasia when compared with patients with no hiatal hernia.[17] However, other studies find contrary results. A 2013 case-control study of approximately 600 patients demonstrated that although the presence of hiatal hernia increased the risk for Barrett's esophagus, it did not increase the risk of neoplastic progression to adenocarcinoma or high-grade dysplasia.[10] Overall, it is unclear if hiatal hernia size is an independent risk factor for neoplastic progression in Barrett's esophagus.

Mucosal Abnormalities

Several mucosal changes within the Barrett's segment are associated with an increased risk of progression to adenocarcinoma or high-grade dysplasia. Erosive esophagitis has emerged as a potential risk factor for esophageal adenocarcinoma. A Dutch multicenter cohort study found an increased risk of progression to adenocarcinoma or high-grade dysplasia in patients with Barrett's esophagus with esophagitis at baseline endoscopy (risk ratio [RR], 3.5; 95% CI, 1.3–9.5).[12] A Danish cohort study also found an increased standardized incidence ratio for esophageal adenocarcinoma among patients with Barrett's esophagus with erosive esophagitis when compared with the general population (standardized incidence ratio, 5.2; 95% CI, 4.6–5.8).[18]

Ulceration within a Barrett's segment is also associated with an increased risk of neoplastic progression to adenocarcinoma or high-grade dysplasia. The abovementioned population-based case-control study from Northern Ireland also found that patients with ulceration in the Barrett's segment at diagnosis, but not elsewhere in the esophagus, were more likely to progress to cancer or high-grade dysplasia than those without (HR, 1.72; 95% CI, 1.08–2.76).[9]

It is unclear if mucosal abnormalities such as erosive esophagitis or ulceration are in fact risk factors for progression or rather are markers of prevalent adenocarcinoma or high-grade dysplasia, as shown by current endoscopic eradication studies. Overall, it seems that mucosal abnormalities are associated with an increased risk of neoplastic progression in patients with Barrett's esophagus.

Circumferential Position

Early adenocarcinoma and high-grade dysplasia seem to have a predilection to develop in the right hemisphere of the esophagus.[19–22] The author's group found that 85% of patients with adenocarcinoma or high-grade dysplasia referred for endoscopic management had these abnormalities located in the right hemisphere of the esophagus, predominantly in the area between 12-o'clock and 3-o'clock positions.[20] Similar findings were described in an Australian study, where more than 50% of advanced lesions were found between 2-o'clock and 5-o'clock positions.[19] Both of these studies are in line with previous data demonstrating greater chances for esophagitis to be found on the right hemisphere of the esophagus, suggesting a potential inflammatory mechanism to explain this observation.[23]

PATHOLOGIC RISK FACTORS
Intestinal Metaplasia Versus Columnar Metaplasia

At present, there is some disagreement among gastrointestinal (GI) societies as to the definition of Barrett's esophagus. The major difference is whether or not the presence of intestinal metaplasia within the columnar lined esophagus is required for the diagnosis. Early data from Scandinavia suggested that the risk of progression to adenocarcinoma or high-grade dysplasia in the columnar lined esophagus was equivalent in patients with and without intestinal metaplasia.[24] However, multiple subsequent studies have demonstrated an increased risk of neoplastic progression in patients with intestinal metaplasia.

Work from the population-based Northern Ireland Barrett's Esophagus Registry examined the risk of progression to high-grade dysplasia and esophageal adenocarcinoma in 8522 patients diagnosed with Barrett's esophagus defined as a columnar lined esophagus both with and without intestinal metaplasia.[6] The risk of cancer for patients with intestinal metaplasia at index endoscopy was increased compared with that of those without intestinal metaplasia at index endoscopy (0.38% per year vs 0.07% per year; HR, 3.54; 95% CI, 2.09–6.0).

An observational study from the University of Chicago demonstrated that among 379 patients with a columnar lined esophagus without goblet cells on pathologic findings, none progressed to adenocarcinoma or high-grade dysplasia during an average follow-up of 5 years.[25] In contrast, 8.9% of patients with a columnar lined esophagus with goblet cells progressed to adenocarcinoma or high-grade dysplasia.

Although there are not yet enough data to definitively state that intestinal metaplasia is a necessary component to the neoplastic risk of Barrett's esophagus, it does seem that there is an increased risk of neoplastic progression in patients with intestinal metaplasia compared with that in those without intestinal metaplasia.

Dysplasia

Dysplasia remains the single best marker for risk of progression in Barrett's esophagus. For patients with nondysplastic Barrett's esophagus, the risk of neoplastic progression remains low. A 2012 meta-analysis found an incidence of esophageal adenocarcinoma of 1 case per 300 patient-years in patients with nondysplastic Barrett's epithelium.[4] Two large, population-based studies not included in this meta-analysis also support these findings. A cohort study from Denmark evaluated the incidence of adenocarcinoma in more than 11,000 patients with Barrett's esophagus.[26] The incidence rate was 1 case per 1000 person-years in patients with nondysplastic Barrett's esophagus over a median follow-up of 5.2 years. A cohort study from Ireland also had similar low rates of progression in patients with nondysplastic Barrett's esophagus, 0.17% per year.[14]

Recent work of a large US multicenter consortium evaluated the importance of repeated biopsy-proven nondysplastic Barrett's esophagus during surveillance endoscopy.[27] Patients were found to have a lower annual risk of progressing to either adenocarcinoma or high-grade dysplasia if they had multiple endoscopies documenting persistent nondysplastic Barrett's esophagus (0.34% in patients with 5 endoscopies vs 0.75% in patients with 1 endoscopy). Overall, the neoplastic progression risk in nondysplastic Barrett's esophagus seems to be very low.

Low-Grade Dysplasia

Low-grade dysplasia has been extensively studied as a risk factor for progression with highly variable results. Probably due to the interobserver variability in the diagnosis of this lesion, the diagnosis becomes problematic.[28] A large, multicenter outcomes study from the United States investigated 210 patients with low-grade dysplasia to determine the rate of neoplastic progression.[29] There was a 1.83% per year incidence of progression to adenocarcinoma or high-grade dysplasia in this cohort. While the progression to esophageal adenocarcinoma was 0.18% per year if only 1 of 3 pathologists confirmed the diagnosis of low-grade dysplasia, the incidence rate increased to 0.39% per year if all 3 pathologists agreed. Critics of the study point out that there was a low interobserver agreement among the 2 expert pathologists (κ, 0.14).[30] In addition, approximately 1 in 4 of the original low-grade dysplasia samples were subsequently upgraded to high-grade dysplasia in this study, further calling into question the results. In a landmark study from the Netherlands, 293 patients with low-grade dysplasia were assessed.[31] Biopsy samples were confirmed by 2 independent pathologists with extensive experience with dysplasia within Barrett's esophagus from a panel of 6 pathologists. Upon expert review, almost three-quarters of patients were downstaged to either nondysplastic Barrett's esophagus or indefinite for dysplasia. In the patients who were confirmed to have low-grade dysplasia on expert review, the risk of neoplastic progression was 9.1% per patient-year with a median follow-up of over 3 years. The patients with nondysplastic Barrett's esophagus or those who were indefinite for dysplasia had a significantly lower risk of neoplastic progression (0.6%–0.9% per patient-year).

These results are similar to previous reports from the Academic Medical Center group in the Netherlands, which put the risk of progression to adenocarcinoma or high-grade dysplasia at 13.4% per year in patients with confirmed low-grade dysplasia.[32] In the surveillance arm of the SURF study examining radiofrequency ablation for patients with confirmed low-grade dysplasia, 26.5% of patients progressed to adenocarcinoma or high-grade dysplasia during a median follow-up of 30 months.[13] Similarly, a high progression rate was seen in the original clinical trial of radiofrequency ablation for low-grade dysplasia where expert gastrointestinal pathologist confirmation was required: 14% of patients in the sham treatment arm developed high-grade dysplasia at 1 year of follow-up.[33] Finally, in a population-based cohort study from Denmark, the standardized incidence ratio for esophageal adenocarcinoma in patients with low-grade dysplasia was 5.1 per 1000 patient-years (95% CI, 3.0–8.6).[26]

These rates are considerably higher than those described in the most recent meta-analysis, which found a rate of progression from low-grade dysplasia to adenocarcinoma of 0.54% per year (95% CI, 0.32%–0.76%) and to adenocarcinoma or high-grade dysplasia of 1.73% per year (95% CI, 0.99%–2.47%).[34] However, the investigators reported significant heterogeneity between the studies and acknowledged that rates of neoplastic progression were higher in the studies when expert pathologists confirmed low-grade dysplasia.

In summary, low-grade dysplasia is a challenging lesion to diagnose but seems to be a risk factor for neoplastic progression when confirmed by multiple pathologists with expertise in GI pathology.

Biomarkers of Increased Risk

Given the low rate of neoplastic progression in Barrett's esophagus and the inherent limitations of current endoscopic surveillance programs, there has long been interest in identifying biomarkers of increased risk in patients with Barrett's esophagus. Although multiple biomarkers have been studied, a select few are discussed here.

One of the best studied biomarkers is the tumor suppressor gene p53. In patients with Barrett's esophagus, loss of heterozygosity (LOH) for p53 (RR, 16; CI, 6.2–39.0) as well as overexpression of p53 (OR, 8.42; 95% CI, 2.37–30.0) are associated with progression to adenocarcinoma or high-grade dysplasia.[35,36] A nested case-control study demonstrated similar results; loss of p53 (RR, 14.0; 95% CI, 5.3–37.2) and over-expression of p53 (RR, 5.6; 95% CI, 3.1–10.3) were associated with a higher risk of progression to adenocarcinoma or high-grade dysplasia.[37] In addition, biopsies with both low-grade dysplasia and aberrant p53 expression seem to have higher rates of neoplastic progression.[37,38]

Other tumor suppressor genes (ie, p16), cell-cycle-related proteins (ie, cyclin A, cyclin D1), growth factor receptors (ie, epidermal growth factor receptor), and flow cytometry for DNA abnormalities (ie, aneuploidy and tetraploidy) have been studied at length. Despite some promising results, none of these potential biomarkers are appropriate for clinical practice at this time.

Considerable efforts have also gone into developing panels of these biomarkers that may assist in the identification of patients at increased risk for progression. A combination of 17p LOH, 9p LOH, and aneuploidy/tetraploidy was found to have a relative risk of 38.7 (95% CI, 10.8–138.5) for neoplastic progression and a 10-year cumulative incidence of adenocarcinoma of nearly 80%.[39] In patients with none of these biomarkers, only 12% progressed to adenocarcinoma. A panel of methylation biomarkers for 8 different genes (including p16, RUNX3, HPP1) had sensitivity for detection of progression of less than 50%.[40] The panel of just p16, RUNX3, and HPP1 has also been studied.[41,42] Finally, a nested case-control study from the Northern Ireland Barrett's Esophagus Registry evaluated a combination of biomarkers and anatomic pathology.[43] The panel of low-grade dysplasia, DNA aneuploidy/tetraploidy detected by image cytometry, and *Aspergillus oryzae* lectin demonstrated an increasing OR for each component of the panel that was present (OR, 3.73 per biomarker; 95% CI, 2.43–5.79).

Biomarkers and biomarker panels may in the future assist in determining who is likely to progress to adenocarcinoma or high-grade dysplasia. At the present time, there are multiple limitations that need to be addressed before these biomarkers are incorporated into daily clinical practice.

EPIDEMIOLOGIC RISK FACTORS
Age

The incidence of esophageal adenocarcinoma increases with age, regardless of sex or race.[44,45] Between the ages of 50 and 59 years, white males have an esophageal adenocarcinoma incidence rate of 8.44 per 100,000 person-years (95% CI, 8.05–8.85), which increases to 26.31 per 100,000 person-years (95% CI, 25.27–27.38) between ages 70 and 79 years.[44] The most recent publication of the Surveillance, Epidemiology, and End Results (SEER) registry reaffirms the increase in esophageal adenocarcinoma with age.[45] Starting at age 40 years and continuing until 79 years, the incidence rates of esophageal adenocarcinoma continue to rise. Beyond the age of 80 years, the incidence rate seems to level off in most groups.

In patients with Barrett's esophagus, most studies suggest an increase in the risk of neoplastic progression with increasing age. A Dutch population-based study found that the risk of progression increased with increasing age at diagnosis, with a marked increase in risk after the age of 75 years (HR, 12; 95% CI, 8.0–18).[46] Similarly, in the

Danish Barrett's esophagus population-based study, the incidence of adenocarcinoma or high-grade dysplasia increased progressively with age and was greatest in patients older than 70 years.[26]

Race

White race is a known risk factor for esophageal adenocarcinoma.[47–49] There is a fourfold increase in the incidence rate of esophageal adenocarcinoma in white males compared with black males and twofold increase compared with that of Hispanic males.[50] Similar patterns are also seen in women, although with lower incidence rates in all races. While the cause of this difference is unclear, a recent study of patients with Barrett's esophagus found a higher rate of dysplasia (7% vs 0%) and of long-segment Barrett's esophagus (26% vs 12%) at the time of endoscopy in Caucasians compared with black patients.[51] As both dysplasia and long-segment Barrett's esophagus are independent risk factors for esophageal adenocarcinoma, this may be an avenue worthy of further study.

Sex

Male gender is another well-documented risk factor for esophageal adenocarcinoma with a 6- to 10-fold risk increase compared with that of women.[45,52] However, both genders have seen a dramatic increase in the number of esophageal cancers. Newer data from the SEER registry have demonstrated the largest gender difference exists largely in the earlier-age cancers (ie, younger than 65 years).[45] Furthermore, the age-adjusted incidence rate in women older than 80 years continues to increase, whereas the rate in men plateaus. This difference may relate to estrogen exposure. Previously, estrogen exposure was suggested as a protective mechanism against both gastric and colon cancers and was demonstrated to reduce apoptosis and cell growth in esophageal adenocarcinoma.[53–55] As women age, there is a significant decrease in estrogen, which may explain the delayed increase in esophageal adenocarcinoma incidence, as seen in the SEER database data. Studies examining how risk factors with possible male predominance, including gastroesophageal reflux disease (GERD), obesity, and tobacco, may affect neoplastic progression risk have not yet provided a clear mechanistic answer to this epidemiologic difference.[56] Among patients with Barrett's esophagus, male gender is also a clearly recognized risk factor for progression to esophageal adenocarcinoma.[4,10,46]

Family History/Genetic Risk

Familial aggregation of Barrett's esophagus and esophageal adenocarcinoma has suggested a potential genetic component to these disease entities. Much of the work in this area has come from Chak and colleagues[57] who initially found that a positive family history (first- or second-degree relative with Barrett's esophagus, esophageal adenocarcinoma, or esophagogastric junction carcinoma) was higher among case subjects than among GERD controls (24% vs 5%). On multivariate analysis, a positive family history for Barrett's esophagus, adenocarcinoma of the esophagus, or esophagogastric junction was associated with an increased risk of developing these lesions when compared with patients with GERD alone (OR, 12.23; 95% CI, 3.34–44.76).

A subsequent segregation analysis by the same group found an incomplete autosomal dominant inheritance pattern for familial aggregations of Barrett's esophagus, esophageal adenocarcinoma, and gastroesophageal junction carcinoma.[58] Finally, in multiplex aggregations characterized by 3 or more members of a family with Barrett's esophagus and/or esophageal adenocarcinoma, the median age for the diagnosis of adenocarcinoma was approximately 5 years less than that in duplex families or sporadic cases.[59] Others have found an increased prevalence of Barrett's esophagus in first-degree relatives of patients with adenocarcinoma.[60]

Last, examination of germline mutations in patients with Barrett's esophagus and esophageal adenocarcinoma has yielded interesting results. In a model-free linkage analysis comparing both concordant sibling pairs with Barrett's and esophageal adenocarcinoma and discordant sibling pairs, 3 genes were identified with significant mutations (MSR1, ASCC1, and CTHRC1).[61] MSR1 was associated with the presence of both Barrett's esophagus and esophageal adenocarcinoma. A genome-wide association study from the BEACON (Barrett's and Esophageal Adenocarcinoma Consortium) group of more than 1500 cases of esophageal adenocarcinoma and 2300 cases of Barrett's esophagus found a high genetic correlation between Barrett's esophagus and adenocarcinoma as well as between multiple shared genes underlying the development of both.[62]

Taken together, these data suggest that there is a genetic component to neoplastic progression in some patients with Barrett's esophagus. More data are still needed to fully characterize this risk.

Tobacco

Tobacco use is a clear risk factor for the development of both Barrett's esophagus and esophageal adenocarcinoma.[63,64] A pooled analysis evaluating approximately 3000 cases of either esophageal adenocarcinoma or esophagogastric junctional adenocarcinoma found an OR of 1.67 (95% CI, 1.04–2.67) for developing esophageal adenocarcinoma in patients with tobacco use, with a significant increase with increased number of pack-years smoking.[65] Current or prior tobacco use also increases the risk of neoplastic progression in patients with Barrett's esophagus.[66,67] A population-based cohort study from the Northern Ireland Barrett's Esophagus Registry demonstrated an increased risk of neoplastic progression to adenocarcinoma or high-grade dysplasia in current smokers when compared with nonsmokers (HR, 2.03; 95% CI, 1.29–3.17).[66] Overall, tobacco is an established risk factor for progression to esophageal adenocarcinoma.

Obesity

Obesity is a well-described risk factor for esophageal adenocarcinoma.[68,69] A 2013 meta-analysis of more than 8000 cancers examined the relationship between body mass index (BMI), calculated as the weight in kilograms divided by the height in meters squared, and esophageal and gastric cardia adenocarcinoma.[69] The relative risk for developing esophageal adenocarcinoma increased with an increasing BMI; the relative risk was 1.71 (95% CI, 1.50–1.96) for a BMI in the range 25 to 30 and 2.34 (95% CI, 1.95–2.81) for a BMI greater than 30. An observational study from England showed a significant increase in esophageal adenocarcinoma with a BMI greater than 35 (HR, 4.95), but only an upward trend at lower BMIs.[70] This finding corresponds to earlier data suggesting that the largest risk was in patients with BMI greater than 35.[68] It would seem that male pattern central obesity is the key component of this risk, with a 2013 meta-analysis reporting an OR of 2.51 (95% CI, 1.56–4.04) for developing esophageal adenocarcinoma in patients with central adiposity.[71]

The impact of obesity and abdominal adiposity specifically on neoplastic progression of Barrett's esophagus to adenocarcinoma is a bit more unclear. A small cross-sectional analysis from Seattle Barrett's Esophagus Project demonstrated an increasing risk of histologic and genetic abnormalities associated with a high likelihood of neoplastic progression in patients with a predominantly abdominal fat distribution.[72] However, a recent cohort study of more than 400 patients with Barrett's esophagus found no relation between higher waist-hip ratios and neoplastic progression to adeno-carcinoma.[67] Although the role of neoplastic progression in Barrett's esophagus is not fully known, it is clear that obesity and specifically abdominal adiposity are associated with an increased overall risk of esophageal adenocarcinoma.

The exact mechanism underlying this risk is not fully known but may involve increased levels of insulinlike growth factor 1, insulin resistance, and adipokines such as leptin.[73–75] These relationships are explored at length by Chandar and Iyer, elsewhere in the issue.

PROTECTIVE FACTORS
Medications

There is emerging evidence that statins may have a protective effect for multiple cancers, including esophageal adenocarcinoma (**Table 2**). In vitro studies of statins have demonstrated multiple potential mechanisms for chemoprevention including antiproliferation, antiangiogenesis, and proapoptotic effects.[76–78] Two studies have demonstrated that regular statin use results in decreased malignant transformation from Barrett's esophagus to esophageal adenocarcinoma or high-grade dysplasia.[79,80] A cohort study from the United Kingdom found an inverse relationship between regular statin use of any dose (10+ months) and developing esophageal adenocarcinoma (OR, 0.58; 95% CI, 0.39–0.87).[81] The protective effect of statins seems to become more apparent with longer-term use. Overall, it seems that statins are protective against neoplastic progression.

Nonsteroidal antiinflammatory drugs (NSAIDs) have also been investigated as potential protective agents against neoplastic progression in Barrett's esophagus. In Barrett's esophagus, there is an increase in cyclooxygenase-2 (COX-2) expression as disease progresses from nondysplastic Barrett's esophagus to adenocarcinoma or high-grade dysplasia.[82] As such, the effect of NSAIDs, including aspirin, on prostaglandin E_2 production via the COX-2 pathways may serve as a potential protective mechanism against neoplastic progression. A pooled analysis by the BEACON group of 6 studies totaling 1226 patients with esophageal adenocarcinoma and 1140 patients with esophagogastric junctional adenocarcinoma examined the impact of aspirin and/or NSAID use on the development of these cancers.[83] "Anytime users" of NSAIDs or aspirin had reduced risk of esophageal adenocarcinoma compared with nonusers (OR, 0.68; 95% CI, 0.56–0.83). The OR improved further with daily use for 10 or more years (OR, 0.56; 95% CI, 0.43–0.73) in patients. For aspirin, the overall OR for developing esophageal adenocarcinoma in anytime users was 0.77 (95% CI, 0.60–0.97).

Table 2	
Protective factors against neoplastic progression to esophageal adenocarcinoma	
Dietary	Significant fruits and vegetables
	Fiber
Medications	Statins
	NSAIDs
	Aspirin
Acid suppression	PPIs
H pylori infection	

Abbreviations: NSAIDs, nonsteroidal antiinflammatory drugs; PPIs, proton pump inhibitors.

Multiple studies have examined the impact of NSAID and/or aspirin use on neoplastic progression of Barrett's esophagus. Work from the Seattle Barrett's Esophagus Project found a decreased HR for progression to adenocarcinoma in current NSAID users (HR, 0.32; 95% CI, 0.14–0.70) over an average follow-up of 65 months.[84] In addition, a multicenter, prospective cohort from the Netherlands showed a reduced risk of progression to cancer in patients with Barrett's esophagus taking NSAIDs (HR, 0.47; 95% CI, 0.24–0.93).[85] This study showed an additive benefit when both NSAIDs and statins were used (HR, 0.22; 95% CI, 0.06–0.85). Finally, a meta-analysis found an overall reduced risk of adenocarcinoma or high-grade dysplasia among patients with Barrett's esophagus taking COX inhibitors (RR, 0.64; 95% CI, 0.53–0.77) or aspirin (RR, 0.63; 95% CI, 0.43–0.94) reaffirming the protective effects of NSAIDs and aspirin against neoplastic progression.[86]

The seminal work by Lagergren and colleagues[87] demonstrated a striking association between more frequent, more severe, and more persistent reflux symptoms and esophageal adenocarcinoma. Thus it makes sense that the effect of acid suppression on neoplastic progression in Barrett's esophagus has been studied. Multiple small studies have suggested a reduced risk of neoplastic progression in patients with Barrett's esophagus who use proton pump inhibitors (PPIs).[79,88] Furthermore, a 2014 meta-analysis demonstrated an adjusted OR of 0.29 (95% CI, 0.12–0.79) for neoplastic progression in patients with Barrett's esophagus taking PPIs.[89] There was no benefit noted from histamine2 antagonists. However, a recent Danish case-control study of 140 patients with Barrett's esophagus found no benefit for PPI long-term users.[90] As such, it is still unclear if PPIs themselves reduce the risk of neoplastic progression in patients with Barrett's esophagus, although there seems to be no role for histamine2 antagonists.

Helicobacter pylori

As treatment and eradication rates of H pylori have increased, the rates of esophageal adenocarcinoma have also increased, prompting investigators to examine the potential relationship between the 2 observations. Multiple studies have demonstrated an inverse relationship between H pylori infection and development of Barrett's esophagus.[91,92] These observations have also suggested a possible protective effect of H pylori infection against the development of esophageal adenocarcinoma. A recent meta-analysis of 13 studies, pooling 1145 esophageal cases with 3453 controls, demonstrated a protective benefit of H pylori against developing adenocarcinoma (OR, 0.57; 95% CI, 0.44–0.73).[93] This study did not specifically address patients with Barrett's esophagus.

Overall, it does seem that H pylori infection has some protective benefit against developing both Barrett's esophagus and esophageal adenocarcinoma. However, the effect of neoplastic progression in patients with Barrett's esophagus has yet to be studied.

Diet

High consumption of fruits and vegetables seems to decrease the risk of adenocarcinoma in patients with Barrett's esophagus.[10,94] A National Institutes of Health study examined dietary patterns in the general population, finding a decreased risk for developing esophageal adenocarcinoma in patients reporting a positive Healthy Eating Index, which puts a premium on vegetables and fruits (HR, 0.75; 95% CI, 0.57–0.98).[95] On the other hand, increased meat consumption, particularly processed red meats, seems to increase the risk of esophageal adenocarcinoma.[96–98] These studies did not address neoplastic progression in patients with Barrett's esophagus.

Multiple different vitamins and supplements have also been studied. The most consistent data, although limited, suggest that fiber may play a protective role against adenocarcinoma.[99,100] Mixed data exist regarding the potential benefit of using a daily multivitamin, folate, or vitamin B_{12}.[100–104] Overall, a healthy diet including significant consumption of fruits and vegetables likely decreases the risk of developing esophageal adenocarcinoma.

SUMMARY

As the prevalence of esophageal adenocarcinoma increases, research has discovered epidemiologic, endoscopic, and pathologic factors that may help determine the risk for neoplastic progression. It is hoped that algorithms can be developed to risk stratify patients in the future to tailor optimal therapy and intervention to prevent the development of adenocarcinoma.

REFERENCES

1. Lepage C, Drouillard A, Jouve JL, et al. Epidemiology and risk factors for oesophageal adenocarcinoma. Dig Liver Dis 2013;45:625–9.
2. Pennathur A, Gibson MK, Jobe BA, et al. Oesophageal carcinoma. Lancet 2013; 381:400–12.
3. Verbeek RE, Leender M, Ten Kate FJ, et al. Surveillance of Barrett's esophagus and mortality from esophageal adenocarcinoma: a population-based cohort study. Am J Gastroenterol 2014;109:1215–22.
4. Desai TK, Krishnan K, Samala N, et al. The incidence of oesophageal adenocarcinoma in non-dysplastic Barrett's oesophagus: a meta-analysis. Gut 2012;61: 970–6.
5. Yousef F, Cardwell C, Cantwell MM, et al. The incidence of esophageal cancer and high-grade dysplasia in Barrett's esophagus: a systematic review and meta-analysis. Am J Epidemiol 2008;168:237–49.
6. Sikkema M, de Jonge PJ, Steyerberg EW, et al. Risk of esophageal adenocarcinoma and mortality in patients with Barrett's esophagus; a systematic review and meta-analysis. Clin Gastroenterol Hepatol 2010;8:235–44.
7. Milind R, Attwood SE. Natural history of Barrett's esophagus. World J Gastroenterol 2012;18(27):3483–91.
8. Gatenby P, Caygill C, Wall C, et al. Lifetime risk of esophageal adenocarcinoma in patients with Barrett's esophagus. World J Gastroenterol 2014;20(28):9611–7.
9. Coleman HG, Bhat SK, Murray LJ, et al. Symptoms and endoscopic features at Barrett's esophagus diagnosis: implications for neoplastic progression risk. Am J Gastroenterol 2014;109:527–34.
10. Pohl H, Wrobel K, Bojarski C, et al. Risk factors in the development of esophageal adenocarcinoma. Am J Gastroenterol 2013;108:200–7.
11. Anaparthy R, Gaddam S, Kanakadandi V, et al. Association between length of Barrett's esophagus and risk of high-grade dysplasia or adenocarcinoma in patients without dysplasia. Clin Gastroenterol Hepatol 2013;11:1430–6.
12. Sikkema M, Looman CW, Steyerberg EW, et al. Predictors of neoplastic progression in patients with Barrett's esophagus: a prospective cohort study. Am J Gastroenterol 2011;106:1231–8.
13. Phoa KN, van Vilsteren FGI, Weusten BL, et al. Radiofrequency ablation vs endoscopic surveillance for patients with Barrett esophagus and low-grade dysplasia. JAMA 2014;311(12):1209–17.

14. Bhat S, Coleman HG, Yousef F, et al. Risk of malignant progression in Barrett's esophagus patients: Results form a large population based study. J Natl Cancer Inst 2011;103:1049–57.
15. Andrici J, Tio M, Cox MR, et al. Hiatal hernia and the risk of Barrett's esophagus. J Gastroenterol Hepatol 2013;28:415–31.
16. Avidan B, Sonnenberg A, Schnell TG, et al. Hiatal hernia size, Barrett's length, and severity of acid reflux are all risk factors for esophageal adenocarcinoma. Am J Gastroenterol 2002;97:1930–6.
17. Weston AP, Sharma P, Mathur S, et al. Risk stratification of Barrett's esophagus: Updated prospective multivariate analysis. Am J Gastroenterol 2004;99: 1657–66.
18. Erichsen R, Robertson D, Farkas DK, et al. Erosive reflux disease increases risk for esophageal adenocarcinoma, compared with nonerosive reflux. Clin Gastroenterol Hepatol 2012;10:475–80.
19. Kariyawasam VC, Bourke MJ, Hourigan LF, et al. Circumferential location predicts the risk of high-grade dysplasia and early adenocarcinoma in short-segment Barrett's esophagus. Gastrointest Endosc 2012;75:938–44.
20. Enestvedt BK, Lugo R, Guarner-Argente C, et al. Location, location, location: does early cancer in Barrett's esophagus have a preference. Gastrointest Endosc 2013;78:462–7.
21. Pech O, Gossner L, Manner H, et al. Prospective evaluation of the macroscopic types and location of early Barrett's neoplasia in 380 lesions. Endoscopy 2007; 39:588–93.
22. Cassani L, Sumner E, Slaughter JC, et al. Directional distribution of neoplasia in Barrett's esophagus is not influenced by distance from the gastroesophageal junction. Gastrointest Endosc 2013;77:877–82.
23. Edebo A, Vieth M, Tam W, et al. Circumferential and axial distribution of esophageal mucosal damage in reflux disease. Dis Esophagus 2007;20:232–8.
24. Gatenby PA, Ramus JR, Caygill CP, et al. Relevance of the detection of intestinal metaplasia in non-dysplastic columnar-lined oesophagus. Scand J Gastroenterol 2008;43:524–30.
25. Westerhoff M, Hovan L, Lee C, et al. Effects of dropping the requirement for goblet cells from the diagnosis of Barrett's esophagus. Clin Gastroenterol Hepatol 2012;10:1232–6.
26. Hvid-Jensen F, Pedersen L, Drewes AM, et al. Incidence of adenocarcinoma among patients with Barrett's esophagus. N Engl J Med 2011;365:1375–83.
27. Gaddam S, Singh M, Gokulakrishnan B, et al. Persistence of nondysplastic Barrett's esophagus identifies patients at lower risk for esophageal adenocarcinoma: results from a large multicenter cohort. Gastroenterology 2013;145:548–53.
28. Montgomery E, Broner MP, Goldblum JR, et al. Reproducibility of the diagnosis of dysplasia in Barrett esophagus: a reaffirmation. Hum Pathol 2001;32:368–78.
29. Wani S, Falk GW, Post J, et al. Risk Factors for progression of low-grade dysplasia in patients with Barrett's esophagus. Gastroenterology 2011;141:1179–86.
30. Bergman J, Vieth M. Let's not jump to conclusions regarding low-grade dysplasia in Barrett's esophagus. Gastroenterology 2012;142(5):e18–9.
31. Duits L, Phoa KN, Curvers WL, et al. Barrett's oesophagus patients with low-grade dysplasia can be accurately risk-stratified after histological review by an expert pathology panel. Gut 2014. [Epub ahead of print].
32. Curvers WL, ten Kate FJ, Krishnadath KK, et al. Low-grade dysplasia in Barrett's esophagus: overdiagnosed and underused. Am J Gastroenterol 2010;15: 1523–30.

33. Shaheen NJ, Sharma P, Overholt BF, et al. Radiofrequency ablation in Barrett's esophagus with dysplasia. N Engl J Med 2009;360:2277–88.
34. Singh S, Manickmam P, Amin AV, et al. Incidence of esophageal adenocarcinoma in Barrett's esophagus with low-grade dysplasia: a systematic review and meta-analysis. Gastrointest Endosc 2014;79:897–909.
35. Reid BJ, Prevo LJ, Galipeau PC, et al. Predictors of progression in Barrett's esophagus II: baseline 17p (p53) loss of heterozygosity identifies a patient subset at increased risk for neoplastic progression. Am J Gastroenterol 2001;96: 2839–48.
36. Murray L, Sedo A, Scott M, et al. TP53 and progression from Barrett's metaplasia to oesophageal adenocarcinoma in a UK population cohort. Gut 2006;55: 1390–7.
37. Kastelein F, Biermann K, Steyerberg EW, et al. Aberrant p53 protein expression is associated with an increased risk of neoplastic progression in patients with Barrett's oesophagus. Gut 2013;62:1676–83.
38. Kaye PV, Haider SA, Ilyas M, et al. Barrett's dysplasia and the Vienna classification: reproducibility, prediction of progression and impact of consensus reporting and p53 immunohistochemistry. Histopathology 2009;54(6):699–712.
39. Galipeau PC, Li X, Blount PL, et al. NSAIDs modulate cdkn2a, tp53, and DNA content risk for progression to esophageal adenocarcinoma. PLoS Med 2007; 4(2):e67.
40. Jin Z, Cheng Y, Gu W, et al. A multi-center, double-blinded validation study of methylation biomarkers for progression prediction in Barrett's esophagus. Cancer Res 2009;69:4112–5.
41. Sato F, Jin Z, Schulmann K, et al. Three-tiered risk stratification model to predict progression in Barrett's esophagus using epigenetic and clinical features. PLoS One 2008;101:1193–9.
42. Schulmann K, Sterian A, Berki A, et al. Inactivation of p16, RUNX3, and HPP1 occurs early in Barrett's associated neoplastic progression and predicts progression risk. Oncogene 2005;24:4138–48.
43. Bird-Lieberman EL, Dunn JM, Coleman HG, et al. Population-based study reveals new risk-stratification biomarker panel for Barrett's esophagus. Gastroenterology 2012;143:927–35.
44. Nordenstedt H, El-Serag H. The influence of age, sex, and race on the incidence of esophageal cancer in the United States (1992–2006). Scand J Gastroenterol 2011;46:597–602.
45. Mathieu LN, Kanark NF, Tsai HL, et al. Age and sex differences in the incidence of esophageal adenocarcinoma: results from the Surveillance, Epidemiology, and End Results (SEER) registry (1973–2008). Dis Esophagus 2014;27:757–63.
46. de Jonge PJ, van Blankenstein M, Looman CW, et al. Risk of malignant progression in patients with Barrett's oesophagus: a Dutch nationwide cohort study. Gut 2010;59:1030–6.
47. Coupland VH, Lagergren J, Konfortion J, et al. Ethnicity in relation to incidence of oesophageal and gastric cancer in England. Br J Cancer 2012;107:1908–14.
48. Ashktorab H, Nouri Z, Nouraie M, et al. Esophageal carcinoma in African Americans: a five-decade experience. Dig Dis Sci 2011;56:3577–82.
49. Sadler GJ, Jothiamni D, Zanetta U, et al. The effect of ethnicity on the presentation and management of oesophageal and gastric cancers: a UK perspective. Eur J Gastroenterol Hepatol 2009;21:996–1000.
50. Kubo A, Corley DA. Marked multi-ethnic variation of esophageal and gastric cardia carcinomas within the United States. Am J Gastroenterol 2004;99:582–8.

51. Khoury JE, Chisholm S, Jamal MM, et al. African Americans with Barrett's esophagus are less likely to have dysplasia at biopsy. Dig Dis Sci 2012;57: 419–23.

52. El-Serag HB, Mason AC, Petersen N, et al. Epidemiological differences between adenocarcinoma of the oesophagus and adenocarcinoma of the gastric cardia in the USA. Gut 2002;50:368–72.

53. Camargo MC, Goto Y, Zabaleta J, et al. Sex hormones, hormonal interventions, and gastric cancer risk: a meta-analysis. Cancer Epidemiol Biomarkers Prev 2012;21:20–38.

54. Chlebowski RT, Wactawski-Wende J, Ritenbaugh C, et al. Estrogen plus progestin and colorectal cancer in postmenopausal women. N Engl J Med 2004;350: 991–1004.

55. Sukocheva OA, Wee C, Ansar A, et al. Effect of estrogen on growth and apoptosis in esophageal adenocarcinoma cells. Dis Esophagus 2012;26(6): 628–35.

56. Rutegård M, Nordenstedt H, Lu Y, et al. Sex-specific exposure prevalence of established risk factors for oesophageal adenocarcinoma. Br J Cancer 2010;103: 735–40.

57. Chak A, Lee T, Kinnard MF, et al. Familial aggregation of Barrett's oesophagus, oesophageal adenocarcinoma, and oesophagogastric junctional adenocarcinoma in Caucasian adults. Gut 2002;51:323–8.

58. Sun X, Elston R, Barnholtz-Sloan J, et al. A segregation analysis of Barrett's esophagus and associated adenocarcinomas. Cancer Epidemiol Biomarkers Prev 2010;19:666–74.

59. Chak A, Chen Y, Vengoechea J, et al. Variation in age at cancer diagnosis in familial versus nonfamilial Barrett's esophagus. Cancer Epidemiol Biomarkers Prev 2012;21:376–83.

60. Juhasz A, Mittal SK, Lee TH, et al. Prevalence of Barrett esophagus in first-degree relatives of patients with esophageal adenocarcinoma. J Clin Gastroenterol 2011;45(10):867–71.

61. Orloff M, Peterson C, He X, et al. Germline mutations in MSR1, ASCC1, and CTHRC1 in patients with Barrett esophagus and esophageal adenocarcinoma. JAMA 2011;206(4):410–9.

62. Weronica E, Levine DM, D'Amato M, et al. Germline genetic contributions to risk for esophageal adenocarcinoma, Barrett's esophagus, and gastroesophageal reflux. J Natl Cancer Inst 2013;105:1711–8.

63. Cook MB, Shaheen NJ, Anderson LA, et al. Cigarette smoking increases risk of Barrett's Esophagus: an analysis of the Barrett's and Esophageal Adenocarcinoma Consortium. Gastroenterology 2012;142(4):744–53.

64. Tramacere I, La Vecchia C, Negri E. Tobacco smoking and esophageal and gastric cardia adenocarcinoma. Epidemiology 2011;22(3):344–9.

65. Cook MB, Kamangar F, Whiteman DC, et al. Cigarette smoking and adenocarcinomas of the esophagus and esophagogastric junction: a pooled analysis from the International BEACON Consortium. J Natl Cancer Inst 2010;102: 1344–53.

66. Coleman HG, Bhat S, Johnston BT, et al. Tobacco smoking increases the risk of high-grade dysplasia and cancer among patients with Barrett's esophagus. Gastroenterology 2012;142:233–40.

67. Hardikar S, Onstad L, Blount PL, et al. The role of tobacco, alcohol, and obesity in neoplastic progression to esophageal adenocarcinoma: a prospective study of Barrett's Esophagus. PLoS One 2013;8(1):e52192.

68. Abnet CC, Freedman ND, Hollenbeck AR, et al. A prospective study of BMI and risk of oesophageal and gastric adenocarcinoma. Eur J Cancer 2008;44:465–71.
69. Turati F, Tramacere I, La Vecchia C, et al. A meta-analysis of body mass index and esophageal and gastric cardia adenocarcinoma. Ann Oncol 2013;24:609–17.
70. Yates M, Cheong E, Luben R, et al. Body mass index, smoking, and alcohol and risks of Barrett's esophagus and esophageal adenocarcinoma: a UK prospective cohort study. Dig Dis Sci 2014;59:1552–9.
71. Singh S, Sharma AN, Murad MH, et al. Central adiposity is associated with increased risk of esophageal inflammation, metaplasia, and adenocarcinoma: a systematic review and meta-analysis. Clin Gastroenterol Hepatol 2013;11:1399–412.
72. Vaughan TL, Kristal AR, Blount PL, et al. Nonsteroidal anti-inflammatory drug use, body mass index, and anthropometry in relation to genetic and flow cytometric abnormalities in Barrett's esophagus. Cancer Epidemiol Biomarkers Prev 2002;11:745–52.
73. Doyle SL, Donohoe CL, Finn SP, et al. IGF-1 and its receptor in esophageal cancer: association with adenocarcinoma and visceral obesity. Am J Gastroenterol 2012;107:196–204.
74. Alexandre L, Long E, Beales IL. Pathophysiological mechanism linking obesity and esophageal adenocarcinoma. World J Gastrointest Pathophysiol 2014;5(4):534–49.
75. Ogunwobi O, Mutungi G, Beales IL. Leptin stimulates proliferation and inhibits apoptosis in Barrett's esophageal adenocarcinoma cells by cycloxygenase-2-dependent, prostatglandin-E2-mediated transactivation of the epidermal growth factor receptor and c-Jun NH2-terminal kinase activation. Endocrinology 2006;147:4505–16.
76. Ogunwobi OO, Beales IL. Statins inhibit proliferation and induce apoptosis in Barrett's esophageal adenocarcinoma cells. Am J Gastroenterol 2008;103:825–37.
77. Sadaria MR, Reppert AE, Yu JA, et al. Statin therapy attenuates growth and malignant potential of human esophageal adenocarcinoma cells. J Thorac Cardiovasc Surg 2011;142:1152–60.
78. Konturek PC, Burnat G, Hahn EG. Inhibition of Barrett's adenocarcinoma cell growth by simvastatin: involvement of COX-2 and apoptosis-related proteins. J Physiol Pharmacol 2007;58(Suppl 3):141–8.
79. Nguyen DM, Richardson P, El-Serag HB. Medications (NSAIDs, statins, proton pump inhibitors) and the risk of esophageal adenocarcinoma in patients with Barrett's esophagus. Gastroenterology 2010;138:2260–6.
80. Beales IL, Vardi I, Dearman L. Regular statin and aspirin use in patients with Barrett's oesophageal adenocarcinoma. Eur J Gastroenterol Hepatol 2012;24:917–23.
81. Alexandre L, Clark AB, Bhutta HY, et al. Statin use is associated with reduced risk of histologic subtypes of esophageal cancer: a nested case-control analysis. Gastroenterology 2014;146:661–8.
82. Morris CD, Armstrong GR, Bigley G, et al. Cyclooxygenase-2 expression in the Barrett's metaplasia-dysplasia-adenocarcinoma sequence. Am J Gastroenterol 2001;96:990–6.
83. Liao LM, Vaughan TL, Corley DA, et al. Nonsteroidal anti-inflammatory drug use reduces risk of adenocarcinomas of the esophagus and esophagogastric junction in a pooled analysis. Gastroenterology 2012;142:442–52.
84. Vaughan TL, Dong LM, Blount PL, et al. Non-steroidal anti-inflammatory drugs and risk of neoplastic progression in Barrett's oesophagus: a prospective study. Lancet Oncol 2005;6:945–52.

85. Kastelein F, Spaander MC, Biermann K, et al. Nonsteroidal anti-inflammatory drugs and statins have chemopreventative effects in patients with Barrett's esophagus. Gastroenterology 2011;141:2000–8.

86. Zhang S, Zhang XQ, Ding XW, et al. Cyclooxygenase inhibitors use is associated with reduced risk of esophageal adenocarcinoma in patients with Barrett's esophagus: a meta-analysis. Br J Cancer 2014;110:2378–88.

87. Lagergren J, Bergstrom R, Lindren A, et al. Symptomatic Gastroesophageal reflux as a risk factor for esophageal adenocarcinoma. N Engl J Med 1999; 340(11):825–31.

88. Kastelein F, Spaander MC, Steyerberg EW, et al. Proton pump inhibitors reduce the risk of neoplastic progression in patients with Barrett's esophagus. Clin Gastroenterol Hepatol 2013;11:382–8.

89. Singh S, Garg SK, Singh PP, et al. Acid-suppressive medications and risk of oesophageal adenocarcinoma in patients with Barrett's oesophagus: a systematic review and meta-analysis. Gut 2014;63(8):1229–37.

90. Hvid Jensen F, Pedersen L, Funch-Jensen P, et al. Proton pump inhibitor use may not prevent high-grade dysplasia and oesophageal adenocarcinoma in Barrett's oesophagus: a nationwide study of 9883 patients. Aliment Pharmacol Ther 2014;39:984–91.

91. Rubenstein JH, Inadomi JM, Scheiman J, et al. Association between Helicobacter pylori and Barrett's esophagus, erosive esophagitis, and gastroesophageal reflux symptoms. Clin Gastroenterol Hepatol 2014;12:239–45.

92. Corley DA, Kubo A, Levin TR, et al. Helicobacter pylori infection and the risk of Barrett's oesophagus: a community-based study. Gut 2007;57:727–33.

93. Nie S, Chen T, Yang X, et al. Association of Helicobacter pylori infection with esophageal adenocarcinoma and squamous cell carcinoma: a meta-analysis. Dis Esophagus 2014;27:645–53.

94. Steevens J, Schouten LJ, Goldbohm RA, et al. Vegetables and fruits consumption and risk of esophageal and gastric cancer subtypes in the Netherlands cohort study. Int J Cancer 2011;129:2681–93.

95. Li WQ, Park Y, Wu JW, et al. Index-based dietary patterns and risk of esophageal and gastric cancer in a large cohort study. Clin Gastroenterol Hepatol 2013;11:1130–6.

96. Zhu HC, Yang X, Xu LP, et al. Meat consumption in associated with esophageal cancer risk in a meat- and cancer-histological-type dependent manner. Dig Dis Sci 2014;59:664–73.

97. Salehi M, Moradi-Lakeh M, Salehi MH, et al. Meat, fish, and esophageal cancer risk: a systematic review and dose-response meta analysis. Nutr Rev 2013; 71(5):257–67.

98. O'Doherty MG, Cantwell MM, Murray LJ, et al. Dietary fat and meat intakes and risk of reflux esophagitis, Barrett's esophagus, and esophageal adenocarcinoma. Int J Cancer 2011;129:1493–502.

99. Coleman HG, Murray LJ, Hicks B, et al. Dietary Fiber and the risk of precancerous lesions and cancer of the esophagus: a systematic review and meta-analysis. Nutr Rev 2013;71(7):474–82.

100. Mayne ST, Risch HA, Dubrow R, et al. Nutrient Intake and risk of subtypes of esophageal and gastric cancer. Cancer Epidemiol Biomarkers Prev 2001;10: 1055–62.

101. Dong LM, Sanchez CA, Rabinovitch PS, et al. Dietary supplement use and risk of neoplastic progression in esophageal adenocarcinoma: a prospective study. Nutr Cancer 2008;60(1):39–48.

102. Dawsey SP, Hollenbeck A, Schatzkin A, et al. A prospective study of vitamin and mineral supplement use and the risk of upper gastrointestinal cancers. PLoS One 2014;9(2):e88774.
103. Sharp L, Carsin AE, Cantwell MM, et al. Intakes of dietary folate and other B vitamins are associated with risks of esophageal adenocarcinoma, Barrett's esophagus, and reflux esophagitis. J Nutr 2013;143:1966–73.
104. Xiao Q, Freedman ND, Ren J, et al. Intakes of folate methionine, vitamin b6, and vitamin b12 with a risk of esophageal and gastric cancer in a large cohort study. Br J Cancer 2014;110:1328–33.

Endoscopic Mucosal Resection and Endoscopic Submucosal Dissection for Endoscopic Therapy of Barrett's Esophagus-related Neoplasia

Shivangi Kothari, MD, Vivek Kaul, MD*

KEYWORDS

- Barrett's esophagus • Esophageal cancer • Dysplasia • Ablation • Resection • EMR
- ESD • Endotherapy

KEY POINTS

- Endoscopic mucosal resection (EMR) and endoscopic submucosal dissection (ESD) are indispensable endoscopic resection (ER) interventions in patients with dysplastic Barrett's esophagus (BE) and esophageal adenocarcinoma, having diagnostic (staging) and therapeutic (curative) value.
- ER interventions are frequently combined with endoscopic ablation to manage dysplastic BE.
- For mucosal (HGD and T1a) disease, continued endoscopic management is recommended.
- For T1b (submucosal involvement) or higher stage, esophagectomy is still the standard of care.
- ER is the most accurate intervention that helps with the above stratification.

INTRODUCTION

Barrett's esophagus (BE) is characterized by a change in the lining of the esophagus from stratified squamous epithelium to a metaplastic columnar epithelium (IM) that has a low, but real, malignant potential. The progression of BE to carcinoma occurs in a stepwise fashion from IM through dysplasia (low grade to high grade [HGD]). Endoscopic surveillance is recommended for patients with BE to detect and manage

---

Disclosure Statements: None relevant.
Division of Gastroenterology & Hepatology, Center For Advanced Therapeutic Endoscopy, University of Rochester Medical Center & Strong Memorial Hospital, 601 Elmwood Ave, Box 646, Rochester, NY 14642, USA
* Corresponding author.
E-mail address: vivek_kaul@urmc.rochester.edu

Gastroenterol Clin N Am 44 (2015) 317–335
http://dx.doi.org/10.1016/j.gtc.2015.02.006
0889-8553/15/$ – see front matter © 2015 Elsevier Inc. All rights reserved.

gastro.theclinics.com

dysplasia before malignant transformation. The annual risk of BE progressing to adenocarcinoma is estimated at 0.1% to 0.5%.[1,2] However, this risk increases to 10% per year with HGD.[3] Esophagectomy was conventional treatment for patients with HGD and early esophageal adenocarcinoma (EAC). However, this is associated with significant morbidity (and some mortality), even in high-volume centers. For this reason, endoscopic management of dysplastic BE and EAC has become extremely popular. This article focuses specifically on the role of endoscopic mucosal resection (EMR) and endoscopic submucosal dissection (ESD) in patients with dysplastic BE and EAC.

ENDOSCOPIC THERAPY OF BARRETT'S ESOPHAGUS: PARADIGM SHIFT

In recent years, a significant paradigm shift has taken place in the realm of esophageal dysplasia/early neoplasia management. The treatment of esophageal HGD and EAC has shifted from surgery (esophagectomy) to an organ-sparing, comprehensive endoscopic management approach. With the advent of endoscopic ablation technologies such as radiofrequency ablation and cryotherapy, and resection techniques like EMR and ESD, endoscopic therapy has now become the standard of care for management of dysplastic BE and EAC.[4,5] Endoscopic resection (ER) not only is used for curative intent but also allows a definitive histologic diagnosis, accurate pathologic staging, and potential cure, with a minimally invasive approach. Several studies have reported the efficacy and safety of endotherapy in the management of HGD and early EAC, with outcomes comparable to esophagectomy.[6–8]

ENDOSCOPIC EVALUATION AND MULTIDISCIPLINARY APPROACH

Patients with HGD and early EAC should undergo further evaluation at a high-volume tertiary center, in a multidisciplinary setting, by providers who have expertise in this entity.[9] A multidisciplinary approach is a key factor in managing these patients with close collaboration between the endoscopists, surgeons, and gastrointestinal pathologists. The endoscopist should have training and expertise in a comprehensive array of endoscopic technologies and interventions that may be required for multimodal management of dysplastic BE and EAC (**Boxes 1** and **2**). The ability to manage immediate and delayed procedure-related complications and the discipline to follow protocol-driven care cannot be overemphasized. Meticulous endoscopic evaluation and rigorous adherence to data-driven guidelines achieve the best patient outcomes.[10,11]

An expert gastrointestinal pathologist should confirm the diagnosis of HGD or EAC. Repeat tissue sampling should be considered when there is doubt, often with adjunct modalities like wide area transepithelial sampling and/or in vivo advanced imaging for confocal endomicroscopy, optical coherence tomography to minimize the chance of diagnostic error, which may lead to suboptimal or unnecessary interventions.

INITIAL STAGING AND ENDOSCOPIC THERAPY OPTIONS FOR DYSPLASTIC BARRETT'S ESOPHAGUS AND ESOPHAGEAL ADENOCARCINOMA
Role of Endoscopic Resection

A variety of endoscopic therapeutic modalities are available for the management of dysplastic BE (see **Box 2**). Resection techniques like EMR and ESD provide significantly more tissue for analysis than a biopsy sample. ER helps with tumor staging and can often be a minimally invasive, curative intervention when low burden neoplasia is encountered in the esophagus.[12,13] As such, ER can play both a "diagnostic" and a "therapeutic role."

Box 1
Initial endoscopic evaluation of dysplastic Barrett's esophagus and early esophageal cancer: technologies and techniques

A. Tissue acquisition

   1. Regular forceps biopsy, modified Seattle protocol

   2. Jumbo/multibite forceps biopsy

   3. Wide area transepithelial sampling

   4. Cytosponge

   5. EMR (pathologic staging possible)

   6. ESD (pathologic staging possible)

B. Endoscopic imaging

   1. Chromoendoscopy

   2. High-definition white light endoscopy

   3. Narrow band imaging, Fujinon intelligent chromoendoscopy, i-scan

   4. Endoscopic ultrasound

     a. Miniprobe

     b. Dedicated echoendoscope (radial or curvilinear)

   5. Confocal laser endomicroscopy

   6. Optical coherence tomography

   7. High magnification endoscopy

EMR is indicated for resection of nodular lesions in BE, short-segment dysplastic BE, early superficial (T1a) EAC (limited to the muscularis mucosa without lymph node or distant metastasis), and esophageal squamous cell carcinoma. ESD can also be used in the above-mentioned situations and may be preferred for resection of larger (>2 cm) lesions and more widespread areas of dysplasia or neoplasia.[4]

ER provides information that complements other staging modalities like endoscopic ultrasound (EUS) and cross-sectional imaging. In fact, ER can be the final diagnostic step in the endoscopic evaluation of HGD and EAC in BE. If only HGD or intramucosal carcinoma (ImCa) is found at ER, then computed tomography (CT) and PET have a low yield for metastatic disease. EUS has limited to no value in the setting of BE with HGD alone.

EUS can help detect tumor depth and local lymph node metastasis, although its accuracy varies by stage of tumor. CT and PET-CT are more useful in diagnosing regional and distant metastases in T1b (tumor invading into the submucosa) or higher-stage esophageal malignancies.

The risk of lymph node involvement or metastatic disease is low in patients with EAC limited to the muscularis mucosa with no lymph-vascular invasion, negative deep margin, and well to moderately differentiated (G1 and G2) tumor biology. It is in this subgroup of patients (pT1a + favorable histologic features) whereby ER provides the maximal chance of a durable curative intervention.

If ER reveals T1b disease (or if poor histologic features are present in a T1a lesion), then surgery is recommended because of a high (up to 30%) risk for subsequent lymph node metastasis. Because of this significant change in treatment approach in T1a versus T1b lesions, it is imperative to accurately diagnose, stage, and treat patients who are candidates for curative endotherapy. ER enables us to do exactly that.

Box 2
Endoscopic therapeutic techniques for dysplastic Barrett's esophagus and early esophageal cancer

A. Endoscopic resection

   1. Endoscopic mucosal resection

      a. Single Band EMR

      b. Multiband mucosectomy

      c. Widespread-EMR

      d. Complete Barrett's eradication

      e. Cap-assisted EMR

   2. Endoscopic submucosal dissection

B. Endoscopic ablation

      a. Radiofrequency ablation

      b. Cryotherapy

         i. Liquid nitrogen spray cryotherapy

         ii. Carbon dioxide cryotherapy

         iii. Cryotherapy balloon device

      c. Photodynamic therapy

      d. Laser

      e. Argon plasma coagulation

      f. Multipolar electrocoagulation

ENDOSCOPIC MUCOSAL RESECTION

Since its inception in Japan for the management of early gastric cancer, EMR has been successfully applied to the treatment of esophageal, duodenal, and colonic neoplasia. The assessment of the depth of invasion of the lesion is a key factor before considering EMR due to the increased risk of lymph node involvement with infiltrating lesions. This increased risk can be assessed based on the endoscopic evaluation of the target lesion ("nonlifting" sign with saline injection) and also by performing EUS before EMR.

The risk of lymph node involvement in the case of EAC depends on the depth of invasion and tumor stage (<5% in T1a lesions and up to 30% in T1b or higher stage lesions or lesions with lymph-vascular invasion).[14,15]

Various tumor classification systems have been developed based on endoscopic appearance of the lesion (**Boxes 3** and **4**, **Table 1**). In the Vienna classification, there are 5 categories of esophageal dysplasia/neoplasia.[16] The Vienna classification is the most commonly used classification in clinical practice in the United States.

UTILITY OF ENDOSCOPIC ULTRASOUND BEFORE ENDOSCOPIC MUCOSAL RESECTION

High-frequency probe EUS (20 MHz, 30 MHz) can identify the mucosal (m1, m2, m3) and submucosal (sm1, sm2, sm3) esophageal wall layers in detail. A recent systematic review evaluating the risk of lymph node metastases in BE patients reported virtually no risk of lymph node metastasis in the setting of HGD and an overall risk

---

Box 3
JSGE (Japanese Society for Gastrointestinal Endoscopy) lesion classification

Type I lesions are polypoid or protuberant and are subcategorized as:

- Ip: Pedunculated
- Ips/sp: Subpedunculated
- Is: Sessile

Type II lesions are flat and are further subcategorized as:

- IIa: Superficial elevated
- IIb: Flat
- IIc: Flat depressed
- IIc+IIa lesions: Elevated area within a depressed lesion
- IIa+IIc lesions: Depressed area within an elevated lesion

Type III lesions: Ulcerated

Type IV lesions: Lateral spreading

---

of 1% to 2 % in patients with ImCa.[17] Factors that predict the risk of node metastasis are as follows[18]:

1. The depth of invasion of the tumor (sm1 and deeper)
2. Tumor diameter greater than 3 cm
3. Presence of lymph vascular invasion on ER specimen
4. The degree of differentiation of the tumor (poorly differentiated or G3 tumor biology more likely to metastasize).

The reported incidence of lymph node metastases has been 9% to 20% in patients with sm1 tumors and as high as 24% to 50% in patients with sm3 tumors.[17]

EUS is widely used for locoregional staging of esophageal tumors but its role in tumor staging of BE with HGD or EAC is unclear. High-frequency miniprobes can be used for pre-EMR staging, but these cannot satisfactorily evaluate nodal disease.

Although some studies report limited value for EUS in superficial lesions once an expert endoscopist has estimated the tumor depth, other reports have shown EUS to have a high negative predictive value for the absence of nodal disease in EAC, while

---

Box 4
Paris classification

- Type 0-I lesions: Polypoid and subcategorized into:
  - Type 0-Ip: Protruded, pedunculated
  - Type 0-Is: Protruded, sessile
- Type 0-II lesions: Nonpolypoid and subcategorized into:
  - Type 0-IIa: Slightly elevated (elevation of lesion above the mucosa <2.5 mm)
  - Type 0-IIb: Flat
  - Type 0-IIc: Slightly depressed
- Type 0-III: Excavated (ulcer)

Table 1
Esophageal dysplasia and neoplasia in Barrett's esophagus: Vienna classification

Category 1	No neoplasia/dysplasia
Category 2	Indefinite for neoplasia/dysplasia
Category 3	Low-grade intraepithelial neoplasia (low-grade adenoma/dysplasia)
Category 4	Noninvasive high grade neoplasia 4.1. High-grade adenoma/dysplasia 4.2. Carcinoma in situ 4.3. Suspicion of invasive carcinoma
Category 5	Invasive neoplasia 5.1. Intramucosal carcinoma 5.2. Submucosal carcinoma or beyond

still others have identified lymph node metastases in up to 20% of such patients (see Fig. 1A–C).[19–21]

Thus, EUS can be considered in conjunction with EMR if there is any concern for lymph node metastasis or if the tumor has any high-risk features, as discussed above.

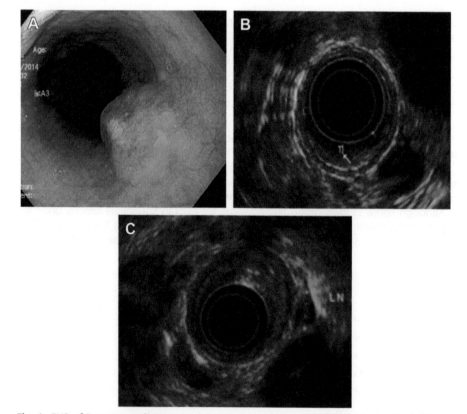

Fig. 1. EUS of Barrett's malignant nodule staged at T1N1. (*A*) Neoplastic nodule arising at proximal edge of Barrett's esophagus. (*B*) EUS of BE nodule staged as a T1 lesion. (*C*) Lymph Node positive for metastatic carcinoma by EUS-FNA (in a patient with T1 nodular lesion in BE): Final stage: T1N1.

ENDOSCOPIC MUCOSAL RESECTION
Indications

EMR is used for the superficial focal or circumferential resection of a BE nodule or visible lesion for diagnostic or therapeutic intent or for short segment Barrett's resection.

The JSGE have described criteria for lesions in Barrett's with HGD that are considered suitable for EMR[22]:

a. Lesions 2 cm or less in diameter in size
b. Lesion involving less than one-third of the circumference of the esophagus
c. Lesions limited to the mucosa (ImCa)

However, recent studies have shown successful resection of larger lesions and also complete Barrett's eradication with EMR as a safe and effective treatment option for BE with HGD/ImCa.[23] Studies have shown no significant difference in cumulative 5-year survival in patients undergoing EMR and ablative therapy for EAC when compared with esophagectomy.[24] Risk of stricture formation is higher when the resection involves more than three-fourths of the circumference of the esophagus.

PATIENT AND PROCEDURE PREPARATION

EMR can be performed safely under moderate sedation or general anesthesia. The latter is preferred in high-risk patients, in difficult to sedate patients, or when a prolonged procedure is anticipated. High-definition white light examination (HD-WLE) combined with electronic chromo-endoscopy (eg, narrow band imaging) is essential to achieve a high-quality examination. In addition to the EMR tools, some other accessories that may be needed are specimen retrieval nets, coaptation/coagulation forceps for hemostasis, and endoclips for bleeding control or closure of microperforations.

ENDOSCOPIC MUCOSAL RESECTION TECHNIQUES
Band-Ligation Assisted Endoscopic Mucosal Resection (Suck-Band-Ligate-Resect)
Single band resection technique
The traditional method of "suck band ligate and resect" involves resection of the target lesion using a standard variceal band ligator without prior submucosal injection. The lesion is suctioned into the banding device and a band is deployed across the captured tissue. The band captures the mucosa and superficial submucosa but typically not the muscularis propria. After creating a "pseudopolyp," the endoscope is withdrawn and the banding device is disassembled. The endoscope is reinserted and, using a standard electrocautery snare, the lesion is resected either above or below the band (**Fig. 2**A, B).

Multiband resection (mucosectomy) technique
The multiband mucosectomy (MBM) technique uses a slightly modified banding device (Duette Multi-Band Mucosectomy Device; Wilson-Cook, Winston-Salem, NC), which contains 6 bands and a dedicated hexagonal snare that passes through the endoscope working channel. The multiband device is available in several sizes that fit endoscopes with outer diameters of 9.5 to 14 mm (**Table 2**), (**Fig. 3**A, B).

After the banding device is loaded onto the appropriate endoscope, the target lesion is suctioned into the banding cap; the rubber band is deployed, and a "pseudopolyp" is created. The snare is then passed through the working channel of the endoscope and placed across the base of the pseudopolyp, and the lesion resected either above or below the band. Multiple areas can be resected without the need to remove the gastroscope out of the patient (**Fig. 4**A–C). MBM allows for piecemeal resection of

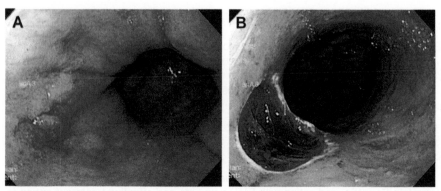

Fig. 2. Single band resection of a nodule in Barrett's esophagus. (*A*) Nodule in Barrett's esophagus. (*B*) Nodule site status-post single band resection (single EMR).

lesions greater than 2 cm, ensuring contiguous resection margins with each resection, making the process more efficient for the endoscopist and more comfortable and quicker for the patient.

A study reviewing 1060 MBM resections reported no perforations despite the absence of submucosal lifting.[25]

Multiband mucosectomy

Advantages:

1. Does not require submucosal injection or need to seat snare within cap
2. Multiple resections can be performed quickly using the same device
3. Lower perforation risk (compared to cap EMR)
4. Endoscope does not need to be withdrawn between resections

Disadvantage:

1. Larger lesions need piecemeal resection, which may result in incomplete resection, possible recurrence, and positive lateral margins.

Table 2
Devices used for endoscopic mucosal resection and multiband mucosectomy

Device	Endoscope Outer Diameter (mm)	Endoscope Working Channel (mm)	Sheath Size	Company
DT-6-5F	9.5–13	2.8 mm	5 Fr	Cook Medical Inc, Winston-Salem, NC
DT-6	9.5–13	3.7 mm	7 Fr	Cook Medical Inc, Winston-Salem, NC
DT-6-XL	11–14	3.7 mm	7 Fr	Cook Medical Inc, Winston-Salem, NC
EMR Kit (with cap, injection needle, spray catheter, and crescent snare)	9.3–10	2.0 mm for snare 2.8 mm for injection needle and spray catheter		Olympus America Inc, Center Valley, PA

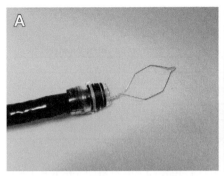
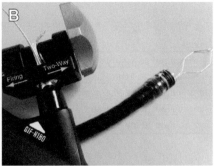

Fig. 3. Multiband mucosectomy (MBM) device with hexagonal snare for EMR in BE. (A) Gastroscope loaded with multiband mucosectomy device & proprietary hexagonal snare. (B) Gastroscope accessory channel showing MBM device and snare loaded.

Large Cap Resection

In the large cap resection method, the target lesion is raised with submucosal injection (saline or another solution) using an injection needle and then resected using a clear cap and snare cautery. A clear EMR cap (soft or hard; oblique or straight) is first fitted over the endoscope tip (**Table 3; Fig. 5**A, B). The endoscope is then advanced to the lesion and submucosal injection is performed. Next, a dedicated crescent-shaped

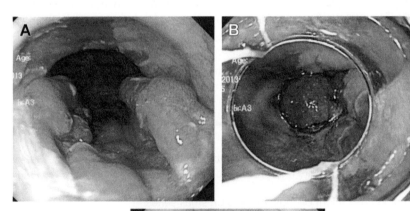
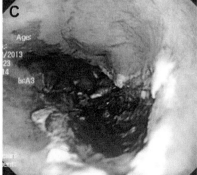

Fig. 4. Multiband mucosectomy of nodular Barrett's esophagus lesion. (A) Long segment of nodular Barrett's esophagus. (B) Multiband mucosectomy in progress (see "pseudopolyp" in distance). (C) Multiband resection completed.

Table 3	
Available caps for cap-assisted endoscopic mucosal resection	
Device	**Endoscope Outer Diameter (mm)**
Hard straight 13.9-mm cap	10–11
Hard straight 14.9-mm cap	9.3–10
Hard wide oblique 16.1-mm cap	8.6–11
Hard straight 12.9-mm cap	8.6–9.2
Soft oblique 18-mm cap	9.1–11.8

snare is passed through the endoscope working channel and seated into a notch at the distal edge of the cap, which requires some practice and experience with the device. The lesion is then suctioned into the cap, creating a "pseudopolyp." With the lesion suctioned into the cap, the snare is closed across the base of the captured tissue and the lesion is resected using cautery at the desired setting (**Fig. 6A–G**).[26] The oblique caps are commonly used in the esophagus to compensate for the parallel position of the scope in regard to the lesion.

Peters and colleagues[27] reported a study of 216 endoscopic cap-assisted resections for EAC in BE using the standard hard cap and large flexible cap. They reported a mean specimen diameter of 20 mm using the standard cap (23 mm with the large flexible cap). Bleeding (24%) was the most common complication, all managed endoscopically. Two perforations were reported, which were treated conservatively.

Large cap endoscopic mucosal resection

Advantages:
1. En-bloc resection of lesions with a diameter up to 2 cm (or greater) can be performed
2. More effective when scar tissue present

Disadvantages:
1. Requires a submucosal injection
2. Adjusting the snare in the cap notch can be tedious
3. Multiple resections require repeat submucosal injection, reseating the snare in the notch (time-consuming)
4. Perforation rates might be higher based on small series

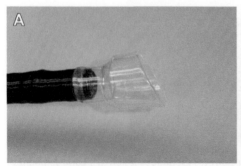
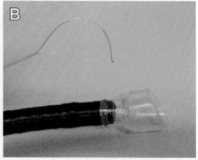

Fig. 5. Large oblique EMR cap with crescent snare shown. (*A*) Large oblique soft EMR cap shown loaded on gastroscope. (*B*) Large soft oblique EMR cap with proprietary snare shown.

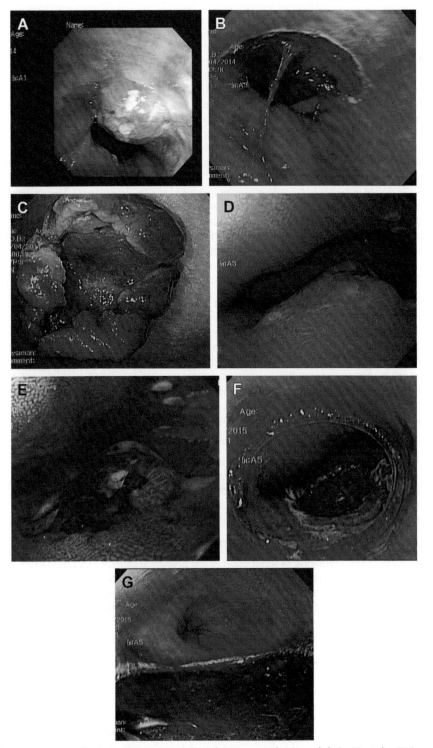

Fig. 6. Large cap EMR of a Barrett's nodule. (*A*) Large neoplastic nodule in BE at the GE junction. (*B*) BE Nodule site status-post large cap single EMR. (*C*) EMR specimen after large cap resection. (*D*) Nodule in BE. (*E*) Nodule in BE, NBI (narrow band imaging) view. (*F*) Lesion status-post large cap EMR. (*G*) Lesion status-post two contiguous large cap EMR (complete resection).

A study comparing endoscopic cap resection (with submucosal injection) to the band-resection technique reported no significant differences in resected specimen size. There were no severe complications in either group.[28]

In a study comparing MBM and large cap resection, MBM was found to be a cheaper and quicker option for piecemeal resection of ImCa lesions. MBM resulted in slightly smaller specimens when compared with cap resection (18 mm vs 20 mm), but there was no significant difference in depth of resection. Perforation rate was lower with MBM despite lack of any submucosal injection (3 perforations with cap and 1 with MBM).[29]

Thus, MBM appears to be safe and effective for piecemeal widespread lesion resection in BE. It is a cheaper and faster option when compared with cap resection and appears to have a lower perforation rate (compared with cap resection). The cap technique may be more effective if patients have previously undergone photodynamic therapy or EMR because the scarring could make band-based EMR more difficult.[30]

POSTPROCEDURE CONSIDERATIONS

EMR is usually performed on an outpatient basis. Patients can be admitted for monitoring in case of any intraprocedural bleeding or perforation or if a large area of resection was undertaken. High-dose acid suppression is maintained in the preprocedure, intraprocedure, and postprocedure periods. The authors advise a liquid diet for 1 day after the procedure and then advance the diet slowly as tolerated. Anticoagulation issues are managed in consultation with the patient's cardiologist and primary care provider after carefully weighing the risks and benefits in each case. Significant chest or abdominal pain after EMR is uncommon, but, if present, warrants immediate investigation. Further treatment is planned based on pathology results.

Contraindications to Endoscopic Mucosal Resection

a. Presence of lymph node or distant metastasis
b. Significant coagulopathy or collagen vascular disorder
c. Submucosal (or deeper) tumor invasion as seen on EUS
d. Failure of the lesion to "lift" with submucosal injection suggests infiltration, scarring, or submucosal invasion, and EMR is not advised

Limitations of Endoscopic Mucosal Resection

One of the major imitations of focal EMR is the presence of multifocal neoplasia and thereby the risk for development of synchronous or metachronous lesions in the residual BE.[6] Lesions larger than 2 cm require piecemeal EMR, and higher recurrence rates have been reported with piecemeal resection.[31] Some studies have thus proposed the technique of complete ER of BE to mitigate this problem.[23,32] Finally, EMR can be more difficult to perform in the setting of underlying scar tissue.

ENDOSCOPIC SUBMUCOSAL DISSECTION

ESD was developed in Japan for performing en-bloc resection of early gastric cancer. Because of its success, this technique has been applied to cancers in the esophagus and rectum. En-bloc resection provides an accurate evaluation of the deep and lateral resection margins. It has high technical success, and this leads to low recurrence rates and high cure rates.[33]

However, ESD is technically challenging and time-consuming and has higher complication rates when compared with EMR. ESD can be used for en-bloc resections of lesions greater than 2 cm. Although ESD has been an established technique for management of esophageal squamous cell cancer, the data for ESD in BE-HGD and EAC are relatively limited.[34] As with EMR, after performing ESD of a lesion in BE, postresection ablation of the residual BE is required to decrease the risk of developing metachronous lesions.

PREPARATION

Because of the procedure time and complexity, ESD should be performed under deep sedation or general anesthesia. Learning and performing ESD requires a thorough understanding of the technique and the tools used for submucosal dissection as well as the ability to manage procedure related complications. A recent European position paper recommends a series of steps to be undertaken by the endoscopist before initiating ESD procedures.[35] Experience with performing a minimum of 50 procedures in easier locations (distal stomach, rectum) before performing the procedure in the esophagus is recommended.[36]

Equipment and Tools

High-definition endoscopes with water jet and narrow band imaging (or similar technology) should be used. A clear cap is usually placed at the distal end of the endoscope to facilitate dissection. A variety of ESD "knives" are used, which are discussed later. Coagulation forceps can be used for hemostasis of small submucosal vessels that can bleed during the procedure. Traditional endoclips and the newer over-the-scope clips can be used to close small perforations.

TECHNIQUE

Accurate identification, mapping, and demarcation of the target lesion are of utmost importance before starting ESD. The lesion is first marked circumferentially with cautery or argon plasma coagulation (APC), approximately at a 3- to 5-mm distance from the edges of the target lesion. The lesion is then "lifted" (away from the muscularis propria) with submucosal injection of saline, 0.5% hyaluronate, or glycerin (and diluted epinephrine). Indigo carmine may be added to the injection solution for easier identification of the submucosal layer.

A circumferential incision is then made into the submucosa using one of several specialized electrocautery-based ESD knives (insulation tip knife, hook knife, triangle-tipped knife, hybrid knife).

The dissection proceeds proximally to distally in the submucosal plane in a careful and meticulous fashion, ensuring that the deeper muscle layer is not breached and the visual field is kept as clear as possible by controlling any bleeding. The aim of ESD is to resect the lesion en bloc, regardless of its size (**Fig. 7**A–C); often though, it may not be possible and piecemeal resection is then performed. A simplified approach has been proposed to reduce the time and tedium associated with ESD in the esophagus: with the Universal ESD technique, the raised, circumferentially incised and isolated lesion is resected en bloc with an electrocautery snare, thereby eliminating the time-consuming and risky submucosal dissection portion of the procedure.[37]

After ESD, patients are usually admitted for overnight monitoring and kept on high-dose acid suppression and allowed nothing by mouth. Liquid diet can be started the next day. Depending on the pathology, surveillance endoscopy should be performed at 2 to 3 months after initial resection, at which point further therapy can be planned as needed.[38]

ESD requires significant experience and technical skill, and its role in the management of dysplastic BE and EAC has not yet been well established. The learning

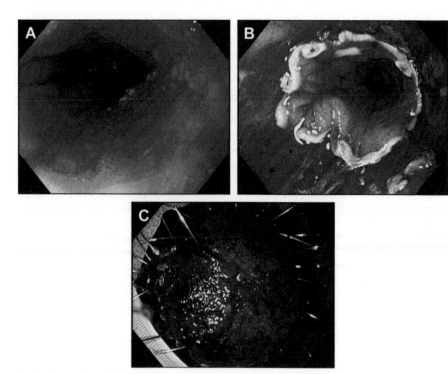

Fig. 7. Circumferential ESD of squamous cell esophageal cancer. (*A*) Circumferential Esophageal Squamous Cell Lesion. (*B*) Esophageal appearance after complete, circumferential ESD. (*C*) Resected specimen status-post ESD. (*Courtesy of* Truptesh Kothari, MD & Gregory Haber, MD, Lenox Hill Hospital, New York, NY.)

curve for ESD can be very steep and the cost (and complications) higher than EMR. With these issues in mind, the advantages of ESD over EMR in BE may be limited.[39]

ESD Advantages:
1. Allows en-bloc resection of large lesions
2. Better curative resection rates when compared with EMR[40]
3. Lower incidence of local recurrence[40]

Disadvantages:
1. Technically difficult
2. Time-consuming and costly
3. Requires experience, steep learning curve
4. Increased risk of perforation (compared with EMR)
5. Higher rate of esophageal stenosis with ESD

COMPLICATIONS OF ENDOSCOPIC MUCOSAL RESECTION AND ENDOSCOPIC SUBMUCOSAL DISSECTION

The most common complications associated with EMR and ESD are bleeding, perforation, and stricture formation.[25,41]

The risk of early and delayed bleeding in a study reporting more than 1000 MBM procedures performed in 243 patients was 2.9% and 2.1%, respectively. No perforations were reported, and all adverse events were managed endoscopically.[25] Other studies have reported only minor bleeding with EMR in 11% to 32% of patients.[31,42] ESD has been reported to have significantly higher bleeding rates when compared with EMR.[33] Most bleeding can be controlled endoscopically. Most bleeding occurs during the procedure or within the first 24 to 72 hours.

Esophageal perforation with EMR has been reported in less than 1% to 5% of cases.[43,44] Reported risk is higher when piecemeal resection is performed.[45] A meta-analysis comparing EMR versus ESD for superficial esophageal cancer reported perforation rates of 4% with ESD and 1.34% with EMR.[40] Recent studies have reported an esophageal perforation rate of 0% to 4%[46–48] with ESD. Small perforations recognized during the procedure can be managed endoscopically with excellent outcomes.[44] Pneumomediastinum can be seen in up to 30% of patients after ESD.[49] Using CO_2 (instead of air) has been shown to significantly reduce after-procedure pneumomediastinum.[50]

Stricture formation has been reported in 2% to 26% of patients undergoing ER for BE (**Fig. 8**).[51–53] The risk of stricture formation is higher with longer segments treated and with circumferential resection. These strictures are usually managed successfully with endoscopic dilation.[54] The risk of stricture formation may be reduced with triamcinolone injection at the time of resection.[55]

A meta-analysis comparing EMR and ESD in the management of superficial esophageal cancer reported similar bleeding and stricture rates, but a significantly higher rate of perforation with ESD. The recurrence rates were found to be significantly lower with ESD compared with EMR but no difference was seen in the recurrence rates when the lesion was smaller than 20 mm.[40] A systematic review reported significantly higher stricture formation rates with ESD when compared with EMR.[56]

ENDOSCOPIC RESECTION: EFFICACY

Multiple studies have reported the safety and long-term efficacy of ER in BE with HGD and EAC, with outcomes comparable to surgery, and fewer overall complications.[6,23,24,31,42,57,58] Complete eradication of neoplasia has been reported in 95% to 100% of patients with 5-year survival rates of 98% to 100%.[6,31,42,43,59,60]

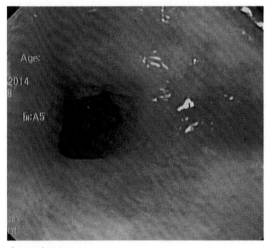

Fig. 8. Post ER esophageal stricture.

Development of metachronous lesions or recurrence of carcinoma after ER has been reported in 6% to 30% of patients.[23,24,31,42,43,57,60–62] Factors associated with recurrence are larger lesions, longer BE segments, piecemeal resection of lesions, presence of multifocal neoplasia, presence of residual dysplasia, and failure to ablate the residual BE segment.[6,24,43,61,62] Recurrences are managed endoscopically in most patients.[43]

It is due to these robust data and excellent long-term results that endoscopic therapy has gained significant traction in the last decade and has now emerged as the new standard for treatment of dysplastic BE and EAC.

SUMMARY

Endoscopic therapy for dysplastic Barrett's and early-stage EAC has essentially replaced surgery for this disease. ER techniques like EMR and ESD are at the center of this treatment revolution and represent a success in endoscopic innovation, technical sophistication, and ingenuity. EMR and ESD are critically essential elements in the algorithm for dysplastic BE and EAC management. These techniques have heralded a new era of "endoscopic surgery." In modern medicine, there are few better examples where such a major, successful paradigm shift has occurred, with such a profound effect on the care and outcome of each individual patient.

REFERENCES

1. Sharma P. Clinical practice. Barrett's esophagus. N Engl J Med 2009;361: 2548–56.
2. Buttar NS, Wang KK, Sebo TJ, et al. Extent of high-grade dysplasia in Barrett's esophagus correlates with risk of adenocarcinoma. Gastroenterology 2001;120: 1630–9.
3. Weston AP, Sharma P, Topalovski M, et al. Long-term follow-up of Barrett's high-grade dysplasia. Am J Gastroenterol 2000;95:1888–93.
4. ASGE Standards of Practice Committee, Evans JA, Early DS, et al. The role of endoscopy in the assessment and treatment of esophageal cancer. Gastrointest Endosc 2013;77:328–34.
5. Bennett C, Vakil N, Bergman J, et al. Consensus statements for management of Barrett's dysplasia and early-stage esophageal adenocarcinoma, based on a Delphi process. Gastroenterology 2012;143:336–46.
6. Pech O, Behrens A, May A, et al. Long-term results and risk factor analysis for recurrence after curative endoscopic therapy in 349 patients with high-grade intraepithelial neoplasia and mucosal adenocarcinoma in Barrett's oesophagus. Gut 2008;57:1200–6.
7. Nijhawan PK, Wang KK. Endoscopic mucosal resection for lesions with endoscopic features suggestive of malignancy and high-grade dysplasia within Barrett's esophagus. Gastrointest Endosc 2000;52:328–32.
8. Galey KM, Wilshire CL, Watson TJ, et al. Endoscopic management of early esophageal neoplasia: an emerging standard. J Gastrointest Surg 2011;15: 1728–35.
9. Cameron GR, Jayasekera CS, Williams R, et al. Detection and staging of esophageal cancers within Barrett's esophagus is improved by assessment in specialized Barrett's units. Gastrointest Endosc 2014;80:971–83.e1.
10. van Vilsteren FG, Pouw RE, Herrero LA, et al. Learning to perform endoscopic resection of esophageal neoplasia is associated with significant complications even within a structured training program. Endoscopy 2012;44:4–12.

11. Kara MA, Peters FP, Rosmolen WD, et al. High-resolution endoscopy plus chromoendoscopy or narrow-band imaging in Barrett's esophagus: a prospective randomized crossover study. Endoscopy 2005;37:929–36.

12. Mino-Kenudson M, Hull MJ, Brown I, et al. EMR for Barrett's esophagus-related superficial neoplasms offers better diagnostic reproducibility than mucosal biopsy. Gastrointest Endosc 2007;66:660–6 [quiz: 767, 769].

13. Peters FP, Brakenhoff KP, Curvers WL, et al. Histologic evaluation of resection specimens obtained at 293 endoscopic resections in Barrett's esophagus. Gastrointest Endosc 2008;67:604–9.

14. Manner H, May A, Pech O, et al. Early Barrett's carcinoma with "low-risk" submucosal invasion: long-term results of endoscopic resection with a curative intent. Am J Gastroenterol 2008;103:2589–97.

15. Alvarez Herrero L, Pouw RE, van Vilsteren FG, et al. Risk of lymph node metastasis associated with deeper invasion by early adenocarcinoma of the esophagus and cardia: study based on endoscopic resection specimens. Endoscopy 2010; 42:1030–6.

16. Schlemper RJ, Riddell RH, Kato Y, et al. The Vienna classification of gastrointestinal epithelial neoplasia. Gut 2000;47:251–5.

17. Dunbar KB, Spechler SJ. The risk of lymph-node metastases in patients with high-grade dysplasia or intramucosal carcinoma in Barrett's esophagus: a systematic review. Am J Gastroenterol 2012;107:850–62 [quiz: 863].

18. Buskens CJ, Westerterp M, Lagarde SM, et al. Prediction of appropriateness of local endoscopic treatment for high-grade dysplasia and early adenocarcinoma by EUS and histopathologic features. Gastrointest Endosc 2004;60: 703–10.

19. May A, Gunter E, Roth F, et al. Accuracy of staging in early oesophageal cancer using high resolution endoscopy and high resolution endosonography: a comparative, prospective, and blinded trial. Gut 2004;53:634–40.

20. Pouw RE, Heldoorn N, Alvarez Herrero L, et al. Do we still need EUS in the workup of patients with early esophageal neoplasia? A retrospective analysis of 131 cases. Gastrointest Endosc 2011;73:662–8.

21. Shami VM, Villaverde A, Stearns L, et al. Clinical impact of conventional endosonography and endoscopic ultrasound-guided fine-needle aspiration in the assessment of patients with Barrett's esophagus and high-grade dysplasia or intramucosal carcinoma who have been referred for endoscopic ablation therapy. Endoscopy 2006;38:157–61.

22. Takeshita K, Tani M, Inoue H, et al. Endoscopic treatment of early oesophageal or gastric cancer. Gut 1997;40:123–7.

23. Chennat J, Konda VJ, Ross AS, et al. Complete Barrett's eradication endoscopic mucosal resection: an effective treatment modality for high-grade dysplasia and intramucosal carcinoma–an American single-center experience. Am J Gastroenterol 2009;104:2684–92.

24. Prasad GA, Wu TT, Wigle DA, et al. Endoscopic and surgical treatment of mucosal (T1a) esophageal adenocarcinoma in Barrett's esophagus. Gastroenterology 2009;137:815–23.

25. Alvarez Herrero L, Pouw RE, van Vilsteren FG, et al. Safety and efficacy of multiband mucosectomy in 1060 resections in Barrett's esophagus. Endoscopy 2011; 43:177–83.

26. Inoue H, Endo M, Takeshita K, et al. A new simplified technique of endoscopic esophageal mucosal resection using a cap-fitted panendoscope (EMRC). Surg Endosc 1992;6:264–5.

27. Peters FP, Brakenhoff KP, Curvers WL, et al. Endoscopic cap resection for treatment of early Barrett's neoplasia is safe: a prospective analysis of acute and early complications in 216 procedures. Dis Esophagus 2007;20:510–5.

28. May A, Gossner L, Behrens A, et al. A prospective randomized trial of two different endoscopic resection techniques for early stage cancer of the esophagus. Gastrointest Endosc 2003;58:167–75.

29. Pouw RE, van Vilsteren FG, Peters FP, et al. Randomized trial on endoscopic resection-cap versus multiband mucosectomy for piecemeal endoscopic resection of early Barrett's neoplasia. Gastrointest Endosc 2011;74:35–43.

30. Tomizawa Y, Iyer PG, Wong Kee Song LM, et al. Safety of endoscopic mucosal resection for Barrett's esophagus. Am J Gastroenterol 2013;108:1440–7 [quiz: 1448].

31. Ell C, May A, Gossner L, et al. Endoscopic mucosal resection of early cancer and high-grade dysplasia in Barrett's esophagus. Gastroenterology 2000;118:670–7.

32. Giovannini M, Bories E, Pesenti C, et al. Circumferential endoscopic mucosal resection in Barrett's esophagus with high-grade intraepithelial neoplasia or mucosal cancer. Preliminary results in 21 patients. Endoscopy 2004;36:782–7.

33. Cao Y, Liao C, Tan A, et al. Meta-analysis of endoscopic submucosal dissection versus endoscopic mucosal resection for tumors of the gastrointestinal tract. Endoscopy 2009;41:751–7.

34. Kagemoto K, Oka S, Tanaka S, et al. Clinical outcomes of endoscopic submucosal dissection for superficial Barrett's adenocarcinoma. Gastrointest Endosc 2014;80:239–45.

35. Deprez PH, Bergman JJ, Meisner S, et al. Current practice with endoscopic submucosal dissection in Europe: position statement from a panel of experts. Endoscopy 2010;42:853–8.

36. Yamamoto S, Uedo N, Ishihara R, et al. Endoscopic submucosal dissection for early gastric cancer performed by supervised residents: assessment of feasibility and learning curve. Endoscopy 2009;41:923–8.

37. Soetikno R, Kaltenbach T, Sanchez-Yague A, et al. Resections of difficult Barrett's cancer using universal-endoscopic submucosal dissection (U-ESD). Gastrointest Endosc 2012;74:AB107.

38. Hammad H, Kaltenbach T, Soetikno R. Endoscopic submucosal dissection for malignant esophageal lesions. Curr Gastroenterol Rep 2014;16:386.

39. Bergman JJ. How to justify endoscopic submucosal dissection in the Western world. Endoscopy 2009;41:988–90.

40. Guo HM, Zhang XQ, Chen M, et al. Endoscopic submucosal dissection vs endoscopic mucosal resection for superficial esophageal cancer. World J Gastroenterol 2014;20:5540–7.

41. Isomoto H, Yamaguchi N, Minami H, et al. Management of complications associated with endoscopic submucosal dissection/endoscopic mucosal resection for esophageal cancer. Dig Endosc 2013;25(Suppl 1):29–38.

42. Ell C, May A, Pech O, et al. Curative endoscopic resection of early esophageal adenocarcinomas (Barrett's cancer). Gastrointest Endosc 2007;65:3–10.

43. Pech O, May A, Manner H, et al. Long-term efficacy and safety of endoscopic resection for patients with mucosal adenocarcinoma of the esophagus. Gastroenterology 2014;146:652–60.e1.

44. Gerke H, Siddiqui J, Nasr I, et al. Efficacy and safety of EMR to completely remove Barrett's esophagus: experience in 41 patients. Gastrointest Endosc 2011;74:761–71.

45. Soetikno RM, Gotoda T, Nakanishi Y, et al. Endoscopic mucosal resection. Gastrointest Endosc 2003;57:567–79.

46. Higuchi K, Tanabe S, Azuma M, et al. A phase II study of endoscopic submucosal dissection for superficial esophageal neoplasms (KDOG 0901). Gastrointest Endosc 2013;78:704–10.

47. Oyama T, Tomori A, Hotta K, et al. Endoscopic submucosal dissection of early esophageal cancer. Clin Gastroenterol Hepatol 2005;3:S67–70.

48. Toyonaga T, Man-i M, East JE, et al. 1,635 Endoscopic submucosal dissection cases in the esophagus, stomach, and colorectum: complication rates and long-term outcomes. Surg Endosc 2013;27:1000–8.

49. Tamiya Y, Nakahara K, Kominato K, et al. Pneumomediastinum is a frequent but minor complication during esophageal endoscopic submucosal dissection. Endoscopy 2010;42:8–14.

50. Maeda Y, Hirasawa D, Fujita N, et al. A pilot study to assess mediastinal emphysema after esophageal endoscopic submucosal dissection with carbon dioxide insufflation. Endoscopy 2012;44:565–71.

51. Larghi A, Lightdale CJ, Memeo L, et al. EUS followed by EMR for staging of high-grade dysplasia and early cancer in Barrett's esophagus. Gastrointest Endosc 2005;62:16–23.

52. Seewald S, Akaraviputh T, Seitz U, et al. Circumferential EMR and complete removal of Barrett's epithelium: a new approach to management of Barrett's esophagus containing high-grade intraepithelial neoplasia and intramucosal carcinoma. Gastrointest Endosc 2003;57:854–9.

53. Peters FP, Kara MA, Rosmolen WD, et al. Stepwise radical endoscopic resection is effective for complete removal of Barrett's esophagus with early neoplasia: a prospective study. Am J Gastroenterol 2006;101:1449–57.

54. Katada C, Muto M, Manabe T, et al. Esophageal stenosis after endoscopic mucosal resection of superficial esophageal lesions. Gastrointest Endosc 2003; 57:165–9.

55. Hashimoto S, Kobayashi M, Takeuchi M, et al. The efficacy of endoscopic triamcinolone injection for the prevention of esophageal stricture after endoscopic submucosal dissection. Gastrointest Endosc 2011;74:1389–93.

56. Sgourakis G, Gockel I, Lang H. Endoscopic and surgical resection of T1a/T1b esophageal neoplasms: a systematic review. World J Gastroenterol 2013;19: 1424–37.

57. Pech O, Bollschweiler E, Manner H, et al. Comparison between endoscopic and surgical resection of mucosal esophageal adenocarcinoma in Barrett's esophagus at two high-volume centers. Ann Surg 2011;254:67–72.

58. Wu J, Pan YM, Wang TT, et al. Endotherapy versus surgery for early neoplasia in Barrett's esophagus: a meta-analysis. Gastrointest Endosc 2014;79:233–41.e2.

59. Peters FP, Kara MA, Rosmolen WD, et al. Endoscopic treatment of high-grade dysplasia and early stage cancer in Barrett's esophagus. Gastrointest Endosc 2005;61:506–14.

60. Moss A, Bourke MJ, Hourigan LF, et al. Endoscopic resection for Barrett's high-grade dysplasia and early esophageal adenocarcinoma: an essential staging procedure with long-term therapeutic benefit. Am J Gastroenterol 2010;105: 1276–83.

61. Esaki M, Matsumoto T, Hirakawa K, et al. Risk factors for local recurrence of superficial esophageal cancer after treatment by endoscopic mucosal resection. Endoscopy 2007;39:41–5.

62. Yamada M, Oda I, Nonaka S, et al. Long-term outcome of endoscopic resection of superficial adenocarcinoma of the esophagogastric junction. Endoscopy 2013; 45:992–6.

Ablative Endoscopic Therapies for Barrett's-Esophagus-Related Neoplasia

Shajan Peter, MD*, Klaus Mönkemüller, MD, PhD

KEYWORDS

- Barrett's esophagus • Radiofrequency ablation • Cryoablation
- Photodynamic therapy • Dysplasia • Neoplasia

KEY POINTS

- Ablative therapy aims at elimination of Barrett's esophagus (BE) by the induction of superficial tissue necrosis by thermal energy, freezing, or photochemical injury.
- Radiofrequency ablation (RFA) is the most studied method with safe, effective, and durable long-term treatment outcomes.
- Two types of RFA are performed, circumferential ablation (c-RFA) and focal ablation (f-RFA).
- RFA is effective either alone or in combination with endoscopic resection for high-grade dysplasia (HGD).
- The role of RFA in low-grade dysplasia (LGD) is still debated, but it can be offered as an alternate treatment in select patients.
- Cryotherapy, argon plasma coagulation (APC), and photodynamic therapy (PDT) can be offered in select patients when RFA is unavailable, has failed, or is contraindicated.

INTRODUCTION

BE is an acquired condition characterized by a change of the normal esophageal squamous epithelium to columnar epithelium containing goblet cells (**Boxes 1** and **2, Table 1**). This metaplastic change can progress to LGD and HGD, the latter having a 5% to 10% per patient-year risk of developing esophageal adenocarcinoma (EAC).[1-3] On the other hand, the risk of EAC in the general population with nondysplastic BE is only 0.1%– to 0.3% per year.[2,4-6] BE is more common in developed countries, affecting 1% to 2% of the general population, and has a strong association with male gender, white race, and gastroesophageal reflux disease.[7-10] The incidence of EAC

Department of Gastroenterology, Basil I. Hirschowitz Endoscopic Centre of Endoscopic Excellence, University of Alabama at Birmingham, 6th Floor Jefferson Tower, 625 19th Street South, Birmingham, AL 35249, USA
* Corresponding author.
E-mail address: shajan@uab.edu

Gastroenterol Clin N Am 44 (2015) 337–353
http://dx.doi.org/10.1016/j.gtc.2015.02.014   **gastro.theclinics.com**
0889-8553/15/$ – see front matter © 2015 Elsevier Inc. All rights reserved.

Box 1
c-RFA equipment list

Endoscope and equipment

RFA energy generator console

HALO[360] sizing balloon

HALO[360] balloon ablation catheter

HALO cap

Gauze

1% N-acetylcysteine solution

Spray catheter

Savary spring-tipped guidewire of 0.025 or 0.035 in diameter, minimum of 260 cm length; Nitinol-based guidewire (Tracer Metro [Cook Endoscopy, Cook Medical Endoscopy Inc, Winston Salem, NC] or equivalent)

Adapted from Frantz DJ, Dellon ES, Shaheen NJ. Radiofrequency ablation of Barrett's esophagus. Techniques in Gastrointestinal Endoscopy 2010;12:100–7.

---

has increased more than 5-fold over the past decades.[11,12] Ablation by thermal energy, freezing, or photochemical injury achieves complete eradication of dysplasia (CE-D) and complete eradication of specialized intestinal metaplasia (IM) resulting in squamous reepithelialization of esophagus. Endoscopic ablative therapies aim to eradicate dysplasia and IM to prevent the development of EAC. This article focuses on the most published ablative therapies, which are RFA, PDT, and cryoablation.

PRINCIPLES OF MUCOSAL ABLATION IN BARRETT'S ESOPHAGUS

Ablative therapy aims at elimination of BE by the induction of superficial tissue necrosis by thermal energy, freezing, or photochemical injury. Healing ensues in an acid-suppressed state, and the damaged tissue is then replaced by normal squamous mucosa. This reepithelialization, characterized by neosquamous epithelium, remains the main goal of therapy. The exact mechanism that leads to reepithelialization is still not clear. It is theorized that squamous regeneration seems to occur from neighboring squamous cells and bone-marrow-derived stem cells.[13,14] Immunohistology and fluorescent in situ hybridization (FISH) studies of this epithelium show loss of preexisting

---

Box 2
f-RFA equipment list

Endoscope and equipment

RFA energy generator console

HALO[90] ablation device

Gauze

1% N-acetyl cysteine solution

Spray catheter

Adapted from Frantz DJ, Dellon ES, Shaheen NJ. Radiofrequency ablation of Barrett's esophagus. Techniques in Gastrointestinal Endoscopy 2010;12:100–7.

Table 1 Pearls and pitfalls	
Indications	• Careful history, endoscopic findings, pathologic review of records should be done before selection of patients for ablation
Selection of ablation method	• Long-segment circumferential areas should be targeted using the circumferential HALO^{360} device • Short segment and subsequent sessions or "touch-up" of BE can be treated using the focal HALO^{90} device
c-RFA	• Endoscopic identification of landmarks and length on segment based on Prague classification • Sizing of device and selection of balloon ablating catheter • Careful positioning and endoscopic visualization of the catheter and performing the first ablation pass • Cleaning of device externally while performing debridement of tissue using the endoscope and cap • Performing the second ablation pass
f-RFA	• Endoscopic identification of landmarks • Attachment of device to endoscope such that it is in 12'o-clock endoscopic view • Optimal opposition to targeted mucosa and energy delivered using dual technique with continued ablation of all areas • Debridement of tissue, cleaning of device, and second pass of ablation for all areas
Follow-up	• Immediate postprocedure instructions are given regarding food intake, pain management, and antireflux medications • Follow-up after 2 mo for repeat endoscopy, further ablation, or biopsies

From Mulholland MW, Albo D, Dalman R, et al. Operative techniques in surgery. Philadelphia: Lippincott Williams & Wilkins; 2014. p. 215; with permission.

ontogenetic alterations suggesting a low risk for malignant progression.[15] However, ablative treatment approach is limited to superficial flat mucosal tissue, does not provide a tissue specimen for histologic staging or assessment, and therefore is distinct from endoscopic resection techniques. The ablative techniques used in the eradication of BE have been classified as (1) thermal: RFA, APC, laser, and multipolar electrocoagulation (the latter 2 being infrequently used) and (2) nonthermal: cryoablation and PDT.

RADIOFREQUENCY ABLATION

RFA is a safe and effective endoscopic treatment modality for BE. The technique is based on using a bipolar electrode array and a generator that delivers a fixed amount of thermal radiofrequency energy that results in uniform tissue dissipation to a depth of 0.5 mm. The electrode array is available on 2 main delivery device platforms: (1) HALO^{360} circumferential also called Barrx 360 Balloon catheter and (2) HALO^{90} focal or Barrx 90 Focal catheter (Covidien Barrx, Sunnyvale, CA, USA) (**Fig. 1**). Furthermore, 3 modifications of the focal device are available for select patients: Barrx 60 RFA Focal Catheter, Barrx Ultra Long RFA Focal Catheter, and Barrx Channel RFA Endoscopic Catheter.

Selection of patients for RFA requires a multidisciplinary approach consisting of the endoscopist, gastrointestinal (GI) pathologist, and the surgeon. Accurate endoscopic pretreatment staging is essential to ensure optimal long-term outcomes. Endoscopic inspection should be performed with high-definition white light. The extent of BE segment should be defined using the Prague C & M classification including the length

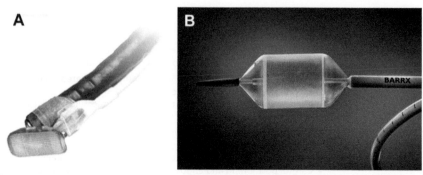

Fig. 1. HALO ablation devices (A) HALO^{90}; (B) HALO^{360}. (*Courtesy of* Barrx, Sunnyvale, CA; with permission.)

of the circumferential segment (C) and the maximal extent (M) of the BE segment (**Fig. 2**).[16] Other imaging modalities that might help in delineating BE are narrow band imaging, standard chromoendoscopy, autofluorescence imaging, and confocal laser endoscopy. Although these methods have not been proven to be superior to white light endoscopy to detect dysplasia, all these techniques might aid in directed or targeted biopsies of suspicious areas. Targeted biopsies are obtained from visible abnormalities, followed by 4-quadrant biopsies of every 1 to 2 cm of the BE segment (Seattle protocol).[17] Nodular lesions or focal visible lesions should be resected and are best staged by doing an endoscopic mucosal resection (EMR) before performing RFA therapy as described by Kaul V and Kothari S, elsewhere in this issue. Before performing RFA, a second, dedicated GI pathologist must confirm the presence of dysplasia on biopsies or resected specimens.[18]

TECHNIQUE OF RADIOFREQUENCY ABLATION
Preoperative Planning

Patients undergo standard esophagoduodenoscopy preprocedure preparation with specific note of sedation and procedural risks. Special attention should be exercised when treating patients with morbid obesity, anatomic variants such as short neck, cervical osteophytes, cricopharyngeal hypertrophy, and prior history of surgery involving the GI tract, radiation, or documentation of previous strictures. No antibiotics are required before any of the ablative therapies. It is desirable to minimize or stop antiplatelet and anticoagulation therapy before the procedure. Procedures are routinely

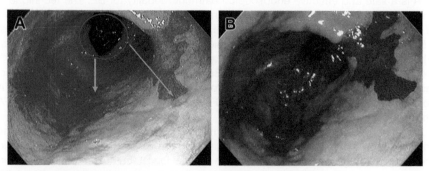

Fig. 2. (A) Endoscopic appearance of BE (*short arrow,* circumferential extent; *long arrow,* maximum extent) (B) Narrow band imaging of the segment.

performed on an outpatient basis using conscious sedation delivered by the endoscopists or by the anesthesia department (ie, monitored anesthesia care). The patient is placed in the left lateral decubitus position and prepared in the same manner as for a routine upper endoscopy.

Circumferential Ablation

c-RFA is done in patients in whom the segment of BE is longer than 2 cm and is circumferential (**Box 1**). The steps include:

1. *Endoscopy with inspection and recording the landmarks*: Measurements are taken to map the extent of the BE showing (a) the Z-line, which is the top of cylindrical epithelium or top of intestinal metaplasia (TIM), (b) the proximal contiguous area of BE (M), as well as (c) the proximal level at which the BE is circumferential (C) and the top of the gastric folds. The top of the gastric folds corresponds to the gastroesophageal junction. Careful inspection should be made to evaluate for hiatal hernia and to rule out prior ulceration, strictures, previous scarring from EMR, or residual nodularity because these may compromise any balloon c-RFA. If strictures are noted, esophageal dilatation should be performed 2 to 3 weeks before ablation. Ideally, before performing RFA, the esophageal mucosa is washed with *N*-acetylcysteine to clear any excess mucus.
2. *Sizing*: After adequate inspection, recording landmarks, a guidewire is passed into the gastric antrum and then the endoscope removed. The sizing balloon is attached to the control unit and then calibrated externally to rule out any leaks (**Fig. 3**). The balloon is then introduced over the guidewire into the body of the esophagus placing it 3 cm proximal to the TIM measurement. Serial measurements are taken at 1-cm intervals, starting proximally and proceeding distally by inflating the device. A technician or nurse then records the displayed measurements. The smallest diameter treatment balloon suggested throughout the sizing is chosen as the appropriate ablation catheter.
3. *Selecting appropriate ablation device*: After sizing, the balloon catheter is removed, keeping the guidewire in place. The smallest diameter treatment balloon suggested throughout the sizing is chosen as the appropriate ablation device and attached to the generator. Balloon catheters are available in several diameters: 18, 22, 25, 28, 31, and 34 mm.
4. *First ablation pass*: The HALO[360] catheter consisting of a 3-cm electrode array encircling a 4-cm-long balloon is then passed over the guidewire into the esophagus (**Fig. 4**). The endoscope is intubated alongside the catheter to visualize the proximal end of the balloon, which is then positioned 1 cm proximal to the TIM.

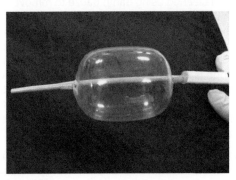

Fig. 3. Sizing balloon for c-RFA.

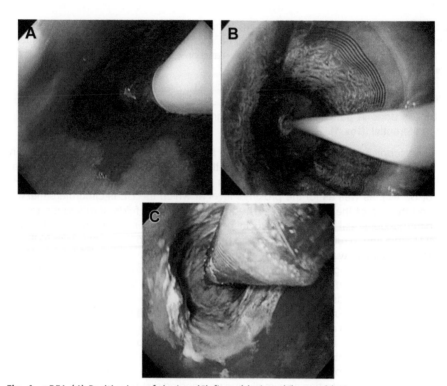

Fig. 4. c-RFA (*A*) Positioning of device; (*B*) first ablation; (*C*) postablation appearance.

The balloon is automatically inflated first, and then energy is delivered by using the foot pedals attached to the control unit. The uniform energy has a density of 12 J/cm^2 and power of 40 W/cm^2 ablating to a depth of 700 to 1000 μm over 3 cm of array. After a second of ablation, the balloon automatically deflates and the circumferential burn is visible. Depending on the length of the segment, an additional 3 cm of c-RFA is performed such that there is minimal overlap (<1 cm) with the previously ablated segment.

5. *Cleaning phase*: The balloon catheter is then removed along with the endoscope, leaving the guidewire in place. After the balloon is taken out of the patient, the balloon is inflated and cleaned using damp gauze to remove any adherent ablated tissue or debris. The treated area is then cleaned of the coagulum using a HALO cap, which is attached to the tip of the endoscope. After reintroduction of the endoscope, the coagulum is gently removed using the edge of the cap, debriding proximal to distally in a circumferential manner and thereafter flushing and cleaning with saline. The endoscope is removed and then the cap discarded.

6. *Second ablation pass*: The cleaned ablation catheter device is then introduced over the guidewire with the endoscope and a second ablation is performed as described previously retreating the area and further coagulating any superficial blood vessels preventing bleeding.

A simplified technique for c-RFA omitting the cleaning phase where the device is not removed or cleaned is also effective as the above-described standard technique. The effectiveness has been demonstrated in a randomized study showing that the mean

BE surface regression at 3 months post-RFA was 83% compared to 88% in the non-cleaning group ($P = .14$).[19] The time was significantly reduced from 20 minutes to 5 minutes, and there was a decrease in the median number of introductions of RFA devices/endoscope from 7 to 4 using this technique.

Focal Ablation

f-RFA is performed for treating shorter segments and tongues or islands of BE, noted during follow-up after initial c-RFA (**Fig. 5**) (**Box 2**). This procedure may also be of special use in treating areas adjacent to the squamocolumnar junction (SCJ). After careful endoscopic examination, the areas are recorded and endoscope removed while externally the HALO[90] device (array measuring 13 × 20 mm, treatment surface area, 2.6 cm^2) is attached to the tip of the scope. The device is positioned such that the back of the thumb-shaped array is located at 12'o-clock position on the endoscopic field of view and can be pivoted easily; it is reintroduced into the esophagus after careful intubation. The esophagus is washed with *N*-acetylcysteine solution. The targeted area of BE is identified and the endoscope is angulated such that the ablation device is tightly opposed to the targeted mucosa. After maintaining optimal contact, the energy is delivered using the foot pedal at energy settings of 15 J/cm^2. While maintaining the same position, a second pulse of energy is given. The device is then moved to the next treatment area and the above-mentioned steps repeated, treating all visualized BE.

A

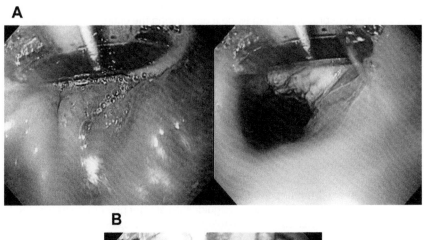

B

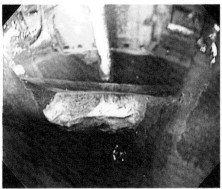

Fig. 5. f-RFA (*A*) Positioning of device; (*B*) ablation.

The coagulum of desiccated mucosa is then removed using a HALO cap as previously described. Also, the tip of the ablation device could be used to scrape the tissue. After gentle debridement, the device is externally cleaned using damp gauze, reintroduced while mounted on the scope, and a second round of 2 applications (2 times) per area are performed in an identical manner. Thus, each targeted area receives a total of 4 energy ablations. A recent multicenter randomized trial suggested that a simplified (3 × 15 J/cm² without cleaning) f-RFA regimen is not inferior to the standard regimen (2 × 2 15 J/cm² with cleaning followed by 2 × 2 15 J/cm²) of the complete endoscopic removal of residual Barrett's islands.[20] This modification may shorten the overall procedural time and limit the number of endoscopic intubations per session.

The smaller f-RFA devices such as the Barrx 60 (treatment surface area 1.6 cm²) and the through the Channel RFA endoscopic catheter (treatment surface area 1.2 cm²) may be useful. The advantage of these smaller f-RFA devices is their smaller size and ability to be advanced through the working channel of the scope, therefore making them useful in patients with difficult esophageal anatomy who require RFA for BE, including those with esophageal stenosis, diverticuli, and pharyngeal pouches.[21,22]

Postprocedural Care and Follow-up

After RFA treatment, patients may experience chest pain and dysphagia for 3 to 4 days. Postcare includes pain management with viscous lidocaine or liquid acetaminophen with narcotic. A liquid diet is advised for 24 hours after treatment, and then the patient can slowly return to normal diet. A maintenance dose of proton pump inhibitors (PPI) such as esomeprazole, 40 mg twice a day, during the entire treatment period for adequate acid suppression is recommended to promote healing. In addition, sucralfate, 1 g 4 times a day for 2 weeks, is prescribed. Patients are usually discharged home on the day of the procedure. On occasion, severe chest pain may require admission for observation and optimizing pain management.

A follow-up for 2 months after the initial ablation is scheduled when patients are reassessed for further treatment or 4-quadrant biopsies if neosquamous epithelium is seen. Particular focus is given to the neo-SCJ (Z-line) and the region distal to this where recurrence seems to be common. Approximately 3 to 4 treatment sessions may be necessary to clear all dysplastic BE, and this depends on the length of segment. After histology has confirmed complete eradication of IM (CE-IM) and/or CE-D, follow-up endoscopies are scheduled at 3, 6, and 12 months and annually thereafter (eg, every 3 months for 1 year, then every 6 months for 1 year, and then every 1 year) (**Table 1**). [23] Clear follow-up guidelines are not present, therefore the frequency of follow-up depends on the histologic grade of dysplasia and other risk factors that might predict recurrence as discussed below.

OUTCOMES

RFA is effective for treatment of HGD and LGD.[3] In a randomized sham controlled trial, complete eradication of HGD (CE-HGD) was noted in 81.0% of the ablation group compared with 19.0% of the control group. Similarly, disease progression was lower in the ablation group (3.6% vs 16.3%).[24] Eradication of LGD was achieved in 90.5% of the ablation group when compared with 22.7% of the control group at the end of 12 months. Durability of RFA was demonstrated with eradication of dysplasia and metaplasia in 98% and 91%, respectively, at the end of 3 years from ablation therapy.[25] However, recent studies have noted recurrence of IM and dysplasia in up to 33% of patients at 2 years underscoring the need for postablation surveillance.[26] Another recent analysis from the US RFA registry showed that the incidence rate of

EAC postablation per 1000 person-years was highest (30.2, 95% confidence interval [CI], 24.1–37.4) in patients treated for HGD with RFA.[27,28]

A multicenter study from Europe looked at predictors of poor response to initial RFA treatment in patients treated for HGD. Four independent baseline predictors of poor response were observed: active reflux esophagitis (odds ratio [OR] 38; 95% CI, 3.2–4.33), endoscopic resection scar regeneration with Barrett's epithelium (OR, 4.7; 95 %CI, 1.1–20.0), esophageal narrowing pre-RFA (OR, 3.9; 95% CI, 1.0–15.1), and years of neoplasia pre-RFA (OR, 1.2; 95% CI, 1.0–1.4). Other risk factors contributing to failure of RFA are longer segment of BE, gastric bypass or large hiatal hernias, baseline histology showing more advanced dysplasia or neoplasia, incomplete healing between treatment sessions, female sex, persistent reflux, and the need for multiple treatment sessions.[28–33] A more recent study of the durability and predictors of successful RFA from the US RFA Registry noted that BE recurred in 20% of patients followed up for an average of 2.4 years after CE-IM. Older age, non-white race, and increasing length of BE segment were independent risk factors.[34] These factors should be taken into consideration when planning the follow-up and further surveillance.

Even though RFA has a short learning curve, the higher endoscopist RFA volume correlates with successful BE eradication. Therefore, better quality measures may be required for performing RFA and improving overall outcomes.[35,36]

COMPLICATIONS AND MANAGEMENT

RFA using the HALO system has a low complication rate. Chest pain and dysphagia are commonly associated symptoms lasting for a period of 3 to 4 days posttreatment and resolve spontaneously to baseline.[37,38] Strictures can occur on follow-up, and the rate varies between 0% and 8% with longer segments and preceding EMR being the greater risk factors for developing them; however, they can be managed by endoscopic dilatation. Bleeding is rare (<1%) and encountered especially in patients on antiplatelet or anticoagulation therapy. No perforations or deaths have been reported after RFA. Fever is also a rare complication and can be managed using antipyretics. Buried IM or glands have been of concern postablation and may not be visible endoscopically; these are less frequently reported after RFA (0.9%) and highlight the need for deep endoscopic biopsies, which need to be carefully reviewed by the dedicated pathologist.[39]

CRYOABLATION

Cryoablation therapy refers to the application of extremely cold temperatures to induce tissue injury. Cryoablation is a noncontact ablative technique using cycles of rapid freezing and thawing resulting in tissue destruction, fracturing of cell membranes, and denaturation of proteins.[40] On endoscopic examination the treatment effect seems minimal at first, with development of cherry red appearance of the mucosa with minimal ooze of blood during reperfusion. However, over time, the tissue sloughs off and heals resulting in neosquamous epithelium.

Devices can deliver either commercially available cyrogens such as liquid nitrogen or carbon dioxide. The authors' personal experience has been with liquid nitrogen using the CryoSpray Ablation System (CSA Medical, Inc., Baltimore, MD, USA). The technique involves the over-the-wire advancement of a 16F-diameter decompression tube, which is essentially a modified orogastric tube with venting ports spanning the distal 12 in, into the antrum. This step allows decompression of the evaporated cryogen from the stomach and esophagus during treatment, thus preventing perforation due to overinsufflation of the lumen. A spray catheter is then advanced through the working channel of the endoscope, and the liquid cryogen is sprayed onto the targeted area (low-pressure liquid nitrogen [<5 psi] at −196°C, with energy delivery of 25 W). Continuous suction is applied to the decompression tube throughout the cryotherapy procedure, which lasts for 20-second cycle of deep freeze followed by thawing for 60 seconds; 2 to 3 cm of BE can be treated while covering about one-third or one-half of luminal circumference. Two to three cycles per area can be performed in between the thaw. Using a transparent endoscopic cap is helpful for targeting the spray delivery and also for preventing the scope lens from frosting. Typically 3 to 4 endoscopy sessions are needed to completely ablate a long segment of BE, and procedures can be performed every 6 to 8 weeks (**Fig. 6**). The adverse events are minimal with reported stricture rates in 3% responding to esophageal dilatation and chest pain in 2% being managed conservatively.

There are no randomized controlled studies assessing the efficacy of cryotherapy in the treatment of dysplastic BE. In a multicenter retrospective study of patients treated with HGD, 97% of patients had CE-HGD and 87% had CE-D.[41] A durability study with 2-year follow-up showed that CE-HGD was 100% and CE-IM was 84% at 2-year follow-up. The investigators noted recurrent HGD in 16%.[42] Recurrent disease was found to mainly involve the area just below the neo-SCJ. A retrospective study for cryotherapy in EAC showed eradication of T1a (mucosal) tumors in 18 (75%) of 24 patients.[43] For T1b (submucosal) tumors, complete eradication was seen in 4 (60%) of 6 patients with a mean follow-up of 11.8 months. There have been no studies comparing cryotherapy to RFA. Similarly, the cost-effectiveness of cryotherapy has not been compared with that of other ablation methods. At present, cryotherapy is being offered to patients in whom RFA might have failed or who are poor candidates for surgery. There is an ongoing Dose-Optimization Study for the Initial Treatment of Dysplastic BE using trūFreeze Spray Cryotherapy (DOSE) (ClinicalTrials.gov Identifier: NCT01845454) that should shed further light on the usefulness of the therapy.

PHOTODYNAMIC ABLATION

PDT uses the photochemical energy of photosensitizer drugs (porphimer sodium [Ps], 4-aminolevulinic acid [ALA], or *m*-tetrahydroxyphenyl chlorine), which are

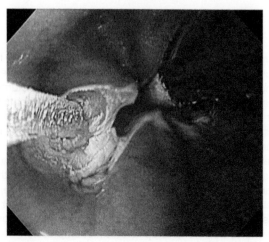

Fig. 6. Cryoablation.

administered systemically. The most widely used is Ps, which is administered intravenously 2 days before the procedure to ensure adequate drug distribution. The porphimers are concentrated in the neoplastic tissue and then are activated by endoscopically delivered laser light of appropriate power and wavelength. The light dose is determined by the type of delivery system such that the balloon catheter system requires 130 J/cm fiber and the bare fiber technique requires 200 J/cm fiber.[14] This activation stimulates a photodynamic reaction where the drug reacts with oxygen to generate free radicals inducing cell damage and apoptosis. This reaction allows for targeted therapy with wide field application and significant depth of tissue penetration. ALA seems to have slightly lesser side effects compared with Ps owing to its shorter half-life and more superficial effect, as shown in a randomized comparative trial.[44]

A large multicenter study comparing PDT to PPI showed that the rate of IM eradication was 52% vs 7%, rate of HGD eradication was 77% vs 39%, and rate of progression to cancer 13% vs 28%, respectively.[45] The same group showed the maintenance of these results after 5 years of follow-up.[46]

Complications during PDT include skin photosensitivity, stricture formation, the need for endoscopic therapy, and odynophagia. The stricture rate can be as high as 36%,[46] and this limits its widespread use. In a comparative nonrandomized study, RFA had less complications and reduced cost compared with PDT for the treatment of BE-related dysplasia.[47]

CURRENT CONTROVERSIES/FUTURE CONSIDERATIONS

A diagnosis of dysplasia in BE increases the risk for malignant progression, and there is strong evidence to support the use of endoscopic eradication therapy in HGD (**Fig. 7**).[48] Ablative therapy is deemed appropriate in patients in whom the disease is limited to the mucosa with no nodal involvement and who have been adequately staged/resected by EMR for visible lesions.[49–53] Among all methods currently available, RFA is the most studied cost-effective ablative treatment modality with a high safety margin.[24,25,54–56] There are not enough head-to-head comparative studies between the available ablative modalities. Therefore, further studies understanding the role of multimodal ablative therapy will be useful.

Treatment in LGD is still not clear because of poor agreement among GI pathologists on its diagnosis and also wide variation in data on long-term outcomes. While progression rates to HGD or intramucosal cancer (IMCa) are less than 1.4% per year,[57,58] data from Europe have documented a 13.4% per year progression rate (confirmed by 2 expert pathologists).[59] The European data support the notion that confirmed LGD has a higher risk of developing into cancer. A meta-analysis also pointed that there was high likelihood of overdiagnosis for LGD.[60] Nonetheless, a decision Markov model concluded that ablation of LGD could be a cost-effective strategy provided the diagnosis was accurate.[54] In a recent study of patients undergoing RFA for LGD, RFA reduced the risk of progression to HGD or IMCa from 26.5% to 1.5% with an absolute risk reduction of 25%.[61] The stricture rate was 11.8%, although it was resolved with a median of 1 endoscopic dilatation. These studies point to the importance of expert pathologist's review of histology, adequate biopsies to avoid sampling error, as well as appropriate risk stratification considering the length of segment, age, family history, and other important factors before offering RFA immediately.[62]

At present, there is no role for ablative therapy in nondysplastic BE.[63] The efficacy of long-term effects of RFA has not been established in this group. Although the risk of progression to EAC is very low,[5] there could be hidden subsquamous IM and IM can

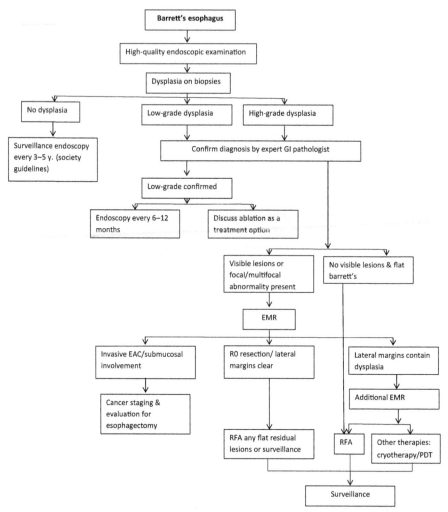

Fig. 7. Algorithm approach for treatment of BE.

recur over time; these factors outweigh the benefits of performing ablative therapy. It is also important to highlight that RFA requires multiple sessions associated with related costs; RFA is associated with stricturing, which is a known complication; and moreover, RFA does not obviate endoscopic surveillance.[64,65]

There is growing evidence that endoscopic treatment may not always result in remission of BE. Biomarkers and improved risk stratification (clinical and histologic) are needed to better identify these patients and plan adequate management and surveillance protocols.[66–68] A recent retrospective study showed that the presence of multiple gains detected by brush cytology specimens and FISH was a negative predictor to response rate for endoscopic therapy.[69] Concomitant treatment of acid reflux with PPIs and continuous surveillance are essential for better success outcomes and maintaining the stability of the neosquamous epithelium. However, prior fundoplication did not improve safety and efficacy outcomes for patients undergoing RFA.[70,71] It is not clear if fundoplication in select individuals will be beneficial in preventing post-RFA recurrence. Future trials will focus on refining ablation therapy such that the numbers of sessions are reduced as well as tailoring therapy to a specific identified risk group. Newer knowledge on the process of epithelialization will help in preventing recurrences as well as optimize the success of ablation.

SUMMARY

At present, endoscopic therapy for BE with dysplasia has established itself as the treatment method of choice. Ablation offers to achieve CE-D and specialized CE-IM of the esophagus resulting in squamous reepithelialization of esophagus. Among the ablative modalities, RFA is the most studied with safe, effective, and durable long-term treatment outcomes. RFA is clearly effective either alone or in combination with endoscopic resection for HGD. The role of RFA in LGD is still in debate, but it can be offered as an alternate treatment in select patients. There is currently no role of ablation in nondysplastic BE. Cryotherapy and PDT can be offered in select patients when RFA has failed. Future research focusing on the natural disease progression, biomarkers, advanced imaging, as well as quality indices both clinical and endoscopic will lead to better clinical outcomes.

REFERENCES

1. Shaheen NJ, Crosby MA, Bozymski EM, et al. Is there publication bias in the reporting of cancer risk in Barrett's esophagus? Gastroenterology 2000;119:333–8.
2. Hvid-Jensen F, Pedersen L, Drewes AM, et al. Incidence of adenocarcinoma among patients with Barrett's esophagus. N Engl J Med 2011;365:1375–83.
3. American Gastroenterological Association, Spechler SJ, Sharma P, et al. American Gastroenterological Association medical position statement on the management of Barrett's esophagus. Gastroenterology 2011;140:1084–91.
4. Desai TK, Krishnan K, Samala N, et al. The incidence of oesophageal adenocarcinoma in non-dysplastic Barrett's oesophagus: a meta-analysis. Gut 2012;61:970–6.
5. Wani S, Falk G, Hall M, et al. Patients with nondysplastic Barrett's esophagus have low risks for developing dysplasia or esophageal adenocarcinoma. Clin Gastroenterol Hepatol 2011;9:220–7 [quiz: e26].
6. Spechler SJ, Souza RF. Barrett's esophagus. N Engl J Med 2014;371:836–45.
7. Zagari RM, Fuccio L, Wallander MA, et al. Gastro-oesophageal reflux symptoms, oesophagitis and Barrett's oesophagus in the general population: the Loiano-Monghidoro study. Gut 2008;57:1354–9.
8. Taylor JB, Rubenstein JH. Meta-analyses of the effect of symptoms of gastro-esophageal reflux on the risk of Barrett's esophagus. Am J Gastroenterol 2010;105:1729, 1730–7. [quiz: 38].
9. Ronkainen J, Talley NJ, Storskrubb T, et al. Erosive esophagitis is a risk factor for Barrett's esophagus: a community-based endoscopic follow-up study. Am J Gastroenterol 2011;106:1946–52.
10. Rastogi A, Puli S, El-Serag HB, et al. Incidence of esophageal adenocarcinoma in patients with Barrett's esophagus and high-grade dysplasia: a meta-analysis. Gastrointest Endosc 2008;67:394–8.
11. Spechler SJ. Barrett esophagus and risk of esophageal cancer: a clinical review. JAMA 2013;310:627–36.
12. Kong CY, Kroep S, Curtius K, et al. Exploring the recent trend in esophageal adenocarcinoma incidence and mortality using comparative simulation modeling. Cancer Epidemiol Biomarkers Prev 2014;23:997–1006.

13. Sarosi G, Brown G, Jaiswal K, et al. Bone marrow progenitor cells contribute to esophageal regeneration and metaplasia in a rat model of Barrett's esophagus. Dis Esophagus 2008;21:43–50.
14. Leggett CL, Gorospe EC, Wang KK. Endoscopic therapy for Barrett's esophagus and early esophageal adenocarcinoma. Gastroenterol Clin North Am 2013;42:175–85.
15. Pouw RE, Gondrie JJ, Rygiel AM, et al. Properties of the neosquamous epithelium after radiofrequency ablation of Barrett's esophagus containing neoplasia. Am J Gastroenterol 2009;104:1366–73.
16. Sharma P, Dent J, Armstrong D, et al. The development and validation of an endoscopic grading system for Barrett's esophagus: the Prague C & M criteria. Gastroenterology 2006;131:1392–9.
17. Levine DS, Haggitt RC, Blount PL, et al. An endoscopic biopsy protocol can differentiate high-grade dysplasia from early adenocarcinoma in Barrett's esophagus. Gastroenterology 1993;105:40–50.
18. ASGE Standards of Practice Committee, Evans JA, Early DS, et al. The role of endoscopy in Barrett's esophagus and other premalignant conditions of the esophagus. Gastrointest Endosc 2012;76:1087–94.
19. van Vilsteren FG, Phoa KN, Alvarez Herrero L, et al. Circumferential balloon-based radiofrequency ablation of Barrett's esophagus with dysplasia can be simplified, yet efficacy maintained, by omitting the cleaning phase. Clin Gastroenterol Hepatol 2013;11:491–8.e1.
20. van Vilsteren FG, Phoa KN, Alvarez Herrero L, et al. A simplified regimen for focal radiofrequency ablation of Barrett's mucosa: a randomized multicenter trial comparing two ablation regimens. Gastrointest Endosc 2013;78:30–8.
21. Peter S, Wilcox CM, Monkemuller K. Radiofrequency ablation of Barrett's esophagus with the channel RFA endoscopic catheter. Gastrointest Endosc 2014;79:1034–5.
22. Allen B, Kapoor N, Willert R, et al. Endoscopic ablation of Barrett's neoplasia with a new focal radiofrequency device: initial experience with the Halo60. Endoscopy 2012;44:707–10.
23. Fitzgerald RC, Rubenstein JH. Oracular guidance on clinical management of early neoplastic Barrett's esophagus. Gastroenterology 2012;143:282–4.
24. Shaheen NJ, Sharma P, Overholt BF, et al. Radiofrequency ablation in Barrett's esophagus with dysplasia. N Engl J Med 2009;360:2277–88.
25. Shaheen NJ, Overholt BF, Sampliner RE, et al. Durability of radiofrequency ablation in Barrett's esophagus with dysplasia. Gastroenterology 2011;141:460–8.
26. Gupta M, Iyer PG, Lutzke L, et al. Recurrence of esophageal intestinal metaplasia after endoscopic mucosal resection and radiofrequency ablation of Barrett's esophagus: results from a US Multicenter Consortium. Gastroenterology 2013;145:79–86 e1.
27. Wolf WA, Dellon ES, Shaheen NJ. Esophageal diseases. Gastrointest Endosc 2014;80:374–9.
28. Wolf WA, Pruitt RE, Ertan A, et al. Sa1452 Predictors of Esophageal Adenocarcinoma in Patients With Prior Radiofrequency Ablation (RFA) for Treatment of Barrett's Esophagus: Results From the U.S. RFA Registry. Gastrointest Endosc 2014;79:AB217.
29. Dunbar KB. Endoscopic eradication therapy for mucosal neoplasia in Barrett's esophagus. Curr Opin Gastroenterol 2013;29:446–53.
30. Bulsiewicz WJ, Kim HP, Dellon ES, et al. Safety and efficacy of endoscopic mucosal therapy with radiofrequency ablation for patients with neoplastic Barrett's esophagus. Clin Gastroenterol Hepatol 2013;11:636–42.

31. Akiyama J, Marcus SN, Triadafilopoulos G. Effective intra-esophageal acid control is associated with improved radiofrequency ablation outcomes in Barrett's esophagus. Dig Dis Sci 2012;57:2625–32.
32. Krishnan K, Pandolfino JE, Kahrilas PJ, et al. Increased risk for persistent intestinal metaplasia in patients with Barrett's esophagus and uncontrolled reflux exposure before radiofrequency ablation. Gastroenterology 2012;143:576–81.
33. Korst RJ, Santana-Joseph S, Rutledge JR, et al. Patterns of recurrent and persistent intestinal metaplasia after successful radiofrequency ablation of Barrett's esophagus. J Thorac Cardiovasc Surg 2013;145:1529–34.
34. Pasricha S, Bulsiewicz WJ, Hathorn KE, et al. Durability and predictors of successful radiofrequency ablation for Barrett's esophagus. Clin Gastroenterol Hepatol 2014;12:1840–7.e1.
35. Zemlyak AY, Pacicco T, Mahmud EM, et al. Radiofrequency ablation offers a reliable surgical modality for the treatment of Barrett's esophagus with a minimal learning curve. Am Surg 2012;78:774–8.
36. Fudman DI, Lightdale CJ, Poneros JM, et al. Positive correlation between endoscopist radiofrequency ablation volume and response rates in Barrett's esophagus. Gastrointest Endosc 2014;80:71–7.
37. Sharma VK. Ablation of Barrett's esophagus using the HALO radiofrequency ablation system. Tech Gastrointest Endosc 2010;12:26–34.
38. van Vilsteren FG, Bergman JJ. Endoscopic therapy using radiofrequency ablation for esophageal dysplasia and carcinoma in Barrett's esophagus. Gastrointest Endosc Clin N Am 2010;20:55–74, vi.
39. Gray NA, Odze RD, Spechler SJ. Buried metaplasia after endoscopic ablation of Barrett's esophagus: a systematic review. Am J Gastroenterol 2011;106:1899–908 [quiz: 909].
40. Greenwald BD, Dumot JA. Cryotherapy for Barrett's esophagus and esophageal cancer. Curr Opin Gastroenterol 2011;27:363–7.
41. Shaheen NJ, Greenwald BD, Peery AF, et al. Safety and efficacy of endoscopic spray cryotherapy for Barrett's esophagus with high-grade dysplasia. Gastrointest Endosc 2010;71:680–5.
42. Gosain S, Mercer K, Twaddell WS, et al. Liquid nitrogen spray cryotherapy in Barrett's esophagus with high-grade dysplasia: long-term results. Gastrointest Endosc 2013;78:260–5.
43. Greenwald BD, Dumot JA, Abrams JA, et al. Endoscopic spray cryotherapy for esophageal cancer: safety and efficacy. Gastrointest Endosc 2010;71:686–93.
44. Dunn JM, Mackenzie GD, Banks MR, et al. A randomised controlled trial of ALA vs. Photofrin photodynamic therapy for high-grade dysplasia arising in Barrett's oesophagus. Lasers Med Sci 2013;28:707–15.
45. Overholt BF, Lightdale CJ, Wang KK, et al. Photodynamic therapy with porfimer sodium for ablation of high-grade dysplasia in Barrett's esophagus: international, partially blinded, randomized phase III trial. Gastrointest Endosc 2005;62:488–98.
46. Overholt BF, Wang KK, Burdick JS, et al. Five-year efficacy and safety of photodynamic therapy with Photofrin in Barrett's high-grade dysplasia. Gastrointest Endosc 2007;66:460–8.
47. Ertan A, Zaheer I, Correa AM, et al. Photodynamic therapy vs radiofrequency ablation for Barrett's dysplasia: efficacy, safety and cost-comparison. World J Gastroenterol 2013;19:7106–13.
48. Rees JR, Lao-Sirieix P, Wong A, et al. Treatment for Barrett's oesophagus. Cochrane Database Syst Rev 2010;(1):CD004060.

49. Kim HP, Bulsiewicz WJ, Cotton CC, et al. Focal endoscopic mucosal resection before radiofrequency ablation is equally effective and safe compared with radiofrequency ablation alone for the eradication of Barrett's esophagus with advanced neoplasia. Gastrointest Endosc 2012;76:733–9.

50. Bennett C, Vakil N, Bergman J, et al. Consensus statements for management of Barrett's dysplasia and early-stage esophageal adenocarcinoma, based on a Delphi process. Gastroenterology 2012;143:336–46.

51. Haidry RJ, Dunn JM, Butt MA, et al. Radiofrequency ablation and endoscopic mucosal resection for dysplastic Barrett's esophagus and early esophageal adenocarcinoma: outcomes of the UK National Halo RFA Registry. Gastroenterology 2013;145:87–95.

52. Fitzgerald RC, di Pietro M, Ragunath K, et al. British Society of Gastroenterology guidelines on the diagnosis and management of Barrett's oesophagus. Gut 2014; 63:7–42.

53. Prasad GA, Buttar NS, Wongkeesong LM, et al. Significance of neoplastic involvement of margins obtained by endoscopic mucosal resection in Barrett's esophagus. Am J Gastroenterol 2007;102:2380–6.

54. Hur C, Choi SE, Rubenstein JH, et al. The cost effectiveness of radiofrequency ablation for Barrett's esophagus. Gastroenterology 2012;143:567–75.

55. Inadomi JM, Somsouk M, Madanick RD, et al. A cost-utility analysis of ablative therapy for Barrett's esophagus. Gastroenterology 2009;136:2101–14.e1–6.

56. Shaheen NJ, Peery AF, Hawes RH, et al. Quality of life following radiofrequency ablation of dysplastic Barrett's esophagus. Endoscopy 2010;42:790–9.

57. Wani S, Falk GW, Post J, et al. Risk factors for progression of low-grade dysplasia in patients with Barrett's esophagus. Gastroenterology 2011;141:1179–86, 1186.e1.

58. Bhat S, Coleman HG, Yousef F, et al. Risk of malignant progression in Barrett's esophagus patients: results from a large population-based study. J Natl Cancer Inst 2011;103:1049–57.

59. Curvers WL, ten Kate FJ, Krishnadath KK, et al. Low-grade dysplasia in Barrett's esophagus: overdiagnosed and underestimated. Am J Gastroenterol 2010;105: 1523–30.

60. Almond LM, Hodson J, Barr H. Meta-analysis of endoscopic therapy for low-grade dysplasia in Barrett's oesophagus. Br J Surg 2014;101:1187–95.

61. Phoa KN, van Vilsteren FG, Weusten BL, et al. Radiofrequency ablation vs endoscopic surveillance for patients with Barrett esophagus and low-grade dysplasia: a randomized clinical trial. JAMA 2014;311:1209–17.

62. Monkemuller K. Radiofrequency ablation for Barrett esophagus with confirmed low-grade dysplasia. JAMA 2014;311:1205–6.

63. Spechler SJ, Sharma P, Souza RF, et al. American Gastroenterological A. American Gastroenterological Association technical review on the management of Barrett's esophagus. Gastroenterology 2011;140:e18–52 [quiz: e13].

64. Spechler SJ. Barrett's esophagus without dysplasia: wait or ablate? Dig Dis Sci 2011;56:1926–8.

65. Dunbar KB, Spechler SJ. Controversies in Barrett esophagus. Mayo Clin Proc 2014;89:973–84.

66. Gregson EM, Fitzgerald RC. Biomarkers for dysplastic Barrett's: ready for prime time? World J Surg 2014;39(3):568–77.

67. Prasad GA, Bansal A, Sharma P, et al. Predictors of progression in Barrett's esophagus: current knowledge and future directions. Am J Gastroenterol 2010; 105:1490–502.

68. Prasad GA, Wang KK, Halling KC, et al. Utility of biomarkers in prediction of response to ablative therapy in Barrett's esophagus. Gastroenterology 2008; 135:370–9.
69. Timmer MR, Brankley SM, Gorospe EC, et al. Prediction of response to endoscopic therapy of Barrett's dysplasia by using genetic biomarkers. Gastrointest Endosc 2014;80:984–91.
70. Shaheen NJ, Kim HP, Bulsiewicz WJ, et al. Prior fundoplication does not improve safety or efficacy outcomes of radiofrequency ablation: results from the U.S. RFA Registry. J Gastrointest Surg 2013;17:21–8 [discussion: p. 28–9].
71. Frantz DJ, Dellon ES, Shaheen NJ. Radiofrequency ablation of Barrett's esophagus. Tech Gastrointest Endosc 2010;12:100–7.

Challenges with Endoscopic Therapy for Barrett's Esophagus

 CrossMark

Sachin Wani, MD[a],*, Prateek Sharma, MD[b]

KEYWORDS

- Barrett's esophagus • Esophageal adenocarcinoma
- Endoscopic eradication therapy • Endoscopic mucosal resection
- Radiofrequency ablation

KEY POINTS

- Endoscopic eradication therapy (EET) has revolutionized the management of Barrett's-related dysplasia and intramucosal cancer, a practice that has essentially replaced esophagectomy as the standard of care for management of this patient population and been endorsed by gastroenterology societal guidelines.
- Candidates for EET are patients with Barrett's-related high-grade dysplasia, intramucosal cancer, and confirmed low-grade dysplasia.
- Evaluation and management should be considered at expert centers and should involve endoscopic mucosal resection of all visible lesions followed by eradication of the remaining Barrett's esophagus.
- Techniques most commonly used for EET include endoscopic mucosal resection, radiofrequency ablation, cryotherapy, and a combination of therapies termed multimodality EET.
- Patients should be enrolled in surveillance programs given the risk of recurrent intestinal metaplasia and dysplasia.

Disclosures: S. Wani was supported by the American Gastroenterological Association Takeda Research Scholar Award in GERD and Barrett's esophagus and University of Colorado Department of Medicine Early Scholars Award. He received grant support from Cook Medical. He is a consultant for Covidien. P. Sharma received grant support from Barrx Medical, CDX Labs, Cook Medical, Ninepoint Medical, and Olympus Inc.
[a] Division of Gastroenterology and Hepatology, University of Colorado Anschutz Medical Campus, Mail Stop F735, 1635 Aurora Court, Room 2.031, Aurora, CO 80045, USA; [b] Division of Gastroenterology and Hepatology, Veterans Affairs Medical Center and University of Kansas, 4801 Linwood Boulevard, Kansas City, MO 64128, USA
* Corresponding author.
E-mail address: sachinwani10@yahoo.com

Gastroenterol Clin N Am 44 (2015) 355–372
http://dx.doi.org/10.1016/j.gtc.2015.02.007
gastro.theclinics.com

INTRODUCTION

Barrett's esophagus (BE) is the only identifiable premalignant condition for esophageal adenocarcinoma (EAC), a cancer that has increased nearly six-fold over the past three decades and is associated with a poor 5-year survival rate of less than 20% (all stages) especially when detected at a symptomatic state.[1–3] BE is believed to progress to EAC in a probabilistic manner through recognizable histologic stages of intestinal metaplasia, low-grade dysplasia (LGD), high-grade dysplasia (HGD), intramucosal cancer, and finally invasive cancer (submucosal invasion and beyond). Endoscopic eradication therapy (EET) has revolutionized the management of Barrett's-related dysplasia and intramucosal cancer, a practice that has essentially replaced esophagectomy as the standard of care for management of this patient population and endorsed by gastroenterology societal guidelines.[4–6] The primary goal of EET is to prevent progression to invasive EAC and ultimately improve survival rates. This is achieved with therapies that focus on removal of neoplastic mucosa by endoscopic mucosal resection (EMR) and ablative techniques (used alone or in combination) followed by acid suppression, which result in re-epithelialization with squamous mucosa.

The basic premise of recommending EET is that patients with cancer limited to the mucosa have a low risk (0%–2%) of lymph node metastasis. A systematic review that included 1350 BE-associated intramucosal cancer cases that underwent esophagectomy and lymph node analysis reported a nodal metastasis rate of 1.9% (95% confidence interval [CI], 1.1–2.6). No lymph node metastasis was found in 524 BE-associated HGD cases that underwent esophagectomy.[7] Patients with submucosal invasion, poorly differentiated cancer, size greater than 2 cm, and lymphovascular infiltration should be referred for surgical resection given the high risk of lymph node metastasis (>20%).[8,9] The basic principles of EET are as follows: (1) resection of all neoplastic visible lesions (lesions typically with the highest grade of neoplasia), (2) eradication of the remaining BE to reduce the risk of metachronous neoplasia[10] (up to 30%), (3) management of adverse events, and (4) enrollment in surveillance programs and address the issue of recurrence of intestinal metaplasia and neoplasia.

With this background, it should be noted that there are several challenges with EET that can be encountered before, during, or after the procedure that are important to understand to optimize the effectiveness and safety of EET and ultimately improve patient outcomes. This article focuses on the challenges with EET discussed under the categories preprocedural, intraprocedural, and postprocedural challenges.

PREPROCEDURAL CHALLENGES
Candidates for Endoscopic Eradication Therapy

Despite all the advances in biomarkers and challenges associated with the diagnosis of dysplasia, the grade of dysplasia is currently the best biomarker to predict progression in patients with BE and is used frequently to determine if a patient is an ideal candidate for EET.

High-grade dysplasia and intramucosal cancer
The diagnosis of HGD in patients with BE is associated with a high yearly rate of progression to EAC (approximately 6% per year based on a meta-analysis with higher rates reported in other prospective randomized controlled trials).[11–13] Coupled with evidence demonstrating efficacy and effectiveness of EET, this is an actionable diagnosis. Similarly, several large cohort studies have demonstrated favorable outcomes with EET in patients with BE-related intramucosal cancer.[14–16] In a series of 1000 consecutive patients who underwent EMR for BE-related intramucosal cancer,

complete eradication of neoplasia was achieved in 96.3% of patients at a mean follow-up of nearly 5 years with a long-term remission rate of 93.8%.[15] Thus, patients with BE-related HGD and intramucosal cancer are ideal candidates for EET.

Low-grade dysplasia

There are several issues regarding the natural history of LGD that make the management of this group of patients highly controversial. First and foremost, several studies have demonstrated significant degree of interobserver variability in the diagnosis of LGD, even among expert gastrointestinal pathologists,[17–19] which has likely contributed to the variable published rates of progression to HGD/EAC.[17,20–24] Consistent with previously published studies addressing interobserver variability with diagnosis of LGD, in a multicenter cohort study, we showed that the interobserver agreement among two expert pathologists for the diagnosis of LGD was slight (kappa = 0.14).[17] These data stress the need for revision of criteria used to make the diagnosis of LGD in clinical practice. In this cohort of patients that included 210 patients with BE with LGD, the annual incidence of EAC was 0.44% (95% CI, 0.2–0.98) and 1.83% (95% CI, 1.23–2.74) for a combined end point of HGD/EAC.[17] Similarly, the Danish population-based cohort study reported an annual incidence of 1.27% (95% CI, 0.9–1.79) for HGD/EAC.[23] In a recent retrospective study that included 293 patients with LGD, expert pathology review resulted in down-staging of LGD diagnosis to non-dysplastic BE (NDBE) or indeterminate for dysplasia in 73% and confirmation of LGD diagnosis in 27% of cases. In patients with confirmed diagnosis of LGD, the risk of progression to HGD/EAC was 9.1% per patient-year compared with 0.6% in patients with NDBE. These data validate the current recommendations that require expert pathologist confirmation of dysplasia in BE especially before making crucial management decisions (EET vs conservative management of surveillance).

With regards to the decision regarding EET, current American Gastroenterological Association recommendations suggest either surveillance at 6 to 12 months or EET, and the concept of shared decision making between the patient and endoscopist is emphasized.[4] However, a recent randomized controlled trial (discussed later) that compared radiofrequency ablation (RFA) with surveillance showed that ablation was associated with a 25% reduction in risk of progression to HGD/EAC.[25] Thus, RFA should be considered in patients with BE with a confirmed diagnosis of LGD on a case-by-case basis (diagnosis confirmed on more than one endoscopy, by expert gastrointestinal pathologists, possibly multifocal LGD, and in centers reporting a high rate of LGD progression).

Nondysplastic Barrett's esophagus

Several arguments have been made for ablation of patients with NDBE, the two most common being lack of impact of endoscopic surveillance on mortality from BE-associated EAC and effectiveness and safety of RFA.[26] The paradigm of surveillance in NDBE was challenged in a recent case-control study that compared the frequency of surveillance endoscopy among 38 cases (BE cases who subsequently died as a result of EAC) with a sample of 101 living cases with BE (control subjects) matched for age, sex, and follow-up evaluation. Endoscopic surveillance was not associated with a decreased risk of death from EAC (adjusted odds ratio, 0.99; 95% CI, 0.36–2.75).[27] However, there are several reasons for not ablating all patients with NDBE: (1) low risk of HGD and cancer in NDBE as demonstrated by several contemporary studies,[22,23,28] (2) prohibitively higher number of cases required to ablate to prevent one case of EAC in patients with NDBE,[29] (3) risk of recurrence of intestinal metaplasia and lack of data on long-term cancer risk postablation, (4) need for ongoing surveillance even postablation and achieving the end point of complete eradication of intestinal metaplasia, (5) ablation is associated with well-defined risks and adverse events, and (6) decision analysis studies have shown that ablation of NDBE is not cost-effective.[30] The authors do not recommend ablation of patients with NDBE and future studies should focus on risk stratification and identifying patients with NDBE at highest risk of progression who might benefit the most from EET.

Treatment Options: Endoscopic Eradication Therapy Versus Esophagectomy

Before embarking on EET, it is critical to not only discuss the indications with the patient but also to review the available treatment options for Barrett's-related neoplasia. Given the high tumor-free survival rates, esophagectomy was long considered as the standard of care for patients with BE-related HGD and early EAC, treatment with which all other therapies are compared.[31–33] However, esophagectomy is associated with an overall operative mortality rate of 2% and a major morbidity rate of 10%; these estimates have been reported from high-volume centers and those with a multidisciplinary care approach.[34,36] It should be noted that there are no randomized controlled trials comparing esophagectomy with EET and neither is such a trial expected in the foreseeable future. In a recent population-based study using the Surveillance, Epidemiology, and End Results (SEER) database that identified 2016 patients with early EAC, comparable 2- and 5-year EAC-specific survival rates were reported between patients undergoing EET and surgical resection. Similar results were reported when analyses were limited to stage T0 and T1a. Cox proportional hazards regression models showed that the hazard ratio for EAC-free survival in the EET group was not different from that of the esophagectomy group (hazard ratio, 1.42; 95% CI, 0.9–2.03).[14] These results are consistent with previous studies reporting no difference in cumulative mortality and survival in patients with BE-related intramucosal cancer and HGD undergoing EET and esophagectomy.[16,36] These results provide confidence that EET is a reasonable and acceptable alternative to esophagectomy in the management of patients with Barrett's-related neoplasia.[14]

Informed Consent and Establishment of Clinical and Procedural Goals

Informed consent

The informed consent process should involve a clear discussion of all treatment options along with the merits and disadvantages of each treatment option. It is recommended that this discussion occur in an office setting and should include discussion of the following points: (1) diagnosis and grade of dysplasia along with natural history estimates regarding progression to HGD/EAC, (2) proposed evaluation plan (endoscopy, endoscopic ultrasound [EUS], and use of advanced imaging techniques), (3) proposed treatment plan and need for multiple sessions every 2 months to achieve the end point of complete remission of dysplasia and intestinal metaplasia (quote personal data if available), (4) discuss the short-term (chest pain, bleeding, perforation, strictures) and long-term (recurrence and progression to cancer) adverse events related to EET, (5) need for ongoing surveillance to address the issue of recurrence and progression to cancer, and (6) need for repeat EET to maintain remission of intestinal metaplasia.

Confirm the diagnosis of dysplasia

Given the significant interobserver variability even among expert gastrointestinal pathologists, the diagnosis of dysplasia should be confirmed by two expert pathologists.[18] If the diagnosis of dysplasia is made at community centers, slides should be obtained and reviewed at expert centers before embarking on EET.

Setting and training
It is well established that esophagectomy for management of EAC should be performed in expert high-volume centers because patient outcomes have been shown to be superior in these centers (lower in-hospital mortality) with a minimum of 15 to 20 esophagectomies per year.[5,37] Similarly, management of Barrett's-related neoplasia should be performed in expert centers with access to endoscopic advanced imaging techniques, multidisciplinary team approach (gastroenterologist, surgeon, expert pathologist, radiologist, oncologist, and nutritionist), and the ability to address adverse events related to EET, including surgery. Although the safety of EMR and ablation has been described from expert centers and endoscopists,[15,38–40] the adverse event rates from community practices and low-volume centers are not known. A recent prospective cohort study compared mucosal lesion and EAC detection rates in patients with Barrett's-related neoplasia between a tertiary care center specializing in BE care and the community. A higher number of patients with visible lesions were noted at the tertiary care center leading to a 56% increased cancer detection rate significantly impacting patient management.[41] In addition, data on learning curves, minimum number of procedures required to attain competence, and minimum number of procedures per year required to maintain competence in EET are scant. A recent study showed that performance of 20 EMRs is not sufficient to reach the peak of the learning curve in EMR.[42] Similarly, results from a retrospective study demonstrated a significant correlation between the endoscopist RFA volume and complete eradication of intestinal metaplasia rates.[43] The British Society of Gastroenterology guidelines recommend a minimum of 30 supervised cases of EMR and 30 cases of endoscopic ablation to attain competence and a minimum of 15 EMRs per year to maintain competence.[5] These estimates need validation in future multicenter studies.

PROCEDURAL CHALLENGES
Accurate Diagnosis and Staging

Given the expanding indications and endoscopic armamentarium for management of patients with Barrett's-related neoplasia, accurate staging is critical.[44] An inaccurate diagnosis could have substantial deleterious consequences for the patient. The goal is to avoid a patient with benign disease being subjected to esophagectomy and a patient with invasive cancer (submucosal invasion or beyond) undergoing EET instead of surgery.

Advanced imaging techniques
The use of high-definition white-light endoscopy (HD-WLE) should be considered as the standard of care and the first critical step in the evaluation of patients with BE. HD-WLE has been shown to have a higher sensitivity for detection of Barrett's-related neoplasia compared with standard endoscopy.[45,46] The rules of BE inspection in patients being considered for EET include use of HD-WLE, cleaning the mucosa using water and/or mucolytic agent, using a distal attachment cap, and spending adequate time to evaluate the BE segment for visible lesions. Most experts believe that HD-WLE detects all lesions that require endoscopic resection.[47] It has been suggested that inspecting the Barrett's segment for more than 1 minute per centimeter length of BE was associated with detection of more patients with suspicious lesions with a trend toward a higher detection rate of HGD/EAC.[48] The extent of BE should be defined using standardized reporting criteria, such as the Prague C&M, criteria and all visible suspicious lesions using the Paris classification.[49,50] Although several advanced imaging techniques, such as dye-based or optical chromoendoscopy, autofluorescence, spectroscopy, confocal laser endomicroscopy, and optical coherence tomography, have been evaluated to improve the yield of current surveillance practices, their role

in guiding EET has not been evaluated adequately in clinical trials. Advanced imaging techniques, such as narrow band imaging, seem to have a role during EET and help delineate margins of areas that harbor early neoplasia and in surveillance post-EET. Costs, limited data from clinical trials demonstrating improved outcomes, lack of standardized classification systems, additional time in busy clinical practices, and need for training are all impediments to widespread clinical application of advanced imaging techniques.

Role of endoscopic ultrasound in accurate staging

EUS is frequently used as a staging modality for patients with Barrett's-related neoplasia who are being considered for EET with the goal of evaluation for advanced cancer (submucosal invasion or beyond and lymph node metastasis).[34] Although the role of EUS in the accurate T and N staging of invasive EAC is well established, the role of EUS in patients with BE with HGD and intramucosal cancer is unclear. A recent population-based study using the SEER-Medicare linked database showed that performance of EUS was associated with improved survival in patients with esophageal cancer for all stages with the exception of stage 0 (HGD only) disease.[51] Results from a multicenter cohort study of patients with BE undergoing EET showed that the accuracy of EUS for determining the depth of invasion using EMR as the gold standard was only 72% (95% CI, 63%–81%).[52] Similarly, a systematic review reported a T-stage concordance rate of 65% using EMR or surgical pathology as the gold standard.[53] Peritumoral inflammation resulting in wall thickening, heterogeneous tissue architectures, anatomic factors in the gastric cardia and distal esophagus, and doubled muscularis mucosae contribute to the limited accuracy rates of EUS in this patient population.[34] A recent meta-analysis that evaluated the use of EUS in patients with BE with HGD and early EAC (N = 656) showed that the overall proportion of patients with advanced disease ($\geq$T1sm or $\geq$N1 disease) detected on EUS was 14% (95% CI, 8%–22%) and 4% (95% CI, 2%–6%) in the absence of nodules.[54] EUS should be considered in the evaluation of patients with Barrett's-related neoplasia, given the potential to alter treatment strategies, albeit in a small proportion of patients.

Endoscopic mucosal resection as a diagnostic and staging modality

EMR has evolved into an important diagnostic/staging and therapeutic tool in the management of patients with Barrett's-related neoplasia (**Fig. 1**).[34] The superiority of EMR compared with biopsy specimens is related to a larger and deeper tissue specimen with limited distortion providing the ultimate proof of invasion depth and in identification of patients with poorly differentiated cancers with lymphovascular invasion. In addition, interobserver agreement among expert gastrointestinal pathologists is superior for EMR specimens compared with biopsy specimens.[18] Results from a recent US multicenter cohort of 138 patients with BE undergoing EET showed that EMR resulted in a change in diagnosis in 31% of patients (upgrade 10%, downgrade 21%).[55] Another recent study reported that a different diagnosis was reported in nearly 50% of cases after initial EMR compared with previous endoscopic biopsy specimens.[38] Although variable rates of change in diagnosis with EMR have been reported in the literature,[38,55–58] the message is clear that EMR is the most accurate staging modality in Barrett's-related neoplasia. This should be performed with therapeutic intent and whenever feasible, all visible lesions should be removed in a single endoscopic procedure.

Technique for endoscopic mucosal resection

Although several techniques for EMR have been described, the two primary techniques used frequently in clinical practice are cap-assisted EMR after saline lift and

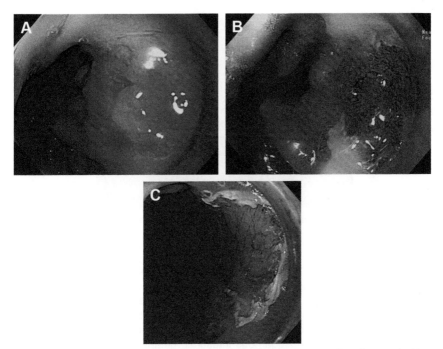

Fig. 1. (*A*) Endoscopic appearance of a visible lesion (Paris class 0-IIa) with outside biopsy showing high-grade dysplasia, seen in the distal esophagus in a patient undergoing surveillance for Barrett's esophagus (Prague C0M1) using high-definition white-light endoscopy. (*B*) Inspection using narrow-band imaging. (*C*) Endoscopic image post endoscopic mucosal resection using the cap technique.

band ligation with snare resection (multiband mucosectomy technique).[34] A randomized controlled trial that compared the two EMR techniques showed a shorter procedure time with multiband mucosectomy compared with cap-assisted EMR (34 vs 50 minutes; $P = .02$). However, specimens obtained using the multiband mucosectomy technique were smaller but no difference in thickness of specimens, resection of submucosa, and adverse event rates was noted.[59] The technique used is a matter of endoscopist preference and both techniques are considered to be equally effective.

Techniques and Modalities for Endoscopic Eradication Therapy

Contemporary treatment options for EET in Barrett's-related neoplasia include complete EMR of the entire Barrett's segment; RFA; cryotherapy; and multimodality therapies, a term used to describe the use of combination of treatment modalities (eg, EMR plus RFA).

Endoscopic mucosal resection of entire Barrett's esophagus

This therapeutic option involves focal EMR of all visible lesions followed by stepwise EMR of the remaining BE to achieve complete eradication (**Fig. 2**). Several case series have reported high complete eradication of neoplasia (85%–100%) and intestinal metaplasia (76%–97%) using this treatment approach.[38,58,60–63] Recently, a single-center US study reported complete eradication of intestinal metaplasia in 86 of 107 (80.4%) based on intention-to-treat analysis. At a mean follow-up of 40.6 months, durability data showed that complete eradication of neoplasia and intestinal

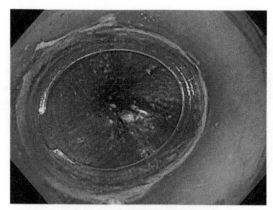

Fig. 2. Endoscopic appearance post complete circumferential resection of Barrett's esophagus.

metaplasia was noted in 100% and 72% of patients, respectively.[38] It is generally believed that 5 cm is the upper limit of effective stepwise complete resection of entire BE and limiting resection to less than 50% of the circumference per treatment session may reduce the risk of strictures.[40] The advantage of this technique is complete histologic correlation along with increased depth of tissue resection, which may decrease the incidence of residual subsquamous intestinal metaplasia (SSIM). However, this technique is associated with high rate of strictures requiring nearly twice the number of endoscopies with its associated adverse events, such as perforation,[38,60] and long-term results are similar to those reported in patients undergoing multimodality therapies. Whether this treatment option should be reserved in a certain subgroup of patients with BE with neoplasia (multifocal disease, diffuse nodularity, deep Barrett's glands, and regenerative tissue) needs to be addressed in future studies.

Radiofrequency ablation

RFA is an ablative technique where the mucosa is heated by bipolar energy that is delivered with a balloon or with a probe attached to the tip of the endoscope (**Fig. 3**). This is the most widely used technique given the evidence base provided

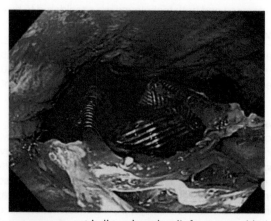

Fig. 3. Endoscopic appearance post balloon-based radiofrequency ablation.

by data from randomized controlled trials (discussed elsewhere in this issue).[12,25] Briefly, results of these randomized controlled trials demonstrate that RFA is associated with a significantly higher rate of eradication of dysplasia and intestinal metaplasia in patients with BE with HGD and LGD. Follow-up data suggest that the treatment is durable with complete eradication of intestinal metaplasia and dysplasia noted in most cases. Of note, a substantial proportion of patients (55%) required repeat ablation treatments after the first year to achieve these high rates of complete eradication.[64] In a systematic review that included 18 studies with 3802 patients reporting efficacy, complete eradication of intestinal metaplasia was achieved in 78% (95% CI, 70%–86%) and complete eradication of dysplasia in 91% (95% CI, 87%–95%) of patients.[65] With regards to the technique, a less labor-intensive RFA treatment regimen that involves no cleaning of mucosa and no use of acetylcysteine between RFA applications was reported.[66] Long-term follow-up studies are required before current treatment technique is altered.

Multimodality endoscopic eradication therapy

The concept of multimodality EET involves EMR of all visible lesions (lesions with the highest histologic grade) followed by eradication of the remaining BE using ablative techniques, such as RFA or cryotherapy.[34,44] This practice and approach has been endorsed by current guidelines.[5,45] Credence to this approach is best provided by data from a randomized controlled trial[60] and long-term outcomes data from observational studies.[10,67–70] A randomized controlled trial that compared stepwise resection of entire BE with EMR of visible lesions followed by RFA of the remaining BE in patients with BE-related HGD and intramucosal cancer showed no difference between the two groups for the end points of complete eradication of intestinal metaplasia (92% and 96%, respectively) and neoplasia (100% and 96%, respectively). However, more strictures were noted (88% vs 14%; $P<.001$), more endoscopies per patient were required (6 vs 3; $P<.001$) and more overall adverse events were noted (24% vs 0%) in the stepwise resection group.[60]

Cryotherapy

This is a catheter-based technique in which either liquid nitrogen or carbon dioxide is delivered by a catheter that sprays cryogen in a noncontact method onto the Barrett's mucosa (**Fig. 4**) in several "freeze-thaw" cycles that results in the formation of extracellular and intracellular ice, which disrupts cell membranes and causes tissue ischemia through vascular thrombosis.[34,71] Although randomized controlled trials and robust long-term results are lacking with this technique, available observational data suggest that the efficacy of cryotherapy may be comparable with RFA for the treatment of BE-related neoplasia.[72,73] Recently, a retrospective study that reported long-term results in 32 patients with BE with HGD treated with liquid nitrogen cryotherapy showed complete eradication of HGD and intestinal metaplasia in 97% and 81% of cases, respectively.[74] In the absence of level 1 evidence, no recommendations can be made regarding use of cryotherapy over RFA. However, this technique is currently being used as the ablative technique of choice by some endoscopists. In addition, cryotherapy can be considered in patients who are refractory to RFA or in patients requiring ablation of intestinal metaplasia beyond a stricture post-EMR.

Persistent neoplasia and intestinal metaplasia

Not all patients achieve the end point of complete eradication of intestinal metaplasia (up to 35%) and dysplasia (up to 15%) despite multiple EET sessions. The understanding of risk factors for unsuccessful EET is limited. Proposed risk factors have included female sex, longer length of BE, need for multiple sessions, incomplete healing

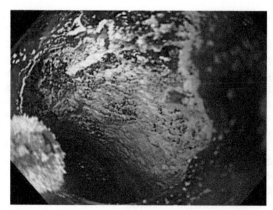

Fig. 4. Endoscopic appearance post cryotherapy using liquid nitrogen.

between treatment sessions, large hiatal hernia, and persistently abnormal acidic or weakly acidic reflux.[75,76] It is unclear if better reflux control, beyond that achieved with high-dose proton pump inhibitor therapy, with antireflux surgery would result in improved outcomes in patients with persistent intestinal metaplasia.

POSTPROCEDURAL CHALLENGES
Adverse Events

Patients and endoscopists need to be well informed of potential adverse events. The most common major adverse events include bleeding (**Fig. 5**A, B), perforation (see **Fig. 5**C, D), and esophageal strictures; rates vary based on the treatment modality. Significant delayed bleeding has been reported in less than 10% of cases undergoing EET predominantly in patients undergoing EMR (uncommon post-RFA, 1%) and perforations in less than 5% of cases.[15,34,38–40,44,65] Strictures post-RFA has been reported in 5% to 12% of patients[25,65] with similar estimates in patients undergoing multimodality EET.[67,68] Higher rates of strictures have been reported in patients undergoing stepwise resection of entire BE (38%–88%).[38,60–62] Chest pain especially post-RFA is frequently reported in nearly 25% to 50% of patients.

Recurrence Post Complete Eradication of Barrett's Esophagus and Need for Surveillance

Recurrence of intestinal metaplasia and dysplasia post complete eradication of BE has been described in several series and not unique to a single treatment modality.[38,61,63,67–69,77,78] A recent retrospective study of 90 patients who underwent complete EMR reported a recurrence of neoplasia and intestinal metaplasia in 6.2% and 39.5% of cases, respectively, with a mean follow-up of 64.8 months. BE length was the only factor significantly associated with recurrence.[63] A US multicenter study reported an overall incidence rate of recurrence of 33% (22% of all recurrences were BE-associated dysplasia) in patients with BE-related neoplasia treated with multimodality EET (EMR and RFA).[67] Similarly, the UK registry study and a cohort study from the Netherlands reported an overall recurrence rate of 9% (47% with dysplasia) and 6% (50% with dysplasia/cancer).[68,69] The Ablation of Intestinal Metaplasia dysplasia trial reported an overall recurrence rate of 13% and of the 119 patients treated with RFA, there were five cases of progression to higher neoplasia grade (two from LGD and HGD to EAC, and three from LGD to HGD; annual rate of progression, 1.4%).[79]

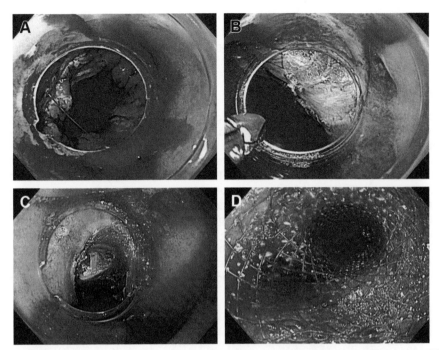

Fig. 5. (*A*) Endoscopic appearance of active bleeding post endoscopic mucosal resection. (*B*) Bleeding controlled with coagulation forceps. (*C*) Perforation noted post endoscopic mucosal resection. (*D*) Perforation closed with covered esophageal self-expanding metallic stent.

Data from the US RFA registry recently reported a recurrence rate of 20%.[80] Although most studies have failed to identify predictors of recurrence, this study reported older age, nonwhite race, and increasing BE length as risk factors for recurrence. In a single center study that included 112 patients who achieved complete eradication of intestinal metaplasia with RFA predominantly, an overall recurrence rate of 7% (4.5% for dysplasia/EAC) was reported. The authors reported an overall recurrence rate of 5.2% per year, HGD/EAC 2.6% per year, and EAC 1.3% per year.[81] These are relevant estimates that should be discussed with patients. A study that included 36 patients with HGD treated with cryotherapy reported a recurrence of neoplasia and intestinal metaplasia in 17% and 30% of cases, respectively, with a median time of recurrence of 6.5 months (range, 3–13).[77] Similarly, another recent study reported a recurrent dysplasia rate of 18% in 32 patients treated with liquid nitrogen cryotherapy.[74] These data justify the current need for enrolling patients in surveillance programs after achieving complete eradication of BE.

Subsquamous Intestinal Metaplasia and Neoplasia

This entity has been reported at variable rates (0%–30%) and with different ablative techniques.[34,44] Variable rates have been attributed to lack of standardized definition, sampling protocol, and inadequate biopsy depth.[82] Limitations of excluding SSIM were highlighted in a study that showed only 37% of all biopsy specimens contained any lamina propria in patients undergoing surveillance post-EET.[82] Proliferation of intestinal metaplasia and neoplastic progression below the neosquamous layer post-EET that escapes endoscopic recognition is a concern. In a systematic review describing results of RFA in 1004 patients, SSIM was found in only nine patients (0.9%).[83] The risk of neoplastic progression associated with SSIM in patients undergoing multimodality EET is unclear (**Fig. 6**).[84]

FUTURE DIRECTIONS

Data from studies evaluating advanced imaging techniques, such as optical frequency domain imaging, a technique that provides high-resolution images of the entire Barrett's segment, are awaited. Whether this and other advanced imaging techniques can help make decisions in real-time related to EET and improve surveillance post-EET should be evaluated in future studies. The role of cryotherapy as an EET modality needs to be clarified in randomized controlled trials and studies reporting long-term outcomes in patients treated with cryotherapy are required. Endoscopic submucosal dissection is a new proposed technique for treatment of Barrett's-related neoplasia and involves en bloc resection of the entire neoplastic area with the goal of achieving R0 (complete) resection. However, this technique is technically challenging compared with EMR and performed at a few expert centers in the United States. Demonstrating difference in clinical outcomes (endoscopic submucosal dissection vs multimodality

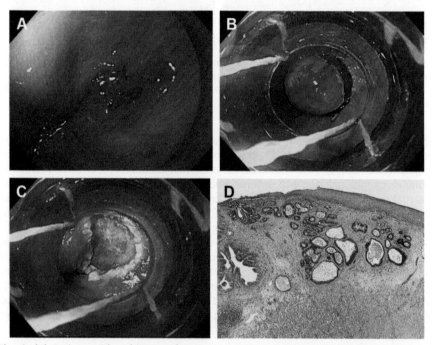

Fig. 6. (*A*) Patient with a history of Barrett's esophagus–related high-grade status post radiofrequency ablation in surveillance noted to have a slightly raised area (5 years post complete eradication of dysplasia and intestinal metaplasia). Biopsy revealed high-grade dysplasia, cannot rule out intramucosal cancer. (*B, C*) Endoscopic mucosal resection with multiband mucosectomy technique and appearance postresection. (*D*) Histology showing the presence of invasive glands in the lamina propria underlying squamous epithelial surface consistent with well-differentiated subsquamous intramucosal cancer. Hematoxylin and eosin stain used for staining. (*Courtesy of* Dr Kalpana Devaraj, University of Colorado, Denver, CO.)

treatment approach) followed by establishment of training programs is critical before wide implementation of endoscopic submucosal dissection in clinical practice for management of Barrett's-related neoplasia can be recommended. Further research is required in understanding the pathophysiology in patients with persistent intestinal metaplasia and dysplasia post-EET. Similarly, recurrence rates and its associated risk factors needs to be defined in future large multicenter trials. Finally, risk stratification tools that include a panel of biomarkers in conjunction with clinical and endoscopic variables are required to answer two main questions: who are the patients with NDBE at high risk for progression and most likely to benefit from EET, and who is least likely to respond to EET and at risk for recurrence of intestinal metaplasia and dysplasia post-EET?

SUMMARY

EET has gained acceptance and replaced esophagectomy as the standard of care for patients with Barrett's-related dysplasia and intramucosal cancer, and has been endorsed by gastroenterology society guidelines. An algorithmic approach to the evaluation and management of BE-related neoplasia is highlighted in **Fig. 7**. The basic principles of EET are detailed inspection of BE with HD-WLE followed by resection of all neoplastic visible lesions, ablation of the remaining BE, ability to manage all adverse events, and finally enrollment in surveillance programs and addressing the issues of recurrence of intestinal metaplasia and dysplasia. Although there are several challenges in EET, following these basic principles ensures optimal results in patients with Barrett's-related neoplasia.

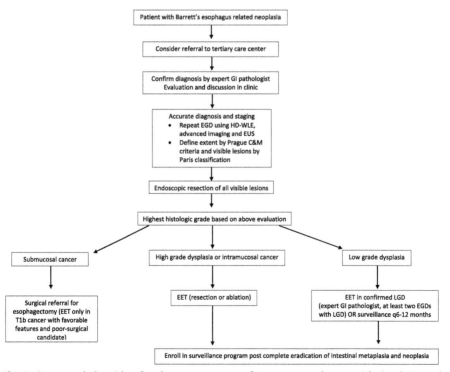

Fig. 7. Suggested algorithm for the management of Barrett's esophagus with dysplasia and intramucosal cancer. EGD, upper endoscopy; GI, gastrointestinal.

REFERENCES

1. Thrift AP, Whiteman DC. The incidence of esophageal adenocarcinoma continues to rise: analysis of period and birth cohort effects on recent trends. Ann Oncol 2012;23:3155–62.
2. Pohl H, Sirovich B, Welch HG. Esophageal adenocarcinoma incidence: are we reaching the peak? Cancer Epidemiol Biomarkers Prev 2010;19:1468–70.
3. Peery AF, Dellon ES, Lund J, et al. Burden of gastrointestinal disease in the United States: 2012 update. Gastroenterology 2012;143:1179–87.e3.
4. American Gastroenterological A, Spechler SJ, Sharma P, et al. American Gastroenterological Association medical position statement on the management of Barrett's esophagus. Gastroenterology 2011;140:1084–91.
5. Fitzgerald RC, di Pietro M, Ragunath K, et al. British Society of Gastroenterology guidelines on the diagnosis and management of Barrett's oesophagus. Gut 2014; 63:7–42.
6. Wang KK, Sampliner RE. Practice Parameters Committee of the American College of G. Updated guidelines 2008 for the diagnosis, surveillance and therapy of Barrett's esophagus. Am J Gastroenterol 2008;103:788–97.
7. Dunbar KB, Spechler SJ. The risk of lymph-node metastases in patients with high-grade dysplasia or intramucosal carcinoma in Barrett's esophagus: a systematic review. Am J Gastroenterol 2012;107:850–62 [quiz: 863].
8. Leers JM, DeMeester SR, Oezcelik A, et al. The prevalence of lymph node metastases in patients with T1 esophageal adenocarcinoma a retrospective review of esophagectomy specimens. Ann Surg 2011;253:271–8.
9. Gockel I, Sgourakis G, Lyros O, et al. Risk of lymph node metastasis in submucosal esophageal cancer: a review of surgically resected patients. Expert Rev Gastroenterol Hepatol 2011;5:371–84.
10. Pech O, Behrens A, May A, et al. Long-term results and risk factor analysis for recurrence after curative endoscopic therapy in 349 patients with high-grade intraepithelial neoplasia and mucosal adenocarcinoma in Barrett's oesophagus. Gut 2008;57:1200–6.
11. Rastogi A, Puli S, El-Serag HB, et al. Incidence of esophageal adenocarcinoma in patients with Barrett's esophagus and high-grade dysplasia: a meta-analysis. Gastrointest Endosc 2008;67:394–8.
12. Shaheen NJ, Sharma P, Overholt BF, et al. Radiofrequency ablation in Barrett's esophagus with dysplasia. N Engl J Med 2009;360:2277–88.
13. Overholt BF, Lightdale CJ, Wang KK, et al. Photodynamic therapy with porfimer sodium for ablation of high-grade dysplasia in Barrett's esophagus: international, partially blinded, randomized phase III trial. Gastrointest Endosc 2005;62: 488–98.
14. Wani S, Drahos J, Cook MB, et al. Comparison of endoscopic therapies and surgical resection in patients with early esophageal cancer: a population-based study. Gastrointest Endosc 2014;79:224–32.e1.
15. Pech O, May A, Manner H, et al. Long-term efficacy and safety of endoscopic resection for patients with mucosal adenocarcinoma of the esophagus. Gastroenterology 2014;146:652–60.e1.
16. Prasad GA, Wu TT, Wigle DA, et al. Endoscopic and surgical treatment of mucosal (T1a) esophageal adenocarcinoma in Barrett's esophagus. Gastroenterology 2009;137:815–23.
17. Wani S, Falk GW, Post J, et al. Risk factors for progression of low-grade dysplasia in patients with Barrett's esophagus. Gastroenterology 2011;141:1179–86, 1186.e1.

18. Wani S, Mathur SC, Curvers WL, et al. Greater interobserver agreement by endoscopic mucosal resection than biopsy samples in Barrett's dysplasia. Clin Gastroenterol Hepatol 2010;8:783–8.

19. Montgomery E, Bronner MP, Goldblum JR, et al. Reproducibility of the diagnosis of dysplasia in Barrett esophagus: a reaffirmation. Hum Pathol 2001;32:368–78.

20. Wani S, Mathur S, Sharma P. How to manage a Barrett's esophagus patient with low-grade dysplasia. Clin Gastroenterol Hepatol 2009;7:27–32.

21. Curvers WL, ten Kate FJ, Krishnadath KK, et al. Low-grade dysplasia in Barrett's esophagus: overdiagnosed and underestimated. Am J Gastroenterol 2010;105:1523–30.

22. de Jonge PJ, van Blankenstein M, Looman CW, et al. Risk of malignant progression in patients with Barrett's oesophagus: a Dutch nationwide cohort study. Gut 2010;59:1030–6.

23. Hvid-Jensen F, Pedersen L, Drewes AM, et al. Incidence of adenocarcinoma among patients with Barrett's esophagus. N Engl J Med 2011;365:1375–83.

24. Duits LC, Phoa KN, Curvers WL, et al. Barrett's oesophagus patients with low-grade dysplasia can be accurately risk-stratified after histological review by an expert pathology panel. Gut 2014. [Epub ahead of print].

25. Phoa KN, van Vilsteren FG, Weusten BL, et al. Radiofrequency ablation vs endoscopic surveillance for patients with Barrett esophagus and low-grade dysplasia: a randomized clinical trial. JAMA 2014;311:1209–17.

26. Ganz RA, Mitlyng B, Leon S. The case for ablating nondysplastic Barrett's esophagus. Gastrointest Endosc 2014;80:866–72.

27. Corley DA, Mehtani K, Quesenberry C, et al. Impact of endoscopic surveillance on mortality from Barrett's esophagus-associated esophageal adenocarcinomas. Gastroenterology 2013;145:312–9.e1.

28. Wani S, Falk G, Hall M, et al. Patients with nondysplastic Barrett's esophagus have low risks for developing dysplasia or esophageal adenocarcinoma. Clin Gastroenterol Hepatol 2011;9:220–7 [quiz: e26].

29. Wani S, Puli SR, Shaheen NJ, et al. Esophageal adenocarcinoma in Barrett's esophagus after endoscopic ablative therapy: a meta-analysis and systematic review. Am J Gastroenterol 2009;104:502–13.

30. Hur C, Choi SE, Rubenstein JH, et al. The cost effectiveness of radiofrequency ablation for Barrett's esophagus. Gastroenterology 2012;143:567–75.

31. Pech O, Bollschweiler E, Manner H, et al. Comparison between endoscopic and surgical resection of mucosal esophageal adenocarcinoma in Barrett's esophagus at two high-volume centers. Ann Surg 2011;254:67–72.

32. Stein HJ, Feith M, Bruecher BL, et al. Early esophageal cancer: pattern of lymphatic spread and prognostic factors for long-term survival after surgical resection. Ann Surg 2005;242:566–73 [discussion: 573–5].

33. Rice TW, Blackstone EH, Goldblum JR, et al. Superficial adenocarcinoma of the esophagus. J Thorac Cardiovasc Surg 2001;122:1077–90.

34. Wani S, Early D, Edmundowicz S, et al. Management of high-grade dysplasia and intramucosal adenocarcinoma in Barrett's esophagus. Clin Gastroenterol Hepatol 2012;10:704–11.

35. Bennett C, Vakil N, Bergman J, et al. Consensus statements for management of Barrett's dysplasia and early-stage esophageal adenocarcinoma, based on a Delphi process. Gastroenterology 2012;143:336–46.

36. Prasad GA, Wang KK, Buttar NS, et al. Long-term survival following endoscopic and surgical treatment of high-grade dysplasia in Barrett's esophagus. Gastroenterology 2007;132:1226–33.

37. Sutton DN, Wayman J, Griffin SM. Learning curve for oesophageal cancer surgery. Br J Surg 1998;85:1399–402.
38. Konda VJ, Gonzalez Haba Ruiz M, Koons A, et al. Complete endoscopic mucosal resection is effective and durable treatment for Barrett's-associated neoplasia. Clin Gastroenterol Hepatol 2014;12:2002–10.e–12.
39. Alvarez Herrero L, Pouw RE, van Vilsteren FG, et al. Safety and efficacy of multiband mucosectomy in 1060 resections in Barrett's esophagus. Endoscopy 2011; 43:177–83.
40. Tomizawa Y, Iyer PG, Wong Kee Song LM, et al. Safety of endoscopic mucosal resection for Barrett's esophagus. Am J Gastroenterol 2013;108:1440–7 [quiz: 1448].
41. Cameron GR, Jayasekera CS, Williams R, et al. Detection and staging of esophageal cancers within Barrett's esophagus is improved by assessment in specialized Barrett's units. Gastrointest Endosc 2014;80:971–83.e1.
42. van Vilsteren FG, Pouw RE, Herrero LA, et al. Learning to perform endoscopic resection of esophageal neoplasia is associated with significant complications even within a structured training program. Endoscopy 2012;44:4–12.
43. Fudman DI, Lightdale CJ, Poneros JM, et al. Positive correlation between endoscopist radiofrequency ablation volume and response rates in Barrett's esophagus. Gastrointest Endosc 2014;80:71–7.
44. Wani S, Sayana H, Sharma P. Endoscopic eradication of Barrett's esophagus. Gastrointest Endosc 2010;71:147–66.
45. Spechler SJ, Sharma P, Souza RF, et al. American Gastroenterological Association technical review on the management of Barrett's esophagus. Gastroenterology 2011;140:e18–52 [quiz: e13].
46. Kara MA, Peters FP, Rosmolen WD, et al. High-resolution endoscopy plus chromoendoscopy or narrow-band imaging in Barrett's esophagus: a prospective randomized crossover study. Endoscopy 2005;37:929–36.
47. Boerwinkel DF, Swager A, Curvers WL, et al. The clinical consequences of advanced imaging techniques in Barrett's esophagus. Gastroenterology 2014; 146:622–9.e4.
48. Gupta N, Gaddam S, Wani SB, et al. Longer inspection time is associated with increased detection of high-grade dysplasia and esophageal adenocarcinoma in Barrett's esophagus. Gastrointest Endosc 2012;76:531–8.
49. Sharma P, Dent J, Armstrong D, et al. The development and validation of an endoscopic grading system for Barrett's esophagus: the Prague C & M criteria. Gastroenterology 2006;131:1392–9.
50. Endoscopic Classification Review Group. Update on the Paris classification of superficial neoplastic lesions in the digestive tract. Endoscopy 2005;37:570–8.
51. Wani S, Das A, Rastogi A, et al. Endoscopic ultrasonography in esophageal cancer leads to improved survival rates: results from a population-based study. Cancer 2014;121(2):194–201.
52. Wani S, Edmundowicz S, Abrams JA, et al. Accuracy of endosocpic ultrasonography (EUS) in staging early neoplasia in Barrett's esophagus (BE): results from a large multicenter cohort study. Gastrointest Endosc 2011;73(Suppl AB):166–7.
53. Young PE, Gentry AB, Acosta RD, et al. Endoscopic ultrasound does not accurately stage early adenocarcinoma or high-grade dysplasia of the esophagus. Clin Gastroenterol Hepatol 2010;8:1037–41.
54. Qumseya BJ, Brown J, Abraham M, et al. Diagnostic performance of EUS in predicting advanced cancer among patients with Barrett's esophagus and high-grade dysplasia/early adenocarcinoma: systemic review and meta-analysis. Gastrointest Endosc 2014. [Epub ahead of print].

55. Wani S, Abrams J, Edmundowicz SA, et al. Endoscopic mucosal resection results in change of histologic diagnosis in Barrett's esophagus patients with visible and flat neoplasia: a multicenter cohort study. Dig Dis Sci 2013;58:1703–9.
56. Larghi A, Lightdale CJ, Memeo L, et al. EUS followed by EMR for staging of high-grade dysplasia and early cancer in Barrett's esophagus. Gastrointest Endosc 2005;62:16–23.
57. Peters FP, Brakenhoff KP, Curvers WL, et al. Histologic evaluation of resection specimens obtained at 293 endoscopic resections in Barrett's esophagus. Gastrointest Endosc 2008;67:604–9.
58. Moss A, Bourke MJ, Hourigan LF, et al. Endoscopic resection for Barrett's high-grade dysplasia and early esophageal adenocarcinoma: an essential staging procedure with long-term therapeutic benefit. Am J Gastroenterol 2010;105:1276–83.
59. Pouw RE, van Vilsteren FG, Peters FP, et al. Randomized trial on endoscopic resection-cap versus multiband mucosectomy for piecemeal endoscopic resection of early Barrett's neoplasia. Gastrointest Endosc 2011;74:35–43.
60. van Vilsteren FG, Pouw RE, Seewald S, et al. Stepwise radical endoscopic resection versus radiofrequency ablation for Barrett's oesophagus with high-grade dysplasia or early cancer: a multicentre randomised trial. Gut 2011;60:765–73.
61. Pouw RE, Seewald S, Gondrie JJ, et al. Stepwise radical endoscopic resection for eradication of Barrett's oesophagus with early neoplasia in a cohort of 169 patients. Gut 2010;59:1169–77.
62. Gerke H, Siddiqui J, Nasr I, et al. Efficacy and safety of EMR to completely remove Barrett's esophagus: experience in 41 patients. Gastrointest Endosc 2011;74:761–71.
63. Anders M, Bahr C, El-Masry MA, et al. Long-term recurrence of neoplasia and Barrett's epithelium after complete endoscopic resection. Gut 2014;63:1535–43.
64. Shaheen NJ, Overholt BF, Sampliner RE, et al. Durability of radiofrequency ablation in Barrett's esophagus with dysplasia. Gastroenterology 2011;141:460–8.
65. Orman ES, Li N, Shaheen NJ. Efficacy and durability of radiofrequency ablation for Barrett's esophagus: systematic review and meta-analysis. Clin Gastroenterol Hepatol 2013;11:1245–55.
66. van Vilsteren FG, Phoa KN, Alvarez Herrero L, et al. Circumferential balloon-based radiofrequency ablation of Barrett's esophagus with dysplasia can be simplified, yet efficacy maintained, by omitting the cleaning phase. Clin Gastroenterol Hepatol 2013;11:491–8.e1.
67. Gupta M, Iyer PG, Lutzke L, et al. Recurrence of esophageal intestinal metaplasia after endoscopic mucosal resection and radiofrequency ablation of Barrett's esophagus: results from a US Multicenter Consortium. Gastroenterology 2013;145:79–86.e1.
68. Haidry RJ, Dunn JM, Butt MA, et al. Radiofrequency ablation and endoscopic mucosal resection for dysplastic Barrett's esophagus and early esophageal adenocarcinoma: outcomes of the UK National Halo RFA Registry. Gastroenterology 2013;145:87–95.
69. Phoa KN, Pouw RE, van Vilsteren FG, et al. Remission of Barrett's esophagus with early neoplasia 5 years after radiofrequency ablation with endoscopic resection: a Netherlands cohort study. Gastroenterology 2013;145:96–104.
70. Guarner-Argente C, Buoncristiano T, Furth EE, et al. Long-term outcomes of patients with Barrett's esophagus and high-grade dysplasia or early cancer treated with endoluminal therapies with intention to complete eradication. Gastrointest Endosc 2013;77:190–9.

71. Greenwald BD, Dumot JA. Cryotherapy for Barrett's esophagus and esophageal cancer. Curr Opin Gastroenterol 2011;27:363–7.
72. Dumot JA, Vargo JJ II, Falk GW, et al. An open-label, prospective trial of cryo-spray ablation for Barrett's esophagus high-grade dysplasia and early esophageal cancer in high-risk patients. Gastrointest Endosc 2009;70:635–44.
73. Shaheen NJ, Greenwald BD, Peery AF, et al. Safety and efficacy of endoscopic spray cryotherapy for Barrett's esophagus with high-grade dysplasia. Gastrointest Endosc 2010;71:680–5.
74. Gosain S, Mercer K, Twaddell WS, et al. Liquid nitrogen spray cryotherapy in Barrett's esophagus with high-grade dysplasia: long-term results. Gastrointest Endosc 2013;78:260–5.
75. Bulsiewicz WJ, Kim HP, Dellon ES, et al. Safety and efficacy of endoscopic mucosal therapy with radiofrequency ablation for patients with neoplastic Barrett's esophagus. Clin Gastroenterol Hepatol 2013;11:636–42.
76. Krishnan K, Pandolfino JE, Kahrilas PJ, et al. Increased risk for persistent intestinal metaplasia in patients with Barrett's esophagus and uncontrolled reflux exposure before radiofrequency ablation. Gastroenterology 2012;143:576–81.
77. Halsey KD, Chang JW, Waldt A, et al. Recurrent disease following endoscopic ablation of Barrett's high-grade dysplasia with spray cryotherapy. Endoscopy 2011;43:844–8.
78. Vaccaro BJ, Gonzalez S, Poneros JM, et al. Detection of intestinal metaplasia after successful eradication of Barrett's esophagus with radiofrequency ablation. Dig Dis Sci 2011;56:1996–2000.
79. Shaheen NJ. More on reports of esophageal cancer with oral bisphosphonate use. N Engl J Med 2009;360:1790–1 [author reply: 1791–2].
80. Pasricha S, Bulsiewicz WJ, Hathorn KE, et al. Durability and predictors of successful radiofrequency ablation for Barrett's esophagus. Clin Gastroenterol Hepatol 2014;12:1840–7.e1.
81. Orman ES, Kim HP, Bulsiewicz WJ, et al. Intestinal metaplasia recurs infrequently in patients successfully treated for Barrett's esophagus with radiofrequency ablation. Am J Gastroenterol 2013;108:187–95 [quiz: 196].
82. Gupta N, Mathur SC, Dumot JA, et al. Adequacy of esophageal squamous mucosa specimens obtained during endoscopy: are standard biopsies sufficient for postablation surveillance in Barrett's esophagus? Gastrointest Endosc 2012; 75:11–8.
83. Gray NA, Odze RD, Spechler SJ. Buried metaplasia after endoscopic ablation of Barrett's esophagus: a systematic review. Am J Gastroenterol 2011;106: 1899–908 [quiz: 1909].
84. Titi M, Overhiser A, Ulusarac O, et al. Development of subsquamous high-grade dysplasia and adenocarcinoma after successful radiofrequency ablation of Barrett's esophagus. Gastroenterology 2012;143:564–6.e1.

Biomarkers in Barrett's Esophagus

Role in Diagnosis, Risk Stratification, and Prediction of Response to Therapy

Ajay Bansal, MD[a],*, Rebecca C. Fitzgerald, MD[b]

KEYWORDS

- Biomarkers • Diagnosis • Screening • Risk stratification • Barrett's esophagus
- High-grade dysplasia • Esophageal adenocarcinoma • Response to therapy

KEY POINTS

- Molecular diagnosis of Barrett's esophagus (BE) can now be performed on nonendoscopic cytology specimens. Trefoil factor 3 is promising. Other markers to test further are microRNA and methylated genes.
- BE can be risk-stratified by measuring global (eg, aneuploidy, multiple gains) or specific (eg, p53 expression) markers. A biomarker panel is likely to be needed.
- Limited data are available on markers that can predict response to therapy. Chromosome and gene loss/gain by fluorescent in situ hybridization may be of value.
- P53 mutational analysis on nonendoscopic cytology specimens can detect prevalent high-grade dysplasia. Thus, the same sample can be used to screen for and risk-stratify BE.

INTRODUCTION

Extensive biomarker research has been conducted to improve the diagnosis and management of Barrett's esophagus (BE). Investigators have worked for many years to discover biomarkers for BE diagnosis, risk stratification, and prediction of response to therapy. The level of evidence required to change clinical practice has generally not been achieved, with the exception of p53; however, more investment and

Conflicts of Interest: Dr A. Bansal has filed a provisional patent application related to microRNA for BE diagnosis and risk stratification. Dr R.C. Fitzgerald is named on patents pertaining to the Cytosponge that has been licensed by the Medical Research Council, UK to Covidien GI Solutions.
^a Division of Gastroenterology and Hepatology, Department of Veterans Affairs Medical Center and the University of Kansas Medical Center, 4801 East Linwood Boulevard, Kansas City, MO 64128-2295, USA; ^b MRC Cancer Unit, Hutchison-MRC Research Centre, University of Cambridge, Hills Road, Cambridge CB2 0XZ, UK
* Corresponding author.
E-mail address: abansal@kumc.edu

collaborative studies are starting to pay dividends.[1] Discovery of clinically applicable biomarkers for BE management has never been more important. The risk of progression of BE to cancer is lower than previously thought.[1–3] Therefore, the resources need to be focused on those BE patients who are most likely to benefit. An important hurdle to clinical application of biomarkers is that specimen acquisition to study biomarkers requires an endoscopy; this has changed recently with the availability of a well-tolerated, easy-to-swallow capsule-based cytology sponge that can collect esophageal cells in an office-based setting.[4] Also, emerging data suggest that blood samples can be used to study the disease status.[5,6] Last, genome-wide next-generation sequencing techniques[7] have significantly added to the understanding of somatic DNA aberrations in BE pathogenesis. All of these factors have created a viable environment for molecular biomarkers of BE and associated risk of cancer to progress to the clinic. In the following sections, important biomarkers to diagnose BE, risk-stratify the patients with BE, and identify those BE patients who are likely to be less responsive to endoscopic therapies are discussed. Where possible, studies published in the last 5 years were the focus.

BIOMARKERS FOR BARRETT'S ESOPHAGUS DIAGNOSIS

Most biomarker research has focused on risk stratification in BE discussed elsewhere in this review. Lately, there has been renewed interest in molecular testing for BE diagnosis. Recent technological developments in esophageal sampling in combination with specific markers have made office-based diagnosis of BE possible. Therefore, widespread application of these tests for BE diagnosis in persons at clinically significant risk for BE may become a viable option. These markers are described in later discussion.

Trefoil Factor 3

Introduction
Trefoil factor 3 (TFF3) is a secretory protein expressed in the goblet cells of the intestinal mucosa that has shown significant promise for molecular BE diagnosis.[4,8]

Studies
To discover BE-specific markers, Lao-Sirieix and colleagues[8] analyzed publicly available microarray datasets that compared normal squamous, BE, and gastric mucosa. Validation by 2 techniques, polymerase chain reaction (PCR) and histochemistry, suggested that TFF3 may be a specific marker for BE-type epithelium. TFF3 as a biomarker for BE diagnosis was tested on specimens acquired via a novel proprietary nonendoscopic cytology sponge within a capsule. After an initial study showed feasibility,[8] the same group of investigators conducted a study in the primary care setting and found the capsule-based cytology sponge to be well tolerated with successful ingestion in 99% of 504 subjects.[4] The sensitivity and specificity of TFF3 expression on cytology samples for diagnosis of circumferential BE 1 cm or longer were 73.3% (95% confidence interval [CI] 44.9%–92.2%) and 93.8% (91.3%–95.8%), respectively. These numbers improved to 90.0% sensitivity (95% CI 55.5%–99.7%) and 93.5% specificity (95% CI 90.9%–95.5%) when BE segments 2 cm or longer were included in the analysis. This approach was recently examined in a larger trial (**Box 1**).

Summary
These results make a strong case for molecular testing on a nonendoscopic cytologic specimen as a practical tool for BE diagnosis in the symptomatic population, most of whom are not investigated. Further studies are ongoing to evaluate the applicability of this strategy to other populations.

Box 1
Trefoil factor 3 for Barrett's esophagus diagnosis

In a recent multicenter case-control study of more than 1000 patients, the sensitivity of TFF3 testing was around 80% (95% CI 76.4%–83.0%) even for short segments (1 cm circumferential) increasing to 90% (95% CI 83.0%–90.6%) in longer segments or when swallowed for a second time with a specificity of 92.4% (95% CI 89.5%–94.7%).[9]

MicroRNA

Introduction

MicroRNAs are novel, noncoding, small RNA molecules shown to be highly tissue-specific in a landmark article that evaluated multiple human cancers[10]; hence, they may have utility as biomarkers.[5]

Studies

Fassan and colleagues[11] used a customized miRNA microarray comprising 326 human miRNAs to compare squamous versus Barrett's epithelium and found 23 miRNAs to be differentially expressed at a P value of less than 0.01. Validation found several of these miRNAs to be significantly different with fold changes of 6 to 63-fold, namely, miR-*215, -192, -194* (all upregulated) and miR-205, miR-203 (both downregulated),[11] and thereby, of potential use for BE diagnosis. Other investigators have examined differential miRNA expression between squamous and BE tissues.[11–16] Although there were some differences in specific miRNAs detected in individual studies, miRNAs *-215, -192, -194, -205,* and *-203* were consistent across multiple studies tissues (**Table 1**).[11–13,15,16] Bansal and colleagues[12] used next-generation sequencing to define the miRNA transcriptome of patients with gastroesophageal reflux disease (GERD) and BE and found several novel miRNAs, including the above-mentioned miRNAs. They subsequently examined the upregulated miRNAs, *-192, -215,* and *-194* for BE diagnosis and found a high sensitivity (91%–100%) and specificity (94%).[17] Systematic analysis by Leidner and colleagues[15] showed that most changes in miRNA expression occurred between squamous versus BE tissues rather than BE versus esophageal adenocarcinoma (EAC) tissues. Garman and colleagues[14] made similar observations that miRNA expression may be more useful for BE diagnosis rather than risk stratification. There are continental differences in BE definition that need to be taken into account however (gastric vs intestinal metaplasia).[1,18] MicroRNAs may be able to differentiate the 2 BE subtypes (**Box 2**).

Summary

Overall, there is good agreement among studies for significantly different miRNAs between the squamous epithelium and the BE epithelium. These early data are promising, but the clinical accuracy of miRNAs for BE diagnosis still needs to be defined in multicenter studies.

DNA Methylation

Introduction

DNA methylation can be defined by the addition of methyl groups to DNA at cytosine bases that typically negatively regulate gene expression.[7] Although initially examined for risk stratification, recent data suggest that methylation abnormalities occur early in BE and thus could be used for BE diagnosis.

Studies

One of the first genes shown to be widely methylated in BE was p16.[19] Subsequently, multiple studies have used candidate and global approaches to demonstrate

Table 1
Candidate miRNAs for Barrett's esophagus diagnosis

Author	Upregulated	Downregulated	Technique
Saad et al,[16] 2013	*-192, -194*	*-205, -203, -31, -21*	Microarray
Fassan et al,[13]	*-192, -215*	*-203, -205, -18a, -20a, -106a*	Microarray
Van Baal et al,[84] 2014	*-192, -215, -194*	-99b	Microarray
Bansal et al,[12]	*-192, -215, -194*	*-205, -203,* -224, -149, -944, -708, -3065	Sequencing
Bansal et al,[17]	*-192, -215, -194*	Not studied	Quantitative real-time PCR
Leidner et al,[15] 2012	*-192, -194, -215,* -7, 199a-5p, -30a	*-203, -205,* -149, -944, -224	Sequencing
Wijnhoven et al,[86] 2010	*-192, -194, -215,* -21, -143, -145	*-203, -205*	Microarray
Garman et al,[14] 2013	-21-, -487b	-27b, -149, -193b	Microarray

MicroRNAs consistently identified in multiple studies have been bolded. For cytologic diagnosis that acquires multiple different cell types, upregulated miRNAs are more likely to be useful.
Data from Refs.[11,12,14–16,62,86].

significant overlap in aberrant methylation signatures between BE and EAC when compared with squamous epithelium.[19–24] Important methylated genes that have been examined in BE are *p16, APC, RUNX3, MGMT, RBP1, SFRP1, TIMP3,* and *CDH13* among others. More recently, aberrant vimentin methylation has been suggested to be a potential marker for BE with tissue expression seen in 90% of BE and 0% among controls.[21] These results were further confirmed on cytology specimens. A study by Xu and colleagues[23] used pyrosequencing to show that the 10 most differentially expressed methylated CpG sites had a sensitivity of 94.8% and a specificity of 91.5% for discriminating BE from normal esophageal tissues. Comparison of methylation of 2 columnar tissues, gastric cardia and BE, with squamous tissues by Verma and colleagues[25] appear to indicate that methylation changes may be specific to BE tissues. Recently, Iyer et al.[26] found methylated genes *NDRG4, SFRP1, BMP3,* and *HPP1* to be highly discriminant between BE tissues and normal controls; at a sensitivity of 100%, the specificity varied 84% to 96%. Expression levels of these markers was dependent on BE length, but not age, sex, inflammation, or the presence of dysplasia.

Summary
To summarize, methylated genes appear to discriminate well between BE and squamous tissues and should be examined further in multicenter trials on BE diagnosis.

Miscellaneous Biomarkers for Barrett's Esophagus Diagnosis
Other markers that have been examined are esophageal stress proteins, such as anterior gradient-2. In a prospective study, anterior gradient-2 had a sensitivity of 65% and specificity of 90% for BE diagnosis.[27] Newer nonendoscopic sampling devices may acquire gastric cardia and fundic mucosa cells. Therefore, markers that are able to differentiate between BE and gastric cardia and fundic tissues will be useful. *Cdx2* and *villin* appear to be highly specific to BE tissues compared with gastric cardia and fundic-type mucosa[28] but may be limited by sensitivity. Further studies that incorporate these markers are needed to define their performance.

Box 2
MicroRNA expression to differentiate Barrett's esophagus subtypes

- A study showed miRNA profiles for both gastric- and intestinal-type BE to be different from squamous epithelium.[13] When the 2 subtypes were compared, miRNAs *-192, -205,* and *-203* were different, whereas *miRNA-215* was similarly expressed.[13]

- Thus, a set of miRNAs may be useful in detection of both gastric- and intestinal-type BE, but specific miRNAs may allow determination of BE subtype.

BIOMARKERS FOR RISK STRATIFICATION IN BARRETT'S ESOPHAGUS

The holy grail of biomarker research in BE is to identify the patients at risk for progression. In this section, biomarkers for risk stratification are discussed.

Chromosomal and Gene Gains and Deletions

Introduction
Chromosomal and gene gains and deletions can be detected by fluorescent in situ hybridization (FISH) that uses a fluorescently labeled probe to detect specific DNA sequences.

Studies
Feasibility of this approach was shown a decade ago when Falk and colleagues[29] found chromosomal gains and loss of p53 and p16 in cytology specimens to have a sensitivity of 95% and a specificity of 100% for diagnosis of high-grade dysplasia (HGD)/EAC. A 4-probe FISH assay (8q24 (C-MYC), 9p21 (P16), 17q12 (HER2), and 20q13) was developed.[30] A subsequent study showed this 4-probe FISH panel to depend on the dysplasia grade with a higher sensitivity for detection of HGD (82%) and EAC (100%) than low-grade dysplasia (LGD, 50%).[31] This initial selection of probes was based on a candidate approach. High-throughput single nucleotide polymorphisms (SNPs) arrays have also been performed.[32] Besides validating the previous targets, frequent gains in several novel candidate genes were identified but need further validation. FISH is readily applied to cytology samples but can be difficult in cut sections from paraffin-embedded tissues due to nuclear truncation.[33] Therefore, separate assays will be needed before data from cytology samples can be directly applied to the paraffin sections. To complicate matters further, low-level copy gains may be missed on standard FISH in 4-μm sections and require thicker sections (16 μm) that need to be evaluated by image analysis.[34] The ideal technique for FISH (cytology vs thin sections vs thick sections) still remains to be defined. Because FISH analysis can be tedious, investigators have attempted to develop automated protocols.[35] A recent large trial examined FISH for risk stratification prospectively (**Box 3**).

Summary
FISH is an important technique for quantitative detection of changes of aneuploidy and specific gene copy numbers during BE transformation. The issue that remains is whether FISH markers are sufficiently discriminatory to be applied in clinical practice.

P53

Introduction
P53 is one of the first biomarkers to show promise for identification of BE progressors.[1,37,38] The focus of this review is on more recent work.

Box 3
Prospective phase 4 study of fluorescent in situ hybridization for risk stratification in Barrett's esophagus

- Krishnadath and colleagues[36] conducted a prospective multicenter trial that used a FISH panel (*P16*, *P53*, *Her-2/neu*, *20q*, and *MYC*, and the chromosomal centromeric probes 7 and 17 to detect aneuploidy) to analyze risk of progression in 428 patients with nondysplastic BE followed for a mean period of 45 months.

- The relative risk of progression with p16 loss or aneuploidy was 3.23 (95% CI 1.32–7.95) after controlling for Barrett's length and age. The absolute risk of progression was 1.83% if the FISH panel was positive versus 0.58% if FISH panel was negative.

Studies

Investigators from the Netherlands analyzed p53 by immunohistochemistry (IHC) on sequential biopsies in patients with BE who ultimately progressed to HGD/EAC.[39] Changes in p53 expression preceded development of HGD/EAC by several years, an important property for a biomarker. P53 expression was an important risk factor for HGD/EAC in a case control study with a hazard ratio (HR) of 6.5 (95% CI: 2.5–17.1).[40] In the largest study of its kind, 2 pathologists independently scored p53 staining in 12,000 biopsies from 635 patients.[41] Results were compelling with both overexpression and complete loss significantly increasing the risk of neoplastic progression after adjusting for age, gender, Barrett length, and esophagitis (relative risk [RR] 5.6 [95% CI 3.1–10.3] and RR 14.0 [95% CI 5.3–37.2], respectively). However, only 49% of patients who progressed had aberrant p53 immunostaining and hence it is specific but not highly sensitive. A nested case control study within a Northern Island registry of BE patients did not find p53 protein overexpression to predict progression in a multivariate analysis.[42] Not all p53 mutations stabilize the protein,[43] and complementary techniques may be needed (**Box 4**).

Summary

Currently, p53 is not routinely recommended for risk stratification but the British Society of Gastroenterology[1] does have a grade B recommendation to test p53 by IHC to

---

Box 4
P53: protein overexpression and loss, mutational analysis and loss of gene locus, all are important and complementary for risk stratification in Barrett's esophagus

- Mutated p53 frequently has a longer half-life and leads to increased p53 immunostaining. *P53* mutations can also result in loss of protein, an absent pattern compared with wild-type.[44] Therefore, both overexpression and loss of p53 appear to have clinical utility.

- Krishnadath and colleagues[45] evaluated p53 expression by immunostaining for protein and FISH for loss of p53 locus and found the combination to detect p53 abnormalities in all patients with LGD, HGD, and EAC. Thus, p53 evaluation by FISH could complement immunostaining for risk stratification in BE.

- Furthermore, p53 mutational status (eg, point mutations and loss of heterozygosity) can be examined directly. Recent whole genome sequencing of esophageal biopsies from normal subjects and patients with BE and BE with HGD found p53 mutations to occur specifically in patients with HGD compared with patients with never dysplastic BE.[46] Evaluation of esophageal samples acquired by the Cytosponge demonstrated that p53 mutations could be successfully detected, albeit with a lower allele frequency than in biopsy samples. The sensitivity and specificity of p53 mutations for prevalent HGD on the cytology samples were 86% and 100%, respectively.

clarify an equivocal histologic diagnosis of dysplasia. The above data also suggest that the same nonendoscopically acquired sample can be molecularly screened not only to diagnose BE but also to risk stratify.

DNA Content Abnormalities

Introduction
There are extensive long-term follow-up data on the measurement of aneuploidy and tetraploidy to identify BE progressors, yet these markers have not made it into clinical practice. An important reason is difficulty with aneuploidy measurements. Initial studies measured aneuploidy using flow cytometry[47] that requires special media and specialized processing. A practical technique may be image cytometry[48] that fares well against flow cytometry (**Box 5**).

Studies
A landmark article by Reid and colleagues[50] led to interest in aneuploidy/tetraploidy as a biomarker. Subsequently, the same investigators found aneuploidy/tetraploidy to have 100% sensitivity and 100% specificity to predict cancer development at 5 years.[51] The ability of aneuploidy to predict progression was less dramatic in other studies in which it was a late marker[39] or it lost predictive ability on multivariate analysis that included LGD as a covariate.[40] More recent data in a population-based nested case-control study showed that the presence of aneuploidy measured by image cytometry increased the odds of progressing to HGD/EAC by 3.2-fold (1.73–6.0), but the overall sensitivity was limited to ~44% (33%–55%).[42] When aneuploidy, again measured by image, was incorporated into a risk score along with staining for Aspergillus oryzae lectin, a score of 1 or more could identify 66% of progressors with nondysplastic BE as baseline histology.[42]

Summary
Current data suggest that aneuploidy alone may not be sufficiently discriminatory to risk-stratify BE patients but may be useful as part of a comprehensive biomarker panel. Measurement will likely need to be based on clinically applicable tests such as image cytometry. Conventional techniques measure DNA content as a whole but do not generally have the resolution to capture the details of gene-specific alterations that are manifest as a result of altered DNA content (**Box 6**). Quantification of somatic chromosomal alterations is an exciting new area of biomarker research that evaluates the BE epithelium at an unprecedented global scale for risk profiling of BE patients.

DNA Methylation

Introduction
Hypermethylation of genes has been extensively studied as a biomarker.

Studies
One of the earliest studies to evaluate methylation in BE was done by Reid and colleagues,[54] who showed p16 methylation to be highly prevalent in EAC. Subsequently, multiple studies have evaluated methylated genes as biomarkers but have

---

Box 5

Comparison of image cytometry versus flow cytometry for aneuploidy measurements

- Investigators evaluated 40-μm sections for aneuploidy by flow and image cytometry in 44 samples from 31 patients.[49] The percentage agreement was 93% and suggests that image cytometry can reliably measure DNA content.

Box 6
Catastrophic genomic events in Barrett's esophagus

- Recent collaborative efforts used genome-wide molecular techniques[52,53] and determined that cancer development can be preceded by a dramatic increase in copy number and catastrophic genomic events in up to 30% of cases.[53] This loss of genomic integrity could be a useful biomarker for progression. Specifically, catastrophic genomic events refer to sudden, punctuated alterations in copy number as a result of chromothripsis (massive genomic rearrangements as a single event) and breakage-fusion-bridge events.

- In addition to the actual copy number and specific loci of structural variants (eg, affecting a specific gene like ErbB2), the degree of copy number variation (termed genetic diversity) between different areas of the Barrett's segment may also be an important risk factor for progression.[52]

- Serial measurements demonstrated that increases in copy number and genetic diversity preceded cancer development by as many as 4 years, providing a window of opportunity for detection.[52]

---

found inconsistent results (hypermethylation of *p16*, *RUNX3*, and *HPP1* in one study[55] but *APC*, *TIMP3*, and *TERT* in another study[56]). Sato and colleagues[57] proposed a tiered risk-stratification model by combining clinical parameters with a composite methylation index for *p16*, *RUNX3*, and *HPP1*. A follow-up study by the same group evaluated additional markers and found an 8-marker panel to have a specificity of 70% at a sensitivity of 80%.[58] Hypermethylation of 2 of the markers (*p16*, *APC*) described earlier were evaluated in a longitudinal study. The panel was found to predict progression (adjusted odds ratio 14.97), but with wide CIs (1.73, infinity).[59] It remained unclear whether methylation was an early or a late event. A group of Australian investigators compared squamous tissues with BE and EAC tissues and elegantly demonstrated that most genes (7 of 9) previously shown to be hypermethylated in EAC were also hypermethylated in metaplastic BE,[22] raising questions about their utility for diagnosis versus risk stratification. Studies discussed earlier used a candidate gene approach, but global methylation profiling is now possible. A group of investigators used methylation microarrays and observed that the number of differentially methylated CpG sites was 10-fold higher for BE versus squamous histology compared with EAC versus BE histology (195 vs 17, $P = .001$).[20] Only 3 sites were different between BE and HGD cases, suggesting that methylation may be less useful as a biomarker for HGD. Methylation was further compared between BE and EAC in a comprehensive study that validated candidate genes using the gold-standard technique of pyrosequencing.[60] A 4-gene methylation signature (*SLC22A18*, *PIGR*, *GJA12*, and *RIN2*) could classify patients into low- (<2 methylated genes), medium- (2 methylated genes), and high-risk (>2 methylated genes) for prevalent dysplasia but needs further validation. Several studies suggest that both hypomethylation and hypermethylation are important during BE development and carcinogenesis (**Box 7**).

Summary
Overall, DNA methylation has been extensively studied and several methylation biomarkers for risk stratification have been identified. However, further validation is still needed to determine which of these markers will be most useful in practice.

MicroRNA

Introduction
Earlier in this review, the role of miRNAs in BE diagnosis was discussed. Here, the utility of miRNA for risk stratification is discussed.

> **Box 7**
> **What is the methylation status in Barrett's esophagus and esophageal adenocarcinoma: is it hypo- or hyper-?**
>
> - Kaz and colleagues.[20] found 75% to 80% of BE and EAC cases to be hypermethylated.
> - Other studies determined that in BE carcinogenesis, widespread hypomethylation predominates[23,25] with hypermethylation at specific loci.
> - Alvi and colleagues[60] compared methylation between BE and EAC by whole-genome methylation profiling and found that of 14, 475 genes, the percentage of hypomethylated versus hypermethylated genes were generally similar, 10.98% versus 12.1%, respectively.
> - These conflicting results regarding the methylation status of BE reflect differences in methylation profiling techniques and quantification of "abnormal" methylation.

Studies

Feber and colleagues[61] conducted one of the original studies to demonstrate the potential utility of miRNAs for differentiating BE epithelium from EAC epithelium. Since then, multiple studies have examined the role of miRNA for differentiating BE and dysplastic tissues with inconsistent results.[11,14–16,62] Fassan and colleagues[11] used a custom miRNA microarray and found a miRNA signature for BE carcinogenesis consisting of 6 upregulated and 7 downregulated miRNAs. Bansal and colleagues[62] found miRNAs -15b, -486-5p, -let-7a, and -203 to differentiate between patients with BE and those with HGD/EAC with a sensitivity and specificity that ranged from 87% to 93% and 55% to 90%, respectively. A retrospective longitudinal phase 3 study found miRNAs -192, -194, -196a, and -196b to have sensitivities of 71% to 85% and specificities of 50% to 71% to identify patients with BE who progressed to EAC versus those who did not.[63]

Summary

Overall, miRNA expression data among studies on risk stratification have been inconsistent. Several of the miRNAs discussed earlier may be dysregulated early in BE[15] and thus more useful for BE diagnosis. An advantage of miRNAs is that they are well preserved in fixed tissues because of their smaller size and can be applied to archival specimens.[64] Further studies are needed to find candidate miRNAs specific to progression of BE to EAC.

MISCELLANEOUS MARKERS

Clonal diversity refers to the presence of multiple cellular clones within a cancerous field with different molecular profiles.[65] Coupled with the process of natural selection, accumulation of mutations may add to the fitness of a clone with an increased likelihood of progression. Maley and colleagues measured clonal diversity and showed that presence of 3 clones doubles the risk of progression.[65] This elegant concept has led to improved understanding of BE carcinogenesis but has not yet been developed as a clinically applicable tool.[66] Proliferation markers such as Ki67[40] and Cyclin A[42] have been studied but are not sufficiently discriminatory to be applied clinically.

Predictive Ability of Biomarkers in Combination with Imaging

Introduction

The idea behind advanced imaging assisted biomarker detection is to enrich for biomarker expression by analyzing biopsies from the abnormal area.

Studies

di Pietro and colleagues[67] performed autofluorescence imaging (AFI) in a prospective cross-sectional study of 157 patients and found the dysplasia yield of the biomarker panel (aneuploidy, p53, and cyclin A) on AFI+ areas to be superior when compared with AFI− areas. The association between AFI status and abnormal biomarker expression persisted after exclusion of dysplasia.

Summary

The combination of imaging-directed biopsies followed by biomarker assessment has the potential to dramatically reduce the number of biopsies required during surveillance; however, further studies are needed.

Risk Stratification of Barrett's Esophagus with Low-Grade Dysplasia

Introduction

Traditionally, molecular biomarkers have been applied to risk-stratify nondysplastic BE. However, European data argue that LGD,[68,69] if confirmed by 2 independent pathologists, is a strong marker for progression. Because BE progresses stepwise via LGD but LGD is a very subjective diagnosis,[68–70] BE with LGD can be risk-stratified by testing biomarkers.

Studies

A few studies have examined the predictive ability of biomarkers in patients with LGD and showed conflicting results. A population-based nested case control study found that aneuploidy in LGD increased the odds of progression to HGD/EAC by 3.74-fold,[42] whereas in another case-control study, p53 overexpression but not aneuploidy was predictive.[40] The positive predictive value of LGD for neoplastic progression in the presence of aberrant p53 expression doubled the positive risk of progression to HGD/EAC compared with that in nondysplastic BE.

Summary

Future studies need to evaluate whether aberrant markers can more easily and objectively identify those LGD patients categorized on consensus by expert pathologists as high risk and therefore should be ablated.

Predictive Biomarkers for Response to Endoscopic Therapy

Introduction

Effective endoscopic therapy is available and is becoming the standard of care for management of patients with confirmed dysplasia and intramucosal cancer in BE. However, in as many as 20% of the patients,[71] BE recurrences can occur. Biomarkers that can identify the subgroup of patients likely to recur will allow for more intensive follow-up and treatment.

Studies

One of the earliest studies evaluated biomarkers to predict recurrence after photodynamic therapy (PDT).[72] Prasad and colleagues[72] evaluated a biomarker panel by FISH (loss of 9p21 (p16) and 17p13.1 (p53) loci; gains of the 8q24 (c-myc), 17q (HER2-neu), and 20q13 (ZNF217) loci; and multiple gains) on cytology specimens collected before and after PDT in 31 patients with HGD/mucosal cancer. In 6 of 31 patients, abnormal expression was present for at least one marker after PDT in the absence of histologic abnormalities. Two of 6 patients with persistent biomarker abnormalities developed recurrent HGD. Using the above FISH panel, the same group prospectively studied patients undergoing PDT.[73] At baseline, 68% of the patients with HGD and 73% with mucosal cancer had FISH abnormalities. On multivariate analysis, p16 loss at baseline predicted lack of response of HGD/mucosal cancer to PDT at 3-month follow-up (0.32, 95% CI 0.10–0.96). The results discussed earlier predict response to PDT, but more recently, endoscopic mucosal resection and radiofrequency ablation have become the primary treatment modalities for BE neoplasia. In a retrospective cohort of 181 patients, the investigators evaluated the same FISH panel as above at baseline and found that the presence of multiple gains predicted complete remission of dysplasia to be less likely (HR 0.57, 95% CI 0.40–0.82).[74] When analysis was restricted to those patients undergoing radiofrequency ablation, multiple gains by FISH again predicted lack of complete remission of dysplasia (0.58, 95% CI 0.31–1.09).

Summary

The above results suggest that patients with BE neoplasia who are less likely to respond to endoscopic therapy can indeed be identified at the onset of treatment. Prospective studies are needed to confirm these results and determine if patients less likely to respond should be treated using a different therapeutic approach.

Serum Biomarkers in Barrett's Esophagus

Introduction

A blood-based assay for diagnosis of EAC and even BE would be useful and widely applicable.[75] Potential serum markers are listed in **Box 8**. At this time, these markers are far from the stage of clinical application.

Studies

Zaidi and colleagues[6] used a proteomics approach to discover a 4-protein panel: biglycan, annexin-A6, myeloperoxidase, and S-100-A9 for the detection of EAC. These markers were then cross-validated in an independent cohort using a Bayesian rule-learning predictive model with an accuracy of 87%. These results are particularly interesting because their discovery was guided by comparison of tissue expression of proteins between BE, HGD, and EAC tissues that indicate biological plausibility. Tissue methylation signatures as a biomarker have been discussed elsewhere but can be detected in cell-free serum DNA.[76] The investigators showed a high degree of correlation between serum DNA methylation and tissue methylation profiles ($r = 0.92$), suggesting that serum DNA methylation profiling could be useful to detect BE and EAC noninvasively. Inflammation is clearly linked to BE diagnosis and risk stratification. Thrift and colleagues[80] developed a multi-biomarker risk model that included clinical

---

Box 8
Potential serum markers for Barrett's esophagus diagnosis and risk stratification

Serum markers includes a myriad of markers

- EAC-specific proteins[6]
- Methylation of cell-free DNA[76]
- Metabolites[77]
- Adipocytokines[78,79]
- Interleukins[25,80]
- Gastrin[81]
- Glycosylation patterns of proteins[79]
- Mesothelin[82]
- MicroRNAs[5,83,84]

Table 2
Current status of biomarkers for diagnosis, risk stratification, and prediction of response to therapy: at a glance

TFF3	• Phase 4 study showed significant promise for diagnosis
FISH	• Phase 3 and 4 studies showed promise for risk stratification, potential candidates studied alone or in combination (8q24 (C-MYC), 9p21 (p16), 17q12 (HER2), 17p13.1 (p53), 20q13, and ZNF217) • Phase 3 and 4 studies showed p16 loss and multiple gains to hold promise for prediction of response to therapy
DNA content abnormalities/Aneuploidy	• Useful in a biomarker panel for risk stratification, may be a late biomarker; image cytometry is the technique of choice for clinical application • Somatic gene diversity can be quantified, a new potential biomarker
Methylation	• Phase 2 studies show that methylation signatures are notably different between squamous and BE tissues, promise for diagnosis; potential candidates to study further are p16, RUNX3, MGMT, SFRP1, TIMP3, and CDH13 among others • Inconsistent data for risk stratification; no dominant methylation marker has emerged from phase 3 and phase 4 studies
MicroRNA	• Phase 2 studies show promise for diagnosis; miRNAs -192, -215, -194, -205, and -203 were consistently different between squamous and BE tissues • Inconsistent data across studies for risk stratification; no dominant miRNA has emerged from limited studies
P53	• Only biomarker recommended to clarify the histologic diagnosis (ie, presence of dysplasia grade in BE) • P53 mutational analysis is feasible on cytologic specimens • Prospective phase 4 data support use of p53 analysis for risk stratification; p53 FISH, immunostaining, and mutational analysis may have additive value • Did not predict response to therapy in a phase 4 study
Clonal diversity	• Phase 2 studies suggest predictive ability for risk stratification but computationally demanding
Proliferation markers	• Limited utility for risk stratification

variables and serum levels of multiple interleukins. Addition of the biomarkers to the variables of GERD frequency and duration improved the ability of this risk prediction score (0.85 vs 0.74, P = .01).[80] An exciting area of research that remains underexplored is evaluation of miRNAs as serum markers for BE and EAC because they are highly stable in harsh conditions,[85] do not require special storage conditions, and are easy to assay. Van Baal and colleagues[84] profiled plasma miRNAs from controls and patients with BE and EAC using PCR arrays and showed promising diagnostic performance of plasma miRNAs *-95, -133a, -136, -194, -382,* and *-451* for the detection of BE and EAC. Bansal and colleagues[83] analyzed serum miRNAs guided by differences in tissue expression between GERD and BE patients and found the panel of serum miRNAs *-15a* and *-196a* to have a sensitivity of 75% and a specificity of 85% for BE diagnosis in GERD patients. The differences in the 2 studies can be ascribed to differences between plasma versus serum and normalization techniques.

Summary

Clearly, noninvasive serum biomarkers for BE diagnosis and risk stratification would be a huge step forward in the management of patients with BE. Much work needs to be done before serum biomarkers for BE become a reality.

SUMMARY

This review has outlined the recent progress made in biomarker research in BE (**Table 2**). To make a real difference to the management of BE patients, highly discriminatory biomarkers that can be tested with noninvasive techniques and are more

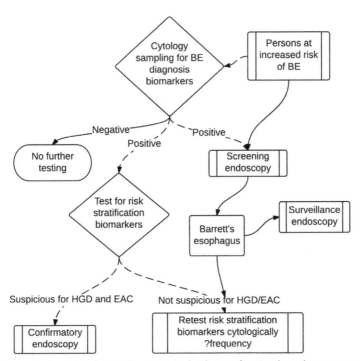

Fig. 1. Proposed algorithm for BE diagnosis and risk stratification based on recent developments. The dotted line depicts the new cytology-based algorithm and the solid line depicts the current endoscopy based algorithm.

comfortable for patients and less expensive for health care systems are needed. These techniques are now becoming available and have been discussed here as a novel algorithm for BE diagnosis and risk stratification (**Fig. 1**). Collaborative studies nationally and internationally on biomarkers are ongoing and will test the recent developments rigorously. For BE investigators who want to improve the outcomes of their patients suffering from EAC, this is a time of hope.

REFERENCES

1. Fitzgerald RC, di Pietro M, Ragunath K, et al. British Society of Gastroenterology guidelines on the diagnosis and management of Barrett's oesophagus. Gut 2014; 63:7–42.
2. Wani S, Falk G, Hall M, et al. Patients With nondysplastic Barrett's esophagus have low risks for developing dysplasia or esophageal adenocarcinoma. Clin Gastroenterol Hepatol 2011;9:220–7.
3. Sharma P. Clinical practice. Barrett's esophagus. N Engl J Med 2009;361:2548–56.
4. Kadri SR, Lao-Sirieix P, O'Donovan M, et al. Acceptability and accuracy of a non-endoscopic screening test for Barrett's oesophagus in primary care: cohort study. BMJ 2010;341:c4372.
5. Lujambio A, Lowe SW. The microcosmos of cancer. Nature 2012;482:347–55.
6. Zaidi AH, Gopalakrishnan V, Kasi PM, et al. Evaluation of a 4-protein serum biomarker panel-biglycan, annexin-A6, myeloperoxidase, and protein S100-A9 (B-AMP)-for the detection of esophageal adenocarcinoma. Cancer 2014;120(24):3902–13.
7. Feero WG, Guttmacher AE, Collins FS. Genomic medicine–an updated primer. N Engl J Med 2010;362:2001–11.
8. Lao-Sirieix P, Boussioutas A, Kadri SR, et al. Non-endoscopic screening biomarkers for Barrett's oesophagus: from microarray analysis to the clinic. Gut 2009;58:1451–9.
9. Ross-Innes CS, Debiram-Beecham I, O'Donovan M, et al. Evaluation of a minimally invasive cell sampling device coupled with assessment of trefoil factor 3 expression for diagnosing Barrett's esophagus: a multi-center case-control study. PLoS Med 2015;12:e1001780.
10. Lu J, Getz G, Miska EA, et al. MicroRNA expression profiles classify human cancers. Nature 2005;435:834–8.
11. Fassan M, Volinia S, Palatini J, et al. MicroRNA expression profiling in human Barrett's carcinogenesis. Int J Cancer 2010;129(7):1661–70.
12. Bansal A, Lee IH, Hong X, et al. Discovery and validation of Barrett's esophagus MicroRNA transcriptome by next generation sequencing. PLoS One 2013;8:e54240.
13. Fassan M, Volinia S, Palatini J, et al. MicroRNA expression profiling in the histological subtypes of Barrett's metaplasia. Clin Transl Gastroenterol 2013;4:e34.
14. Garman KS, Owzar K, Hauser ER, et al. MicroRNA expression differentiates squamous epithelium from Barrett's esophagus and esophageal cancer. Dig Dis Sci 2013;58:3178–88.
15. Leidner RS, Ravi L, Leahy P, et al. The microRNAs, MiR-31 and MiR-375, as candidate markers in Barrett's esophageal carcinogenesis. Genes Chromosomes Cancer 2012;51:473–9.
16. Saad R, Chen Z, Zhu S, et al. Deciphering the unique microRNA signature in human esophageal adenocarcinoma. PLoS One 2013;8:e64463.
17. Bansal A, Hong X, Lee IH, et al. MicroRNA expression can be a promising strategy for the detection of Barrett's Esophagus: A pilot study. Clin Trans Gastroenterol 2014. http://dx.doi.org/10.1038/ctg.2014.17 [in press].

18. American Gastroenterological Association, Spechler SJ, Sharma P, et al. American Gastroenterological Association Medical Position Statement on the Management of Barrett's Esophagus. Gastroenterology 2011;140:1084–91.
19. Wong DJ, Paulson TG, Prevo LJ, et al. p16(INK4a) lesions are common, early abnormalities that undergo clonal expansion in Barrett's metaplastic epithelium. Cancer Res 2001;61:8284–9.
20. Kaz AM, Wong CJ, Luo Y, et al. DNA methylation profiling in Barrett's esophagus and esophageal adenocarcinoma reveals unique methylation signatures and molecular subclasses. Epigenetics 2011;6:1403–12.
21. Moinova H, Leidner RS, Ravi L, et al. Aberrant vimentin methylation is characteristic of upper gastrointestinal pathologies. Cancer Epidemiol Biomarkers Prev 2012;21:594–600.
22. Smith E, De Young NJ, Pavey SJ, et al. Similarity of aberrant DNA methylation in Barrett's esophagus and esophageal adenocarcinoma. Mol Cancer 2008;7:75.
23. Xu E, Gu J, Hawk ET, et al. Genome-wide methylation analysis shows similar patterns in Barrett's esophagus and esophageal adenocarcinoma. Carcinogenesis 2013;34:2750–6.
24. Jin Z, Cheng Y, Olaru A, et al. Promoter hypermethylation of CDH13 is a common, early event in human esophageal adenocarcinogenesis and correlates with clinical risk factors. Int J Cancer 2008;123:2331–6.
25. Alvarez H, Opalinska J, Zhou L, et al. Widespread hypomethylation occurs early and synergizes with gene amplification during esophageal carcinogenesis. PLoS Genet 2011;7:e1001356.
26. Iyer PG, Clemens MA, Yab TC, et al. Highly discriminant methylated DNA markers for detection of Barrett's esophagus. Gastroenterology 2013;144:S-684.
27. Groome M, Lindsay J, Ross PE, et al. Use of oesophageal stress response proteins as potential biomarkers in the screening for Barrett's oesophagus. Eur J Gastroenterol Hepatol 2008;20:961–5.
28. Shi XY, Bhagwandeen B, Leong AS. CDX2 and villin are useful markers of intestinal metaplasia in the diagnosis of Barrett esophagus. Am J Clin Pathol 2008; 129:571–7.
29. Fahmy M, Skacel M, Gramlich TL, et al. Chromosomal gains and genomic loss of p53 and p16 genes in Barrett's esophagus detected by fluorescence in situ hybridization of cytology specimens. Mod Pathol 2004;17:588–96.
30. Brankley SM, Wang KK, Harwood AR, et al. The development of a fluorescence in situ hybridization assay for the detection of dysplasia and adenocarcinoma in Barrett's esophagus. J Mol Diagn 2006;8:260–7.
31. Fritcher EG, Brankley SM, Kipp BR, et al. A comparison of conventional cytology, DNA ploidy analysis, and fluorescence in situ hybridization for the detection of dysplasia and adenocarcinoma in patients with Barrett's esophagus. Hum Pathol 2008;39:1128–35.
32. Wiech T, Nikolopoulos E, Weis R, et al. Genome-wide analysis of genetic alterations in Barrett's adenocarcinoma using single nucleotide polymorphism arrays. Lab Invest 2009;89:385–97.
33. Geppert CI, Rummele P, Sarbia M, et al. Multi-colour FISH in oesophageal adenocarcinoma-predictors of prognosis independent of stage and grade. Br J Cancer 2014;110:2985–95.
34. Rauser S, Weis R, Braselmann H, et al. Significance of HER2 low-level copy gain in Barrett's cancer: implications for fluorescence in situ hybridization testing in tissues. Clin Cancer Res 2007;13:5115–23.

35. Rygiel AM, van Baal JW, Milano F, et al. Efficient automated assessment of genetic abnormalities detected by fluorescence in situ hybridization on brush cytology in a Barrett esophagus surveillance population. Cancer 2007;109: 1980–8.

36. Timmer JL, Rosmolen CT, Meijer W, et al. A FISH biomarker panel for the prediction of high-grade dysplasia and adenocarcinom in non-dysplastic Barrett's esophagus: results from a long-term prospective cohort study. United European Gastroenterol J 2014;2(suppl):A1–131 [abstract].

37. Timmer MR, Sun G, Gorospe EC, et al. Predictive biomarkers for Barrett's esophagus: so near and yet so far. Dis Esophagus 2013;26:574–81.

38. Prasad GA, Bansal A, Sharma P, et al. Predictors of progression in Barrett's esophagus: current knowledge and future directions. Am J Gastroenterol 2010; 105:1490–502.

39. Kerkhof M, Steyerberg EW, Kusters JG, et al. Aneuploidy and high expression of p53 and Ki67 is associated with neoplastic progression in Barrett esophagus. Cancer Biomark 2008;4:1–10.

40. Sikkema M, Kerkhof M, Steyerberg EW, et al. Aneuploidy and overexpression of Ki67 and p53 as markers for neoplastic progression in Barrett's esophagus: a case-control study. Am J Gastroenterol 2009;104:2673–80.

41. Kastelein F, Biermann K, Steyerberg EW, et al. Aberrant p53 protein expression is associated with an increased risk of neoplastic progression in patients with Barrett's oesophagus. Gut 2013;62:1676–83.

42. Bird-Lieberman EL, Dunn JM, Coleman HG, et al. Population-based study reveals new risk-stratification biomarker panel for Barrett's esophagus. Gastroenterology 2012;143:927–35.e3.

43. Alsner J, Jensen V, Kyndi M, et al. A comparison between p53 accumulation determined by immunohistochemistry and TP53 mutations as prognostic variables in tumours from breast cancer patients. Acta Oncol 2008;47:600–7.

44. Kaye PV, Haider SA, James PD, et al. Novel staining pattern of p53 in Barrett's dysplasia–the absent pattern. Histopathology 2010;57:933–5.

45. Davelaar AL, Calpe S, Lau L, et al. Aberrant TP53 detected by combining immunohistochemistry and DNA-FISH improves Barrett's esophagus progression prediction: a prospective follow-up study. Genes Chromosomes Cancer 2015;54(2): 82–90.

46. Weaver JM, Ross-Innes CS, Shannon N, et al. Ordering of mutations in preinvasive disease stages of esophageal carcinogenesis. Nat Genet 2014;46:837–43.

47. Reid BJ, Prevo LJ, Galipeau PC, et al. Predictors of progression in Barrett's esophagus II: baseline 17p (p53) loss of heterozygosity identifies a patient subset at increased risk for neoplastic progression. Am J Gastroenterol 2001;96:2839–48.

48. Yu C, Zhang X, Huang Q, et al. High-fidelity DNA histograms in neoplastic progression in Barrett's esophagus. Lab Invest 2007;87:466–72.

49. Dunn JM, Mackenzie GD, Oukrif D, et al. Image cytometry accurately detects DNA ploidy abnormalities and predicts late relapse to high-grade dysplasia and adenocarcinoma in Barrett's oesophagus following photodynamic therapy. Br J Cancer 2010;102:1608–17.

50. Reid BJ, Blount PL, Rubin CE, et al. Flow-cytometric and histological progression to malignancy in Barrett's esophagus: prospective endoscopic surveillance of a cohort. Gastroenterology 1992;102:1212–9.

51. Reid BJ, Levine DS, Longton G, et al. Predictors of progression to cancer in Barrett's esophagus: baseline histology and flow cytometry identify low- and high-risk patient subsets. Am J Gastroenterol 2000;95:1669–76.

52. Li X, Galipeau PC, Paulson TG, et al. Temporal and spatial evolution of somatic chromosomal alterations: a case-cohort study of Barrett's esophagus. Cancer Prev Res (Phila) 2014;7:114–27.

53. Nones K, Waddell N, Wayte N, et al. Genomic catastrophes frequently arise in esophageal adenocarcinoma and drive tumorigenesis. Nat Commun 2014;5: 5224.

54. Wong DJ, Barrett MT, Stoger R, et al. p16INK4a promoter is hypermethylated at a high frequency in esophageal adenocarcinomas. Cancer Res 1997;57:2619–22.

55. Schulmann K, Sterian A, Berki A, et al. Inactivation of p16, RUNX3, and HPP1 occurs early in Barrett's-associated neoplastic progression and predicts progression risk. Oncogene 2005;24:4138–48.

56. Clement G, Braunschweig R, Pasquier N, et al. Methylation of APC, TIMP3, and TERT: a new predictive marker to distinguish Barrett's oesophagus patients at risk for malignant transformation. J Pathol 2006;208:100–7.

57. Sato F, Jin Z, Schulmann K, et al. Three-tiered risk stratification model to predict progression in Barrett's esophagus using epigenetic and clinical features. PLoS One 2008;3:e1890.

58. Jin Z, Cheng Y, Gu W, et al. A multicenter, double-blinded validation study of methylation biomarkers for progression prediction in Barrett's esophagus. Cancer Res 2009;69:4112–5.

59. Wang JS, Guo M, Montgomery EA, et al. DNA promoter hypermethylation of p16 and APC predicts neoplastic progression in Barrett's esophagus. Am J Gastroenterol 2009;104:2153–60.

60. Alvi MA, Liu X, O'Donovan M, et al. DNA methylation as an adjunct to histopathology to detect prevalent, inconspicuous dysplasia and early-stage neoplasia in Barrett's esophagus. Clin Cancer Res 2013;19:878–88.

61. Feber A, Xi L, Luketich JD, et al. MicroRNA expression profiles of esophageal cancer. J Thorac Cardiovasc Surg 2008;135:255–60 [discussion: 260].

62. Bansal A, Lee IH, Hong X, et al. Feasibility of microRNAs as biomarkers for Barrett's esophagus progression: a pilot cross-sectional, phase 2 biomarker study. Am J Gastroenterol 2011;106(6):1055–63.

63. Revilla-Nuin B, Parrilla P, Lozano JJ, et al. Predictive value of MicroRNAs in the progression of Barrett esophagus to adenocarcinoma in a long-term follow-up study. Ann Surg 2013;257:886–93.

64. Peiro-Chova L, Pena-Chilet M, Lopez-Guerrero JA, et al. High stability of microRNAs in tissue samples of compromised quality. Virchows Arch 2013;463: 765–74.

65. Maley CC, Galipeau PC, Finley JC, et al. Genetic clonal diversity predicts progression to esophageal adenocarcinoma. Nat Genet 2006;38:468–73.

66. Merlo LM, Shah NA, Li X, et al. A comprehensive survey of clonal diversity measures in Barrett's esophagus as biomarkers of progression to esophageal adenocarcinoma. Cancer Prev Res (Phila) 2010;3:1388–97.

67. di Pietro M, Boerwinkel DF, Shariff MK, et al. The combination of autofluorescence endoscopy and molecular biomarkers is a novel diagnostic tool for dysplasia in Barrett's oesophagus. Gut 2014;64(1):49–56.

68. Duits LC, Phoa KN, Curvers WL, et al. Barrett's oesophagus patients with low-grade dysplasia can be accurately risk-stratified after histological review by an expert pathology panel. Gut 2014. [Epub ahead of print].

69. Curvers WL, ten Kate FJ, Krishnadath KK, et al. Low-grade dysplasia in Barrett's esophagus: overdiagnosed and underestimated. Am J Gastroenterol 2010;105: 1523–30.

70. Wani S, Falk GW, Post J, et al. Risk factors for progression of low-grade dysplasia in patients with Barrett's esophagus. Gastroenterology 2011;141:1179–86, 1186.e1.
71. Pasricha S, Bulsiewicz WJ, Hathorn KE, et al. Durability and predictors of successful radiofrequency ablation for Barrett's esophagus. Clin Gastroenterol Hepatol 2014;12(11):1840–7.e1.
72. Prasad GA, Wang KK, Halling KC, et al. Correlation of histology with biomarker status after photodynamic therapy in Barrett esophagus. Cancer 2008;113:470–6.
73. Prasad GA, Wang KK, Halling KC, et al. Utility of biomarkers in prediction of response to ablative therapy in Barrett's esophagus. Gastroenterology 2008;135:370–9.
74. Timmer MR, Brankley SM, Gorospe EC, et al. Prediction of response to endoscopic therapy of Barrett's dysplasia by using genetic biomarkers. Gastrointest Endosc 2014;80(6):984–91.
75. Lao-Sirieix P, Fitzgerald RC. Screening for oesophageal cancer. Nature reviews. Nat Rev Clin Oncol 2012;9:278–87.
76. Zhai R, Zhao Y, Su L, et al. Genome-wide DNA methylation profiling of cell-free serum DNA in esophageal adenocarcinoma and Barrett esophagus. Neoplasia 2012;14:29–33.
77. Zhang J, Bowers J, Liu L, et al. Esophageal cancer metabolite biomarkers detected by LC-MS and NMR methods. PLoS One 2012;7:e30181.
78. Rubenstein JH, Morgenstern H, McConell D, et al. Associations of diabetes mellitus, insulin, leptin, and ghrelin with gastroesophageal reflux and Barrett's esophagus. Gastroenterology 2013;145:1237–44.e1–5.
79. Mechref Y, Hussein A, Bekesova S, et al. Quantitative serum glycomics of esophageal adenocarcinoma and other esophageal disease onsets. J Proteome Res 2009;8:2656–66.
80. Thrift AP, Garcia JM, El-Serag HB. A multibiomarker risk score helps predict risk for Barrett's esophagus. Clin Gastroenterol Hepatol 2014;12:1267–71.
81. Wang JS, Varro A, Lightdale CJ, et al. Elevated serum gastrin is associated with a history of advanced neoplasia in Barrett's esophagus. Am J Gastroenterol 2010;105:1039–45.
82. Rizk NP, Servais EL, Tang LH, et al. Tissue and serum mesothelin are potential markers of neoplastic progression in Barrett's associated esophageal adenocarcinoma. Cancer Epidemiol Biomarkers Prev 2012;21:482–6.
83. Bansal A, Hong X, Lee IH, et al. Serum exosomal microRNA expression can be a novel non-invasive strategy for the screening of Barrett's esophagus. Gastroenterology 2013;144:S-684.
84. Van Baal JW, Kestens C, Ten Kate FT, et al. Comprehensive profiling of plasma MicroRNAs reveals potential biomarkers for Barrett's esophagus and esophageal adenocarcinoma. Gastroenterology 2014;146:S-97.
85. Li Y, Jiang Z, Xu L, et al. Stability analysis of liver cancer-related microRNAs. Acta Biochim Biophys Sin (Shanghai) 2011;43:69–78.
86. Wijnhoven BP, Hussey DJ, Watson DI, et al. MicroRNA profiling of Barrett's oesophagus and oesophageal adenocarcinoma. Br J Surg 2010;97(6):853–61.

Chemoprevention in Barrett's Esophagus
Current Status

Muhammad H. Zeb, MD[a], Anushka Baruah, MD[b],
Sarah K. Kossak, BS[a], Navtej S. Buttar, MD[a],*

KEYWORDS

- Barrett's esophagus • Esophageal adenocarcinoma • Chemoprevention
- Chronic reflux

KEY POINTS

- At present, chemoprevention in Barrett's esophagus is applied only in research settings.
- Identifying pathways that can be targeted by safe, pharmaceutical or natural compounds is key to expanding the scope of chemoprevention.
- Defining meaningful surrogate markers of cancer progression is critical to test the efficacy of chemopreventive approaches.
- Chemopreventive agents that show promise across epidemiologic, preclinical (in vitro and in vivo), and early clinical trials will be more likely to be successful when applied in clinical practice.
- Combinatorial chemoprevention that targets multiple components of the same pathway or parallel pathways could reduce the risk and improve the efficacy of chemoprevention.

INTRODUCTION

Barrett's esophagus (BE) is a premalignant condition in which chronic reflux injury leads to replacement of normal squamous mucosa by metaplastic columnar mucosa. Approximately 1 in 10 to 20 adults with reflux in the United States harbor BE, and based on currently available data, the annual incidence of adenocarcinoma in patients

Disclosures: None.
Author Contributions: Study concept and design; analysis and interpretation of data; drafting of the article (M.H. Zeb, MD); Study concept and design; analysis and interpretation of data; drafting of the article (A. Baruah, MD); Study concept and design; drafting of the article and critical revision of the article (S.K. Kossak); Study concept and design; analysis and interpretation of data, drafting of the article; critical revision of the article for important intellectual content; study supervision (N.S. Buttar, MD).
[a] Division of Gastroenterology and Hepatology, Mayo Clinic, 200 First Street Southwest, Rochester, MN 55905, USA; [b] Department of Internal Medicine, John H. Stroger, Jr. Hospital of Cook County, 1901 W. Harrison Street, Chicago, IL 60612, USA
* Corresponding author.
E-mail address: buttar.navtej@mayo.edu

with BE is estimated to range from 0.3% to 0.5%. Esophageal adenocarcinoma (EAC) is becoming increasingly common in Western countries over the past several decades. Although the incidences of most malignances are trending downward, the rate of EAC is rapidly increasing. The 5-year survival rate for patients with EAC is approximately 17%, and this dismal prognosis has not changed.[1] Although strategies involving early detection of cancer at a potentially curable stage make sense, these approaches are inherently expensive and are based on limited data.[2] Alternatively, novel interventions, such as ablation or resection of dysplastic Barrett's mucosa, are being increasingly used in clinical practice; recurrent metaplasia and neoplasia remain problematic. Here we discuss the role of chemoprevention as an independent or an adjuvant management option in BE-associated EAC.

DEFINITION AND CONCEPT OF CHEMOPREVENTION

Chemoprevention refers to a strategy of using pharmaceutical or nutraceutical compounds to prevent the initiation or progression of dysplasia, as well as blocking the invasion of dysplastic epithelial cells across the basement membrane. To clinically apply this strategy, several factors need to be considered. Is there a cohort of patients with a premalignant lesion that can be easily detected or are there known clinical and or pathophysiological conditions that facilitate neoplastic progression? Are there modifiable molecular, biochemical, or cellular derangements that can be targeted using pharmaceutical or nutraceutical compounds, and if so are there intermediate or definitive endpoints that could assess the efficacy of these compounds? In the following discussion, we review the existing scientific evidence to examine the role of chemoprevention in BE.

RISK STRATIFICATION OF COHORT

Unlike standard therapeutic paradigms in EAC, chemoprevention has to be undertaken in individuals with reflux or Barrett's metaplasia in which the risk of lethal EAC is extremely variable depending on dysplasia grade. Therefore, the potential benefit of an intervention has to be carefully weighed against possible side effects or toxicity associated with the intervention. Additionally, existing comorbidities, patient preferences, and local expertise also have to factor into decision-making. For the purpose of chemoprevention, we discuss risk stratification in the following 3 cohorts.

Gastroesophageal Reflux

Gastroesophageal reflux (GERD) is a key risk factor for the development of BE as well as EAC. Patients with long-standing and severe reflux injury are at 6-fold to 8-fold higher risk of developing BE and 7-fold to 43-fold increased risk of EAC. These observations suggest that the GERD population could be a reasonable cohort for chemoprevention. A Gallup survey demonstrated that 44% of adults in the United States experience heartburn at least once a month. A survey of residents in Olmsted County in Minnesota demonstrated that 18% of respondents experienced heartburn at least weekly.[3] Given that nearly one-fifth of the US population has significant reflux symptoms and there is a lack of reflux symptom correlation with the identifiable premalignant lesion of BE, it makes this population a viable chemoprevention cohort only for interventions that are essentially risk free.

Nondysplastic Barrett's or Barrett's with Low-Grade Dysplasia

Most the patients diagnosed with BE are nondysplastic or have low-grade dysplasia. Overall, the risk of neoplastic progression in nondysplastic BE is very low. In a Danish population-based, cohort study involving 11,028 patients with Barrett's esophagus, the incidence rate for adenocarcinoma was 1.2 cases per 1000 person-years in non-dysplastic Barrett's and 5.1 cases per 1000 person-years in Barrett's with low-grade dysplasia.[4] Another cohort study from Ireland showed a progression rate of 0.17% per year in patients with nondysplastic BE.[5] Similar to these studies, a recent meta-analysis showed the incidence of EAC in patients with nondysplastic Barrett's epithelium to be 1 case per 300 patient years.[6] Based on these results, if a chemopreventive intervention reduces the risk of cancer by 50%, one would need to treat 2000 nondysplastic or 400 patients with low-grade dysplasia to prevent 1 cancer death. Therefore, if the patient is relatively healthy, with such a low-risk of progression, it is reasonable to use chemopreventive agents that have been deemed extremely safe for use. In this patient population, even a moderate reduction in cancer risk by 50% would translate into a significant public health benefit, as most Barrett's patients fall under this category.

Patients with Barrett's with High-Grade Dysplasia and Postablative Barrett's

Unlike nondysplastic Barrett's or patients with low-grade dysplasia in whom the risk of cancer progression is low and it takes several years to progress to EAC, up to 20% patients with high-grade dysplastic Barrett's already have a prevalent EAC. A subset of patients with ablated dysplastic Barrett's are also at higher risk of recurrent dysplastic BE or EAC.[4,5] Because of the relatively high risk of neoplastic transformation, it is important to use more effective chemopreventive agents in this cohort, even if these agents carry a considerably higher risk of adverse effects. Alternatively, in this cohort, it will be reasonable to consider chemoprevention as an adjunctive approach along with other therapy, such as endoscopic ablation.

DRUGGABLE TARGETS

Similar to therapeutic interventions, target discovery is a critical step in chemoprevention. It is important to understand which pathways are deregulated during progression to EAC and if these pathways could be modifiable with the use of nutraceutical or pharmaceutical compounds. Identification of druggable targets largely depends on data derived from epidemiologic associations and through pathophysiological studies using cell culture and/or animal models to see if these associations could be directly implicated in neoplastic transformation. Because the process of carcinogenesis involves host-environment interactions at local and systemic levels, in the following paragraphs we discuss the target identification along these lines.

Luminal

Acid and bile salts
The esophageal mucosa is constantly exposed to luminal contents. In patients with reflux, gastric and duodenal secretions intermittently cover the esophageal mucosa. Bile salts contained in duodenal secretions in a gastric pH dependent manner play a key role in the chronic injury-inflammation-carcinogenesis cascade. There is significantly more gastric acid and duodenal bile reflux in patients with Barrett's complicated by dysplasia or cancer compared with Barrett's without dysplasia.[7] Bile salts that reach the esophagus produce injury over a wide range of pH depending on their pKa. For example, when the reflux is acidic (pH <4), taurine-conjugated bile salts cause injury. When pH is from 4 to 6, glycine-conjugated bile salts cause injury, and unconjugated bile salts cause injury when the pH is neutral or alkaline.[7,8] Interestingly, the levels of taurine-conjugated and unconjugated bile salts are significantly higher in

the esophagus of patients with BE compared with patients with mild or minimal reflux.[8] Even though proton pump inhibitors (PPIs) successfully heal the obvious esophagitis in 80% to 90% of patients, up to one-third of these patients continue to have bile reflux.[9] In addition, chronic use of PPIs deconjugates bile salts by bacterial colonization of the proximal gut.[10] These unconjugated bile salts, in the high-pH environment created by PPIs, are implicated in chronic low-grade inflammation and promote carcinogenesis in BE. Consistent with these epidemiologic associations, chronic reflux of gastric acid and/or duodenal contents in animal models leads to dysplasia and EAC. In canine and rodent models, bile reflux alone induces carcinogenesis in BE.[11,12]

Human studies that simultaneously target acid production along with bile salt modulation, for example a combination of PPIs and ursodeoxycholic could result in prevention of EAC. Other potential targets can be mucosal protectants or agents that could reduce mucosal permeability. Because exposure of esophageal mucosa to acid and/or bile induces oxidative stress, activates proinflammatory pathways, and initiates aberrant repair process in the mucosa, several mechanisms discussed in the following sections identify additional chemoprevention strategies.

Carcinogens

There is only limited information available on the effects of carcinogen exposure in the development of EAC.[13,14] However, a weak association exists between cigarette smoking and progression to adenocarcinoma. In a multivariate analysis, the Rotterdam Esophageal Tumor Study Group noted that compared with nonsmokers, the odds of EAC in smokers were 2.3 times higher.[15] Compared with patients with BE, patients with EAC have higher median duration as well as the number of pack-years of smoking (median 29.5 vs 38.5 years, $P < .003$ and median 15.0 vs 55.25 pack-years, $P < .001$).[16] Other investigators found no clear association between smoking and neoplastic progression in BE.[17,18] The differences could simply be due to variable definition of Barrett's, by including prevalent and incident cases together and inability to control for confounding factors because of small sample size. Preclinical animal studies support a link between carcinogen exposure and EAC.[13,14] The risk of EAC in mice and rodents increases with 2,6-dimethylnitrosomorpholin or N-methyl-N-benzylnitrosamine carcinogen administration.[14] This is clinically relevant because in the latter half of the past century there was marked increase in the nitrate levels in food and water.[19] Nitrates are concentrated by the salivary glands and secreted into the mouth,[20] where oral microbes reduce these nitrates to nitrites.[20] Moreover, achlorhydria induced by PPI use leads to overgrowth of nitrate-reducing bacteria in the stomach,[19,21] and these bacteria convert dietary nitrate to nitrite. Contents of gastroduodenal reflux in the lower esophagus change these nitrites to nitrous acid and eventually to nitric oxide.[22] Nitric oxide, through DNA damage, lipid peroxidation, and mutagenesis, promotes tumorigenesis. Targeting carcinogen metabolism or downstream pathways can therefore provide an alternate strategy to prevent carcinogenesis.[23] Similarly, taking steps toward cessation of smoking in high-risk individuals also may prevent neoplastic transformation.

Mucosal

The mucosal compartment of the esophagus allows complex interactions among epithelial, stromal, and immunoregulatory cells. Among the most studied molecular mechanisms that are dysfunctional during neoplastic transformation include prostaglandin biosynthesis, increased proinflammatory cytokine release, increased expression and binding of growth factor ligands to their receptors followed by upregulation of membrane to nuclear signaling, and polyamine synthesis. These derangements provide numerous potential chemoprevention targets.

Arachidonic acid pathway and prostaglandin synthesis

The arachidonic acid pathway is a key mediator of inflammatory response through prostaglandin synthesis, particularly PGE2. This pathway is upregulated during neoplastic progression in BE.[24,25] PGE2 synthesis is regulated at various steps. The first step is catalyzed by phospholipases to release arachidonic acid from membrane phospholipids. Arachidonic acid is catalyzed by cyclooxygenase (COX) to synthesize PGE2.[26,27] Among phospholipases, cytosolic PLA2α, because of its high selectivity for a particular type of unsaturated fatty acid, is considered the rate-limiting step for PGE2 synthesis.[26] Transcription factor KLF11, an epigenetic regulator, inhibits PGE2 by silencing cPLA2α and thereby downregulates growth of epithelial cells in BE. In addition, in an in vitro study performed on Barrett's cell lines by our laboratory, we found that COX-2 inhibition significantly decreases proliferation of BE cells, whereas treatment of these cells with PGE2 (product of COX-2 activity) restored proliferation of cell lines, suggesting a possible role of COX-2 inhibition for chemoprevention in BE.[19] A preclinical study conducted by us established that the use of selective and nonselective COX-2 inhibitors in a rodent model of chronic reflux produced a statistically significant reduction in relative risk of developing EAC by 55% in rats treated with MF-tricyclic and 79% (P<.01) in those treated with sulindac as compared with the control group. The degree of inflammation was found to be more severe in the control group compared with the study group.[22] In summary, downregulation of PGE2 levels, either by KLF11-mediated inhibition of cPLA2α or through COX2 inhibition, reduces cell growth in vitro and neoplastic transformation in Barrett's and mucosa of animals with reflux injury.[24,25,28,29] These findings, along with epidemiologic evidence of lower risk of EAC in patients who chronically use nonsteroidal anti-inflammatory drugs (NSAIDs), suggest that intercepting prostaglandin biosynthesis through anti-inflammatory drugs or natural epigenetic modifiers could have chemopreventive potential.

Cytokines

In patients with BE, chronic mucosal injury by acid and bile reflux[30] leads to inflammation and release of cytokines and chemokines.[31–35] Through ligand-receptor binding, these factors trigger the activation of membrane to nuclear signaling that deregulate cell growth and differentiation and facilitate neoplastic progression. The mechanism involved here can be targeted to prevent neoplastic progression. Several recent preclinical and clinical studies show deregulation of the proinflammatory cytokine cascade that starts with upregulation of interleukin (IL)-1β and tumor necrosis factor (TNF)-α.[24,25,36–44] In vitro and in vivo work support that IL-1β and TNF-α via the IL-6-STAT3 pathway upregulate oncogenic AKT and COX to drive PGE2 biosynthesis. During carcinogenesis in BE, there is upregulation of TNF-α ligand and receptors, as well as polymorphism of the IL-1β gene. Interestingly, transgenic expression of human IL-1β in the esophagus of mice with bile salt injury leads to abnormal differentiation of pluripotent stem cells, metaplasia, and progression to carcinoma via changes in the stromal microenvironment. Members of this cascade are targets of drugs such as NSAIDs, inhibitors of IL-1β, TNF-α, or STAT3. Therefore, interrupting this pathway at various levels could have chemopreventive potential.[24,25,36–44]

Growth factors

Injury-repair is central to the process of carcinogenesis in BE and is associated with upregulation of many growth factors.[45] If the cells express appropriate receptors, growth factors can facilitate cell growth. The ligand secreted by stromal cells or adjacent cells bind to receptors on epithelial cells modulating growth regulatory cytoplasmic and nuclear signaling as well as changing stromal epithelial interactions in a feed-forward manner.[46]

Neoplastic progression in BE is associated with increased expression of epidermal growth factor (EGF), transforming growth factor α, and EGF receptor (EGFR), raising a potential for autocrine or paracrine signaling.[45,47,48] Transition from Barrett's to cancer is associated with overexpression of c-erb B-2 oncogene that translates into constitutively active EGFR that does not require EGF overexpression. Tumors expressing c-erb B-2 have poor outcomes. Because this is a delayed event during carcinogenesis, it therefore does not appear to be a useful chemoprevention target for primary prevention.[48–51]

The typical growth factor signaling involves activation of downstream membrane to nuclear cascades through kinases that cause posttranslational changes in proteins. In many cancers, ras, src, and myc family of proteins play an important role in transformation. Interestingly, unlike many other cancers, K-ras does not appear to be relevant to neoplastic transformation in Barrett's but H-ras, src, and myc all show progressive increase during carcinogenesis and could be targeted for chemoprevention.[52,60]

Differentiation-related extracellular signaling ligands

The WNT glycoprotein family of extracellular signaling ligands is involved in cell growth, motility, and differentiation.[54] WNT inhibitory factor 1 (WIF1), a WNT antagonist, is silenced by promoter hypermethylation, leading to an increase in cellular proliferation, a phenotype that can be rescued by WIF1 restoration.[55] This suggests that agents that activate WIF1, due to their ability to inhibit WNT signaling, could have chemopreventive potential.[56] Restoration of APC and secreted frizzled-related protein-1 (SFRP1) function by reversing promoter methylation could also inhibit WNT signaling and carcinogenesis.[57,58]

Polyamines

Growth factors, TNF-α, nuclear factor (NF)-kB, and Myc, which are upregulated in neoplastic transformation,[59] activate ornithine decarboxylase (ODC). ODC is the rate-limiting enzyme in polyamine synthesis. Polyamines (putrescine, spermidine, and spermines) have a key role in cell growth. Increased ODC activity and resulting polyamine synthesis is noted during neoplastic progression in BE.[60] Therefore, ODC inhibition by difluoromethylornithine is a reasonable chemopreventive strategy.

Prosurvival and antideath pathways

NF-kB is a proinflammatory, prosurvival transcription factor. There is an upregulation of several members of the NF-kB pathway during cancer development in patients with Barrett's. As discussed previously, TNF-α, an upstream activator of NF-kB, has been shown to be progressively upregulated in Barrett's tissues, and IL-8, a downstream transcriptional target of NF-kB, also has been shown to be upregulated in Barrett's-related adenocarcinomas. In vitro studies using Barrett's epithelial cells show that physiologic concentrations of bile acid deoxycholic acid (DCA) at neutral pH activate NF-kB.[61] Similar results also are noted in patients undergoing infusion of DCA into the esophagus. DCA induces oxidative stress in Barrett's mucosa of patients, which causes genotoxic injury, and it also simultaneously induces activation of the NF-κB pathway, which enables cells with DNA damage to resist apoptosis. These molecular mechanisms point to the chemopreventive potential of NF-kB inhibitors, such as BAY 11-7085, Ad$\mathrm{I\kappa B}$ super repressor, Bortezomib, or curcumin during carcinogenesis in BE.[61]

One of the important concepts during carcinogenesis is uncoupling of cell proliferation from cell death or apoptosis. Several events during carcinogenesis, such as inflammation, generation of reactive oxygen species, lack of antioxidant defenses, and mutagenic pressure exerted by nitroso-compounds, result in hyperproliferation of epithelial cells and mutagenesis. Entry of these mutated cells into further cell division is typically prevented by the tumor suppressor protein p53.[62] Functional p53 induces apoptosis in these abnormal cells if DNA is repaired.[63] Loss of p53 function is a common phenomenon in BE that compromises this protective mechanism. Clonal expansion of these cells with mutated DNA facilitates neoplastic progression in BE.[63] Therefore, pharmacologic measures that upregulate p53 (eg, trans-retinoic acid) may result in chemoprevention by restoration of the apoptotic response.[64] Similar to p53 loss, several other mechanisms help Barrett's epithelial cells evade apoptosis. Bile acid DCA via Erk-1/2 and p38 MAPK-mediated activation of AP-1 transcription factor induces antiapoptotic protein COX-2.[56] Likewise, an increase in the expression of constitutively active splice variant of the cholecyctokinin-2 receptor in Barrett's mucosa also leads to activation of antiapoptotic pathways via PKB/Akt.[57] These findings support targeting these kinases either individually or in combination to achieve chemoprevention.

Epigenetic signals

Chromosomal instability influences various genes that modulate the biological and biochemical processes involved in carcinogenesis. To an extent, these genetic changes are modifiable via epigenetic signals, and in certain situations, epigenetic signals actually facilitate the chromosomal instability. Global hypomethylation along with promoter-specific hypermethylation during carcinogenesis in BE leads to inactivation of tumor suppressor gene p16, thereby nullifying its tumor-suppressive action. Further, there is loss of p16 heterozygosity at 9p21 and inactivation of tumor suppressor p53. Loss of function of these key regulatory tumor-suppressive genes results in uncontrolled cell proliferation.[65] Progressive hypermethylation and epigenetic silencing leading to loss of function of the glutathione peroxidase 3 gene also is observed in BE.[66] This epigenetic silencing results in loss of antioxidant defense against repeated oxidative stress from chronic reflux–induced injury. The end result is accumulation of abnormal esophageal cells with a high degree of chromosomal instability.[65] These observations along with introduction of novel epigenetic drugs in clinical practice open a new field of epigenetic chemoprevention.

Immunosurveillance

Normally Fas ligand (Fas-L) binds to Fas and initiates the cell apoptosis cascade. During neoplastic progression in BE, Fas-L is overexpressed and Fas expression is decreased in the epithelial cells. This protects dysplastic Barrett's epithelial cells from self-destruction and also allows them to evade immune surveillance.[67,68] Moreover, upregulation of Fas-L expression in dysplastic epithelium could induce apoptosis in Fas-expressing lymphocytes that further compromises tumor surveillance in BE.[67,68] Strategies to restore immunosurveillance could positively impact the chemopreventive efforts.

Systemic

The mucosal response to luminal insults and epithelial-stromal interaction are modulated by systemic influences, which are outlined as follows.

Obesity-induced disruption of antireflux mechanisms and altered composition of reflux

Visceral obesity increases intra-abdominal pressure and changes the relationship between the gastroesophageal junction (GEJ) and diaphragmatic antireflux mechanisms. These changes increase reflux that eventually causes injury, BE, and

EAC.[69,70] Twenty-four–hour pH monitoring and motility studies reveal that obese patients have increased incidence of asymptomatic reflux[71] and obesity is associated with significant drop in lower esophageal sphincter (LES) pressure.[72] Pharmacologic agents that change LES pressure may therefore have chemopreventive potential in obese patients. Obesity also is associated with dietary and systemic derangements that could alter reflux composition. In a systematic review, McQuaid et al[73] found that the concentration of carcinogenic bile acid in esophageal aspirate was higher in obese patients. Although compliance with dietary modifications is difficult, changes in dietary composition, such as the use of polyunsaturated fatty acids or targeting the obesity-associated derangements in bile salt synthesis with ursodeoxycholate or protecting esophageal mucosa from bile injury (topical protective barriers), could prevent carcinogenesis in BE.

Obesity-induced systemic inflammatory response

There is increasing evidence that obesity is a systemic endocrine derangement that results in a systemic and local proinflammatory state.[74] Adipocytes release high circulating concentration of cytokines like TNF-α, IL-6, IL-1B, IL-10, C-reactive protein, interferon (INF)-ϒ, monocyte chemotactic protein, plasminogen activator inhibitor-1, and fibrinogen.[74,75] These cytokines create a proinflammatory state, an important connecting link between obesity and various cancers, including EAC.[74] Activated CD8+ T cells in the visceral adipose tissue produce IFN-ϒ resulting in TNF-α production in adipose tissue.[76] Systemic release of this TNF-α acts locally on the subepithelial tissue and switches the stromal macrophage phenotype to modulate inflammation in target tissues such as Barrett's mucosa. This hypothesis is supported by the findings of increased expression of both the ligand and the receptor of TNF-α during carcinogenesis in BE.[31] This suggests that in overweight patients, adipocytes in endocrine manner, by influencing systemic and local inflammatory response, facilitate neoplastic transformation. This proinflammatory state also upregulates inducible nitric oxide synthase (iNOS) and nitric oxide production, which is typically seen during inflammation and carcinogenesis in BE.[42] As alluded to earlier, this proinflammatory state creates oxidative stress and this altered oxidative tissue state favors mutagenesis to promote neoplasia.[66] Interestingly, there is relative deficiency of antioxidant micronutrients like βcarotene, lycopene, and vitamin C in obese patients and consumption of vegetables and fruits rich in natural antioxidants is associated with a decreased risk of esophageal cancer.[77,78] Approaches to alter mucosal response to injury through inhibitors of the previously mentioned pathways (anti–TNF-α or IL-1/iNOS inhibitors or dietary antioxidants) could prevent carcinogenesis in BE.

Pathways deranged in the metabolic syndrome

The metabolic syndrome is a cluster of conditions, including increased blood pressure, a high blood sugar level, excess body fat around the waist, and abnormal cholesterol levels, that occur together, increasing the risk of various cancers. One of the characteristic features of metabolic syndrome is insulin resistance. A diet high in energy and animal fat, and low in fiber in combination with physical inactivity contributes to insulin resistance and resulting hyperinsulinemia.[79–82] Insulin, by activating insulinlike growth factor-1 receptors, stimulates cellular proliferation and inhibits apoptosis via the oncogenic PI3K-AKT-mTOR-S6K1 signaling cascade that facilitates carcinogenesis in BE.[69,83] Next, leptin, as a part of the metabolic syndrome, increases EAC cell survival through PGE2-mediated activation of EGFR and c-Jun NH2-terminal kinase.[84] Metabolic syndrome is also associated with downregulation of adipokine signaling and the expression of adiponectin receptors that has been correlated with

EAC.[85] Thus, obesity, lifestyle changes, and nutritional modification, although difficult to implement, remain important chemopreventive targets in BE.

Hypergastrinemia

Long-term PPI use in patients with BE leads to increased serum gastrin levels.[86–88] Gastrin is a trophic hormone and promotes cell survival in the gastrointestinal tract.[86–89] Gastrin binds to the cholecystokinin (CCK2) receptor that in turn induces EGF and the trefoil peptide expression.[87,88] These gastrin-induced signals lead to COX-2 expression and facilitate carcinogenesis in BE.[87] Interestingly Barrett's mucosa expresses high levels of CCK2 receptors,[87,88] and gastrin exposure is known to increase Barrett's epithelial cell survival.[87,88] Therefore, strategies to combine PPIs with gastrin inhibitors or the inhibitors of downstream signaling could prevent esophageal cancer.

END POINT EVALUATION

Ideally, cancer incidence and associated mortality should be included as primary endpoints in chemoprevention studies, but use of such definitive endpoints is not feasible during neoplastic transformation in Barrett's. Using cancer risk reduction, although ideal and clinically relevant, is impractical because of the need for a lengthy follow-up and large number of trial participants to gather any meaningful information. To overcome these drawbacks, the markers to assess the chemoprevention response are broadly divided into 2 categories. The first set of markers, such as change in the grade of dysplasia, are clinically relevant. The next set of markers examine the effect of chemopreventive changes on the surrogate markers of neoplastic progression and also assess if the molecular pathways intended to be targeted by the chemopreventive agent are indeed downregulated.

Histopathology

Because grade of dysplasia is clinically used to predict the risk of cancer development and guide therapy in BE, one way to monitor chemoprevention would be to evaluate if the use of a chemopreventive agent downgrades the dysplastic changes or prevents progression to dysplasia in BE. Although histologic grade assessment is the principal predictor of Barrett's progression, this approach is subjective. Typically, 20% to 30% of patients progress from nondysplastic to low-grade dysplastic Barrett's and 14% to 28% of patients with high-grade dysplasia progress to cancer within 2 months to 4 years. [Reid, 1988 #1][90] However, only 85% of expert pathologists can confidently differentiate between EAC and high-grade dysplasia from nondysplastic Barrett's and low-grade dysplasia. Moreover, agreement among pathologists regarding low-grade dysplasia diagnosis is dismal.[90,91] In addition, high-grade dysplasia occupies less than 5% of the Barrett's surface area, and a sampling error may erroneously increase the effectiveness of a chemopreventive agent.[92] Use of degree of dysplasia as the chemoprevention endpoint does require complementary surrogate endpoint biomarkers (SEBs).

Surrogate Endpoint Biomarkers

The surrogate biomarkers that objectively correlate with cancer risk in BE are commonly used in chemoprevention trials. Depending on the phase of chemoprevention trial or the degree of dysplasia in the target population, these surrogate markers are used either independently or as complementary to histopathology. An important concept while selecting SEB is that the marker should not be an irreversible genetic event. Choosing such marker, by virtue of being irreversible, will portray a picture of agent inefficacy or failure regardless of whether or not the preventive agent is showing benefit.

Flow cytometery, image cytometry, and fluorescent in situ hybridization (FISH) show that abnormal p16 and p53 expression due to loss of heterozygosity, promotor silencing, or mutations, along with aneuploidy or hyper-tetraploidy could predict progression of neoplasia.[93-100] Prasad and colleagues[101] evaluated a biomarker panel by FISH (loss of 9p21 [p16] and 17p13.1 [p53] loci; gains of the 8q24 [c-myc], 17q [HER2-neu], and 20q13 [ZNF217] loci; and multiple gains) on cytology specimens collected before and after photodynamic therapy (PDT) in 31 patients with high-grade BE (HGD)/mucosal cancer. In 6 of 31 patients, abnormal expression was present for at least one marker after PDT in the absence of histologic abnormalities. Two of 6 patients with persistent biomarker abnormalities developed recurrent HGD. The previously mentioned FISH panel was then prospectively applied to patients undergoing PDT.[102] At baseline, 68% of the patients with HGD and 73% with mucosal cancer had FISH abnormalities. On multivariate analysis, p16 loss at baseline predicted the lack of response of HGD/mucosal cancer to PDT at 3-month follow-up (0.32, 95% confidence interval [CI] 0.10–0.96). In a cohort of 181 patients undergoing radiofrequency ablation, the same FISH panel found that the presence of multiple gains at baseline predicted failure of complete remission of dysplasia (hazard ratio [HR] 0.57, 95% CI 0.40–0.82).[103] As pointed out earlier, if these changes are irreversible, use of these markers may spuriously underestimate the chemopreventive potential of an agent. Contrary to this, epigenetic effects, such as global hypomethylation and promoter-specific hypermethylation that are more dynamic in nature, or microRNA will likely be better markers to assess the efficacy of a chemopreventive agent.[58,104-109]

Recent studies have demonstrated progressive increase in the levels of GLI-1, vascular endothelial growth factor, transcription factor MCM2, COX-2 enzyme, PGE2, polyamine,[3,87] and upregulation of prosurvival NF-kB during oncogenesis in BE.[108] These biochemical and molecular markers of neoplastic progression also can assess if the molecular pathways intended to be targeted by chemopreventive agents are actually being downregulated. In addition to these, markers of increased cellular proliferation, along with elevated pro-oncogenic pathways, provide biologically relevant markers. Commonly used biomarkers for increased cellular proliferation include Ki-67, PCNA, and MCM2. These markers, along with markers of apoptosis, such as caspases and BcL2, determine overall cell survival.[109,110] Another way to assess degree of dysplastic regression in Barrett's patients would be to quantify the ratio between proliferative and apoptotic markers. Decrease in the ratio with use of chemopreventive agents would suggest dysplastic regression. Quantification of this ratio appears to be a practical approach to monitoring chemoprevention agent efficacy.

Many of the SEBs mentioned previously are currently used in phase 1 and 2 clinical trials either individually or as components of a pathway or to complement histopathology. If molecular, biological, and histologic outcomes change in parallel in response to a chemopreventive agent, there will be higher confidence in accepting the efficacy of a chemopreventive agent.

CLINICAL STUDIES AND RANDOMIZED TRIALS

The earlier discussion in this review focused predominantly on target identification and monitoring of chemoprevention. These important concepts need complementary clinical studies to predict or validate the efficacy of chemopreventive agents. Although together the information presented here provides a framework to discuss chemoprevention in clinical settings, chemoprevention at the present time remains an experimental approach.

Acid Suppression and Bile Salt Modification

As outlined earlier, acid and bile reflux initiate a cascade of proinflammatory pathways that are known to promote neoplasia. The caveats are that most patients with BE already use PPIs that change the degree of acid and it requires invasive monitoring to examine the effectiveness of interventions to suppress reflux. Therefore, this premise is mainly tested with case-control or observational studies.

Epidemiologic studies show conflicting evidence regarding chemopreventive potential of acid suppression using PPIs. In Veteran Administration setting, follow-up of 236 patients with BE for more than a decade showed approximately 60% risk reduction of dysplastic changes in patients using PPIs compared with those who did not use PPIs.[110] In a larger Dutch study, a more robust risk reduction (up to 75%) of neoplastic progression in BE was noted with acid suppression.[111] Similarly, a prospective review of surveillance data in 350 Australian patients showed that in the patients who delayed the use of PPIs for more than 2 years after Barrett's diagnosis, there was an increased risk for developing low-grade dysplasia (HR 5.6, 95% CI 2.0–15.7) and high-grade dysplasia or cancer (HR 20.9, 95% CI 2.8–158).[112] However, most of the progression in this study was to low-grade dysplasia, a diagnosis that is commonly contested. Although the clinical relevance of extent of Barrett's mucosa to the risk of neoplastic progression is not clear, studies show more frequent squamous islands or a partial regression of BE in patients who take PPIs.[113]

Contrary to these results, in a recent Danish study of 9883 patients with BE, a high adherence to PPI use was associated with increased relative risk (RR) of developing high-grade dysplasia and cancer (RR 3.4, 95% CI 1.1–10.5).[114] A meta-analysis conducted by Singh and colleagues[115] demonstrated a 71% risk reduction in development of EAC and high-grade dysplasia in patients who were on PPIs for more than 2 to 3 years, whereas patients who received less than 2 years of therapy did not seem to benefit much from PPI use. Congruent with these observations, small clinical trials addressed the question of whether profound acid suppression can have chemopreventive potential in Barrett's mucosa. Epithelial cell proliferation, which correlates with dysplasia,[116,117] decreases during near complete elimination of acid reflux in patients.[118,119] Villin, which is a marker of differentiation, is more strongly expressed after acid reflux normalization in patients.[118] PPI treatment is also associated with fewer abnormalities in mucosal expression of cell cycle regulatory proteins, such as p16, p21, and cyclins D1 and E, as well as decreased DNA damage in Barrett's mucosa.[120,121] In a different patient population of ablated Barrett's epithelium, when mucosal ablation failed during insufficient acid suppression, a more profound acid suppression resulted in successful ablation.[122,123] In a short-term study, however, normalization of acid reflux did not appear to be necessary.[124] On the other hand, recurrence of metaplasia was observed after discontinuation of omeprazole maintenance.[35] Because mucosal ablation studies are typically performed with concomitant acid suppression, they do not clearly address the chemopreventive potential and require more definitive studies.

During reflux injury, bile acids are directly implicated in producing esophageal epithelial damage. Bile salt–related injury is pH dependent and the use of PPIs not only alters the pH, but also decreases the overall quantity of reflux. Interestingly, one-third of the patients on PPI treatment continue to have bile reflux.[9] Moreover, different bile acids inflict injury to the epithelial tissue at different pH, as outlined earlier in this review. The composition of bile acids in duodenal bile is modifiable. In healthy individuals, the bile mainly consists of cytotoxic hydrophobic bile acids, such as deoxycholic acid and cholic acid. These cytotoxic bile acids are largely replaced by tertiary hydrophilic bile acids when treated with ursodeoxycholic acid, thus reducing bile acid–induced injury to the esophagus.[125] Although in animals with reflux, ursodeoxycholic acid use led to suppression of inflammation-metaplasia-neoplasia sequence,[125] in patients with BE, urso failed to change markers of differentiation or proliferation.[126] In samples derived from patients with BE and in preclinical investigations, our laboratory found that bile acids trigger activation of GLI-1, an effector of the Hedgehog pathway, which is upregulated during carcinogenesis in BE. GLI-1, through cell cycle regulator CDK2, promotes Barrett's epithelial cell proliferation. Combination of ursodeoxycholic acid and aspirin via their inhibitory action on GLI-1 downregulate CDK2, decrease cell growth, and prevent cancer in animals.[39] It is therefore possible that if ursodeoxycholic acid is combined with aspirin in patients with BE, it could prevent carcinogenesis.

Nonsteroidal Anti-inflammatory Drugs (Celecoxib)

NSAIDs target COX enzyme, which regulates prostaglandin synthesis from arachidonic acid. COX is implicated in the oncogenic transformation of Barrett's to EAC.[12–15] Compared with nonusers, NSAIDs reduce the risk of development of EAC or esophageal junction adenocarcinomas by 40% ($P<.01$) in patients who take them frequently and for longer durations of time (>10 years).[122] Based on these epidemiologic data and aforementioned in vivo and in vitro studies, a phase IIb multicenter randomized placebo-controlled trial of celecoxib in patients with BE was conducted (Chemoprevention for Barrett's Esophagus Trial or CBET). In this study, 100 Barrett's patients with low-grade or high-grade dysplasia were randomly assigned to treatment (n = 49 to celecoxib 200 mg twice a day) or placebo (n = 51). After 48 weeks of treatment, no difference was observed in the median change in the proportion of biopsy samples with dysplasia or cancer between treatment groups in either the low-grade (median change with celecoxib = −0.09, interquartile range [IQR] = −0.32–0.14 and with placebo = −0.07, IQR = −0.26–0.12; $P = .64$) or high-grade (median change with celecoxib = 0.12, IQR = −0.31–0.55, and with placebo = 0.02, IQR = −0.24–0.28; $P = .88$) stratum. No significant differences in total surface area of the BE; in prostaglandin levels; in COX-1/2 mRNA levels; or in methylation of tumor suppressor genes p16, adenomatous polyposis coli, and E-cadherin were found with celecoxib compared with placebo. The study concluded that 200 mg celecoxib twice daily for 48 weeks of treatment did not prevent progression of Barrett's dysplasia to cancer.[123] The lack of effect could be due to unabated prostaglandin synthesis by COX1 or decreased catabolism of prostaglandin E2 by PGE2 dehydrogenase.

Ornithine Decarboxylase Inhibitors

The polyamines putrescine, spermidine, and spermine, produced during cellular metabolism, are closely associated with inflammation as well as oxidative stress and are signaling molecules for cell growth and differentiation. Ornithine decarboxylase (ODC) is a key enzyme that is involved in the synthesis of polyamines.[127] Patients with BE have markedly increased ODC activity that could potentially promote neoplastic changes in BE. Difluoromethylornithine (DFMO) is an irreversible inhibitor of ODC. Although DFMO prevents growth of Barrett's epithelial cells, there is no correlation between polyamine levels and ODC activity in patients with Barrett's. In a cohort of patients with Barrett's with low-grade dysplasia (n = 10), administration of DFMO (0.5 g/m^2/d) for 6 months significantly reduced the levels of putrescine, spermidine, and the spermidine/spermine ratio.[128] Furthermore, DFMO downregulated

RPL11, which is known to activate tumor suppressor p53 pathway and inhibited KLF5, a transcription factor that promotes cell proliferation. There was also a partial regression of extent of low-grade dysplasia, but clinical relevance of the finding is unclear. In summary, an ODC inhibitor-based chemopreventive approach has mechanistic rationale but only limited success in clinical settings. Combining DFMO with anti-inflammatory drugs, such as NSAIDs or antioxidants, appears to be a reasonable strategy.

Metformin

Metformin lowers serum insulin levels, activates adenosine monophosphate (AMP)-activated protein kinase (AMPK).[129,130] AMPK activation by metformin increases insulin-dependent glucose uptake and inhibits mTOR, resulting in downregulation of ribosomal protein S6 kinase 1(S6K1) that leads to decreased protein synthesis. This decrease in phosphorylated S6K1 (pS6K1) inhibits cell proliferation. Metformin also has AMPK-independent, indirect antiproliferative effects related to lower systemic levels of insulin. Based on these observations, 74 subjects with BE were recruited to test the chemopreventive potential of metformin (2000 mg/d, n = 38) or placebo (n = 36) for 12 weeks. Biopsy specimens were collected at baseline and at week 12. This was a negative trial, as the percent change in median level of pS6K1 did not differ significantly between groups (1.4% among subjects given metformin vs 14.7% among subjects given placebo; 1-sided *P* of .80). Metformin was associated with an almost significant reduction in serum insulin levels (median −4.7% among subjects given metformin vs 23.6% increase among those given placebo, *P* = .80), as well as in homeostatic model assessments of insulin resistance (median −7.2% among subjects given metformin vs 38% among subjects given placebo, *P* = .06). Metformin had no effects on cell proliferation (on the basis of KI67 assays) or apoptosis (on the basis of caspase 3 assays).[131] This study did raise the possibility that the use of metformin in obese patients with Barrett's with a high degree of insulin resistance may have a chemopreventive function.

Statins

Preclinical studies show that statins via 3-hydroxy-3-methylglutaryl-coenzyme A reductase-dependent and independent manner exert chemopreventive potential. By inhibiting posttranslational modification of the Ras/Rho superfamily, statins decrease cell growth.[132] Observational and case-control studies also support the chemopreventive potential of statins. Patients with Barrett's who fill statin prescriptions are at reduced risk of EAC (0.55, 95% CI 0.36–0.86), In the same study a significant trend toward greater risk reduction was noted with longer duration of statin use.[133] In a prospective study of 570 patients with BE in Dutch hospitals during a median follow-up period of 4.5 years, 38 patients (7%) developed high-grade dysplasia or adenocarcinoma. After Barrett's diagnosis, in 209 (37%) patients who used statins, there was a reduced risk of neoplastic progression (HR 0.47, *P* = .030, and HR 0.46, *P* = .048, respectively).[134] In another prospective cohort of 411 patients with Barrett's, after accounting for variation in use during follow-up and adjusting for age, sex, and smoking, the HR for statin use among patients with high-grade dysplasia was 0.31 (95% CI 0.11–0.86).[135]

In a case-control study comparing statin use between patients with an incident EAC (n = 85) and matched nonprogressive Barrett's controls (n = 170), there was significantly lower incidence of EAC in statin users (uncorrected odds ratio [OR] 0.45, 95% CI 0.24–0.84). After correction for confounding variables, including aspirin and NSAID use, statin use was still associated with a reduced incidence of EAC

(OR 0.57, 95% CI 0.28–0.94). Longer duration of statin use and higher doses were both associated with a significantly greater reduction in EAC.[136] Recently, a case-control study was conducted among patients scheduled for elective endoscopy in primary care settings at a Veterans Affairs center. A total of 303 patients with BE were compared with 2 separate sex-matched control groups: 606 elective endoscopy controls and 303 primary care controls without BE. Statin use was associated with a significantly lower risk of BE (adjusted OR 0.57, 95% CI 0.38–0.87) compared with the combined control groups. The risk of BE was especially lower with statin use among obese patients (OR 0.26, 95% CI 0.09–0.71), as was the risk for BE segments of 3 cm or larger (OR 0.13, 95% CI 0.06–0.30). There was no significant association between BE and nonstatin lipid-lowering medications (P = .452).[137] Contrary to these studies, a series of nested case-control studies covering 574 UK general practices with 88,125 cases and 362,254 matched controls, showed that the adjusted OR for any statin use and cancer at any site was 1.01 (95% CI 0.99–1.04). Interestingly, statin use had no significant negative association with EAC.[138]

A recent meta-analysis that included 13 studies (including a post hoc analysis of 22 randomized controlled trials) reporting 9285 cases of esophageal cancer among 1,132,969 patients showed a 28% reduction in the risk of esophageal cancer among patients who took statins (adjusted OR 0.72, 95% CI 0.60–0.86). In a subset of patients known to have BE (5 studies, 312 EAC developed in 2125 patients), statins were associated with a 41% decrease in the risk of EAC, after adjusting for potential confounders (adjusted OR 0.59, 95% CI 0.45–0.78). The number needed to treat with statins to prevent 1 case of EAC in patients with BE was 389.[139] Together these studies suggest a chemopreventive potential of statins in the development of BE and progression to EAC. However, randomized prospective studies are warranted.

Polyunsaturated fatty acids

Obesity is rising in epidemic proportions in Western countries.[140,141] The increased incidence of obesity is attributed to distinct dietary patterns and sedentary life style.[142–145] Subjects with a body mass index (BMI) in the highest quartile have a four-fold increase in the risk of developing EAC compared with subjects with a BMI in the lowest quartile.[143] It appears that the association between being obese and EAC is mediated via central adiposity.[83,146–148] A recent study using computed tomography of the abdomen shows that the excess visceral fat, compared with subcutaneous fat, is more likely to predict EAC risk.[81,84] In a case-control study of 50 BE cases and 50 controls, Nelsen and colleagues[148] found that both visceral fat and GEJ fat were significantly greater in patients with HGD compared with those without HGD, independent of BMI and GERD. It is proposed that diet rich in saturated fatty acids leads to increased visceral obesity that enhances esophageal inflammation by paracrine mechanisms through proinflammatory phenotype macrophage infiltration in Barrett's mucosa.[149] Because epidemiologic data also suggest a reduced risk of EAC in populations with a high consumption of fish, and n−3 fatty acids inhibit experimental carcinogenesis, the effects of dietary supplementation with the n−3 fatty acid eicosapentaenoic acid (EPA) on a number of biological endpoints in BE were examined.[150] Fifty-two patients with Barrett's were randomly assigned to consume EPA capsules (1.5 g/d) or no supplement (controls) for 6 months. There was a significant decline in oncogenic COX-2 protein concentrations in the n−3 group compared with controls (P<.05). The change in COX-2 protein was inversely related to the change in EPA content (P<.05). However, cellular proliferation was not different between the 2 groups.[150] Designing an EPA supplementation trial in patients with visceral obesity or high levels of serum saturated fatty acids may show the chemopreventive potential of polyunsaturated fatty acid such as EPA.

Combinatorial Chemoprevention

Most patients with BE are on acid suppressive therapy,[151] which increases postprandial and fasting serum gastrin levels.[86] Gastrin binds to the cholecystokinin (CCK2) receptor, and the downstream signaling increases COX2 expression, which is known to promote carcinogenesis in BE.[87] In fact, gastrin does increase Barrett's epithelial cell survival by inducing proliferation[87,88] and inactivating proapoptotic factors to promote carcinogenesis.[87,88] In a retrospective, patients with the highest quartile of serum gastrin levels were more likely to have high-grade dysplasia or cancer (OR 5.46, 95% CI 1.2–24.8).[152] Because PPIs suppress acid-reflux–related procarcinogenic signaling, combining them with inhibitors of gastrin-dependent signaling appears to be a novel strategy to prevent the development of esophageal cancer. To address this, a recent multicenter double blind, randomized, placebo-controlled, phase 2 clinical trial recruited 114 patients with nondysplastic or low-grade dysplastic BE. Patients were randomized into 3 groups and received 40 mg esomeprazole with either placebo, low-dose aspirin (81 mg) or high-dose aspirin (325 mg) daily for 28 days. Esophageal endoscopic biopsies were performed before and after intervention to measure PGE2 levels and cell growth. It was found that a higher dose of aspirin combined with esomeprazole significantly reduced tissue concentration of PGE2[1] as well as cell growth (unpublished data) and a low dose of aspirin as well as placebo did not have a significant effect. These findings, along with the ongoing ASPECT trial,[124] could pave the way to use aspirin along with PPI as a chemopreventive strategy in BE in the near future.

SUMMARY

Chemoprevention in BE is currently applied only in research settings. Our understanding of pathways that can be safely targeted and surrogate markers of cancer progression is key to the future success of chemoprevention in BE. The concepts of secondary chemoprevention, adjunctive chemoprevention, and combinatorial chemoprevention are novel and will likely be more practical and direct future research.

REFERENCES

1. Falk GW, Buttar NS, Foster NR, et al. A combination of esomeprazole and aspirin reduces tissue concentrations of prostaglandin E(2) in patients with Barrett's esophagus. Gastroenterology 2012;143(4):917–26.e1.
2. Spechler SJ, Sharma P, Souza RF, et al. American Gastroenterological Association technical review on the management of Barrett's esophagus. Gastroenterology 2011;140:e18–52 [quiz: e13].
3. Shaheen N, Ransohoff DF. Gastroesophageal reflux, Barrett esophagus, and esophageal cancer: scientific review. JAMA 2002;287(15):1972–81.
4. Hvid-Jensen F, Pedersen L, Drewes AM, et al. Incidence of adenocarcinoma among patients with Barrett's esophagus. N Engl J Med 2011;365(15):1375–83.
5. Bhat S, Coleman HG, Yousef F, et al. Risk of malignant progression in Barrett's esophagus patients: results from a large population-based study. J Natl Cancer Inst 2011;103(13):1049–57.
6. Desai TK, Krishnan K, Samala N, et al. The incidence of oesophageal adenocarcinoma in non-dysplastic Barrett's oesophagus: a meta-analysis. Gut 2012; 61(7):970–6.

7. Vaezi MF, Richter JE. Synergism of acid and duodenogastroesophageal reflux in complicated Barrett's esophagus. Surgery 1995;117(6):699–704.

8. Nehra D, Howell P, Williams CP, et al. Toxic bile acids in gastro-oesophageal reflux disease: influence of gastric acidity. Gut 1999;44(5):598–602.

9. Sontag SJ. The medical management of reflux esophagitis. Role of antacids and acid inhibition. Gastroenterol Clin North Am 1990;19(3):683–712.

10. Theisen J, Nehra D, Citron D, et al. Suppression of gastric acid secretion in patients with gastroesophageal reflux disease results in gastric bacterial overgrowth and deconjugation of bile acids. J Gastrointest Surg 2000;4(1):50–4.

11. Goldstein SR, Yang GY, Curtis SK, et al. Development of esophageal metaplasia and adenocarcinoma in a rat surgical model without the use of a carcinogen. Carcinogenesis 1997;18(11):2265–70.

12. Kawaura Y, Tatsuzawa Y, Wakabayashi T, et al. Immunohistochemical study of p53, c-erbB-2, and PCNA in Barrett's esophagus with dysplasia and adenocarcinoma arising from experimental acid or alkaline reflux model. J Gastroenterol 2001;36(9):595–600.

13. Gammon MD, Schoenberg JB, Ahsan H, et al. Tobacco, alcohol, and socioeconomic status and adenocarcinomas of the esophagus and gastric cardia. J Natl Cancer Inst 1997;89(17):1277–84.

14. Mirvish SS. Studies on experimental animals involving surgical procedures and/or nitrosamine treatment related to the etiology of esophageal adenocarcinoma. Cancer Lett 1997;117(2):161–74.

15. Menke-Pluymers MB, Hop WC, Dees J, et al. Risk factors for the development of an adenocarcinoma in columnar-lined (Barrett) esophagus. The Rotterdam Esophageal Tumor Study Group. Cancer 1993;72(4):1155–8.

16. Gray MR, Donnelly RJ, Kingsnorth AN. The role of smoking and alcohol in metaplasia and cancer risk in Barrett's columnar lined oesophagus. Gut 1993;34(6):727–31.

17. Avidan B, Sonnenberg A, Schnell TG, et al. Hiatal hernia size, Barrett's length, and severity of acid reflux are all risk factors for esophageal adenocarcinoma. Am J Gastroenterol 2002;97(8):1930–6.

18. Bani-Hani KE, Bani-Hani BK, Martin IG. Characteristics of patients with columnar-lined Barrett's esophagus and risk factors for progression to esophageal adenocarcinoma. World J Gastroenterol 2005;11(43):6807–14.

19. Forman D, Al-Dabbagh S, Doll R. Nitrates, nitrites and gastric cancer in Great Britain. Nature 1985;313(6004):620–5.

20. Duncan C, Dougall H, Johnston P, et al. Chemical generation of nitric oxide in the mouth from the enterosalivary circulation of dietary nitrate. Nat Med 1995;1(6):546–51.

21. Calmels S, Béréziat JC, Ohshima H, et al. Bacterial formation of N-nitroso compounds from administered precursors in the rat stomach after omeprazole-induced achlorhydria. Carcinogenesis 1991;12(3):435–9.

22. Spechler SJ. Carcinogenesis at the gastroesophageal junction: free radicals at the frontier. Gastroenterology 2002;122(5):1518–20.

23. Liu RH, Hotchkiss JH. Potential genotoxicity of chronically elevated nitric oxide: a review. Mutat Res 1995;339(2):73–89.

24. Buttar NS, Wang KK, Anderson MA, et al. The effect of selective cyclooxygenase-2 inhibition in Barrett's esophagus epithelium: an in vitro study. J Natl Cancer Inst 2002;94(6):422–9.

25. Buttar NS, Wang KK, Leontovich O, et al. Chemoprevention of esophageal adenocarcinoma by COX-2 inhibitors in an animal model of Barrett's esophagus. Gastroenterology 2002;122(4):1101–12.

26. Buttar NS, DeMars CJ, Lomberk G, et al. Distinct role of Kruppel-like factor 11 in the regulation of prostaglandin E2 biosynthesis. J Biol Chem 2010;285(15):11433–44.

27. Buttar NS, Fernandez-Zapico ME, Urrutia R. Key role of Kruppel-like factor proteins in pancreatic cancer and other gastrointestinal neoplasias. Curr Opin Gastroenterol 2006;22(5):505–11.

28. Kaur BS, Triadafilopoulos G. Acid- and bile-induced PGE(2) release and hyperproliferation in Barrett's esophagus are COX-2 and PKC-epsilon dependent. Am J Physiol Gastrointest Liver Physiol 2002;283:G327–34.

29. Souza RF, Shewmake K, Pearson S, et al. Acid increases proliferation via ERK and p38 MAPK-mediated increases in cyclooxygenase-2 in Barrett's adenocarcinoma cells. Am J Physiol Gastrointest Liver Physiol 2004;287:G743–8.

30. Buttar NS, Wang KK. Mechanisms of disease: carcinogenesis in Barrett's esophagus. Nat Clin Pract Gastroenterol Hepatol 2004;1(2):106–12.

31. Tselepis C, Perry I, Dawson C, et al. Tumour necrosis factor-alpha in Barrett's oesophagus: a potential novel mechanism of action. Oncogene 2002;21(39): 6071–81.

32. Jankowski J, Hopwood D, Wormsley KG. Flow-cytometric analysis of growth-regulatory peptides and their receptors in Barrett's oesophagus and oesophageal adenocarcinoma. Scand J Gastroenterol 1992;27(2):147–54.

33. Jankowski J, Coghill G, Tregaskis B, et al. Epidermal growth factor in the oesophagus. Gut 1992;33(11):1448–53.

34. Jankowski J, Hopwood D, Wormsley KG. Expression of epidermal growth factor, transforming growth factor alpha and their receptor in gastro-oesophageal diseases. Dig Dis 1993;11(1):1–11.

35. Nishigaki H, Wada K, Tatsuguchi A, et al. ErbB2 without erbB3 expression in metaplastic columnar epithelium of Barrett's esophagus. Digestion 2004;70(2): 95–102.

36. Quante M, Bhagat G, Abrams JA, et al. Bile acid and inflammation activate gastric cardia stem cells in a mouse model of Barrett-like metaplasia. Cancer Cell 2012;21(1):36–51.

37. Kaur BS, Ouatu-Lascar R, Omary MB, et al. Bile salts induce or blunt cell proliferation in Barrett's esophagus in an acid-dependent fashion. Am J Physiol Gastrointest Liver Physiol 2000;278:G1000–9.

38. Feagins LA, Zhang HY, Zhang X, et al. Mechanisms of oxidant production in esophageal squamous cell and Barrett's cell lines. Am J Physiol Gastrointest Liver Physiol 2008;294:G411–7.

39. Rizvi S, Demars CJ, Comba A, et al. Combinatorial chemoprevention reveals a novel smoothened-independent role of GLI1 in esophageal carcinogenesis. Cancer Res 2010;70(17):6787–96.

40. Yen CJ, Izzo JG, Lee DF, et al. Bile acid exposure up-regulates tuberous sclerosis complex 1/mammalian target of rapamycin pathway in Barrett's-associated esophageal adenocarcinoma. Cancer Res 2008;68(8):2632–40.

41. Song S, Guha S, Liu K, et al. COX-2 induction by unconjugated bile acids involves reactive oxygen species-mediated signalling pathways in Barrett's oesophagus and oesophageal adenocarcinoma. Gut 2007;56(11):1512–21.

42. Fitzgerald RC, Abdalla S, Onwuegbusi BA, et al. Inflammatory gradient in Barrett's oesophagus: implications for disease complications. Gut 2002;51(3): 316–22.

43. Fitzgerald RC, Onwuegbusi BA, Bajaj-Elliott M, et al. Diversity in the oesophageal phenotypic response to gastro-oesophageal reflux: immunological determinants. Gut 2002;50(4):451–9.

44. Dvorakova K, Payne CM, Ramsey L, et al. Increased expression and secretion of interleukin-6 in patients with Barrett's esophagus. Clin Cancer Res 2004; 10(6):2020–8.

45. Jankowski J, McMenemin R, Hopwood D, et al. Abnormal expression of growth regulatory factors in Barrett's oesophagus. Clin Sci (Lond) 1991;81(5):663–8.

46. Venere M, Lathia JD, Rich JN. Growth factor receptors define cancer hierarchies. Cancer Cell 2013;23(2):135–7.

47. van Hagen P, Biermann K, Boers JE, et al. Human epidermal growth factor receptor 2 overexpression and amplification in endoscopic biopsies and resection specimens in esophageal and junctional adenocarcinoma. Dis Esophagus 2015;13(4):665–72.

48. al-Kasspooles M, Moore JH, Orringer MB, et al. Amplification and over-expression of the EGFR and erbB-2 genes in human esophageal adenocarcinomas. Int J Cancer 1993;54(2):213–9.

49. Jankowski J, Coghill G, Hopwood D, et al. Oncogenes and onco-suppressor gene in adenocarcinoma of the oesophagus. Gut 1992;33(8):1033–8.

50. Nakamura T, Nekarda H, Hoelscher AH, et al. Prognostic value of DNA ploidy and c-erbB-2 oncoprotein overexpression in adenocarcinoma of Barrett's esophagus. Cancer 1994;73(7):1785–94.

51. Hardwick RH, Shepherd NA, Moorghen M, et al. c-erbB-2 overexpression in the dysplasia/carcinoma sequence of Barrett's oesophagus. J Clin Pathol 1995; 48(2):129–32.

52. Lagorce C, Fléjou JF, Muzeau F, et al. Absence of c-Ki-ras gene mutation in malignant and premalignant Barrett's oesophagus. Clin Mol Pathol 1995;48: M198–9.

53. Zhang X, Yu C, Wilson K, et al. Malignant transformation of non-neoplastic Barrett's epithelial cells through well-defined genetic manipulations. PLoS One 2010;5 [pii:e13093].

54. Clement G, Braunschweig R, Pasquier N, et al. Alterations of the Wnt signaling pathway during the neoplastic progression of Barrett's esophagus. Oncogene 2006;25(21):3084–92.

55. Clement G, Guilleret I, He B, et al. Epigenetic alteration of the Wnt inhibitory factor-1 promoter occurs early in the carcinogenesis of Barrett's esophagus. Cancer Sci 2008;99(1):46–53.

56. Taniguchi H, Yamamoto H, Hirata T, et al. Frequent epigenetic inactivation of Wnt inhibitory factor-1 in human gastrointestinal cancers. Oncogene 2005;24(53): 7946–52.

57. Zou H, Molina JR, Harrington JJ, et al. Aberrant methylation of secreted frizzled-related protein genes in esophageal adenocarcinoma and Barrett's esophagus. Int J Cancer 2005;116(4):584–91.

58. Clement G, Braunschweig R, Pasquier N, et al. Methylation of APC, TIMP3, and TERT: a new predictive marker to distinguish Barrett's oesophagus patients at risk for malignant transformation. J Pathol 2006;208(1):100–7.

59. Pegg AE, Feith DJ. Polyamines and neoplastic growth. Biochem Soc Trans 2007;35(Pt 2):295–9.

60. Brabender J, Lord RV, Danenberg KD, et al. Upregulation of ornithine decarboxylase mRNA expression in Barrett's esophagus and Barrett's-associated adenocarcinoma. J Gastrointest Surg 2001;5(2):174–81 [discussion: 182].

61. Huo X, Juergens S, Zhang X, et al. Deoxycholic acid causes DNA damage while inducing apoptotic resistance through NF-kappaB activation in benign Barrett's epithelial cells. Am J Physiol Gastrointest Liver Physiol 2011;301:G278–86.

62. Hanas JS, Lerner MR, Lightfoot SA, et al. Expression of the cyclin-dependent kinase inhibitor p21(WAF1/CIP1) and p53 tumor suppressor in dysplastic progression and adenocarcinoma in Barrett esophagus. Cancer 1999;86(5):756–63.
63. Barrett MT, Sanchez CA, Prevo LJ, et al. Evolution of neoplastic cell lineages in Barrett oesophagus. Nat Genet 1999;22(1):106–9.
64. Hormi-Carver K, Feagins LA, Spechler SJ, et al. All trans-retinoic acid induces apoptosis via p38 and caspase pathways in metaplastic Barrett's cells. Am J Physiol Gastrointest Liver Physiol 2007;292:G18–27.
65. Akiyama J, Alexandre L, Baruah A, et al. Strategy for prevention of cancers of the esophagus. Ann N Y Acad Sci 2014;1325(1):108–26.
66. Lee OJ, Schneider-Stock R, McChesney PA, et al. Hypermethylation and loss of expression of glutathione peroxidase-3 in Barrett's tumorigenesis. Neoplasia 2005;7(9):854–61.
67. Younes M, Schwartz MR, Finnie D, et al. Overexpression of Fas ligand (FasL) during malignant transformation in the large bowel and in Barrett's metaplasia of the esophagus. Hum Pathol 1999;30(11):1309–13.
68. Younes M, Lechago J, Ertan A, et al. Decreased expression of Fas (CD95/APO1) associated with goblet cell metaplasia in Barrett's esophagus. Hum Pathol 2000;31(4):434–8.
69. Lagergren J. Influence of obesity on the risk of esophageal disorders. Nat Rev Gastroenterol Hepatol 2011;8(6):340–7.
70. Koppman JS, Poggi L, Szomstein S, et al. Esophageal motility disorders in the morbidly obese population. Surg Endosc 2007;21(5):761–4.
71. Ortiz V, Ponce M, Fernández A, et al. Value of heartburn for diagnosing gastroesophageal reflux disease in severely obese patients. Obesity (Silver Spring) 2006;14(4):696–700.
72. Kuper MA, Kramer KM, Kirschniak A, et al. Dysfunction of the lower esophageal sphincter and dysmotility of the tubular esophagus in morbidly obese patients. Obes Surg 2009;19(8):1143–9.
73. McQuaid KR, Laine L, Fennerty MB, et al. Systematic review: the role of bile acids in the pathogenesis of gastro-oesophageal reflux disease and related neoplasia. Aliment Pharmacol Ther 2011;34(2):146–65.
74. Ryan AM, Duong M, Healy L, et al. Obesity, metabolic syndrome and esophageal adenocarcinoma: epidemiology, etiology and new targets. Cancer Epidemiol 2011;35(4):309–19.
75. Renehan AG, Roberts DL, Dive C. Obesity and cancer: pathophysiological and biological mechanisms. Arch Physiol Biochem 2008;114(1):71–83.
76. Lysaght J, Allott EH, Donohoe CL, et al. T lymphocyte activation in visceral adipose tissue of patients with oesophageal adenocarcinoma. Br J Surg 2011;98(7):964–74.
77. Damms-Machado A, Weser G, Bischoff SC. Micronutrient deficiency in obese subjects undergoing low calorie diet. Nutr J 2012;11:34.
78. Fountoulakis A, Martin IG, White KL, et al. Plasma and esophageal mucosal levels of vitamin C: role in the pathogenesis and neoplastic progression of Barrett's esophagus. Dig Dis Sci 2004;49(6):914–9.
79. Otterstatter MC, Brierley JD, De P, et al. Esophageal cancer in Canada: trends according to morphology and anatomical location. Can J Gastroenterol 2012;26(10):723–7.
80. Turati F, Tramacere I, La Vecchia C, et al. A meta-analysis of body mass index and esophageal and gastric cardia adenocarcinoma. Ann Oncol 2013;24(3):609–17.

81. Beddy P, Howard J, McMahon C, et al. Association of visceral adiposity with oesophageal and junctional adenocarcinomas. Br J Surg 2010;97(7):1028–34.

82. El-Serag HB, Kvapil P, Hacken-Bitar J, et al. Abdominal obesity and the risk of Barrett's esophagus. Am J Gastroenterol 2005;100(10):2151–6.

83. Kendall BJ, Macdonald GA, Hayward NK, et al. The risk of Barrett's esophagus associated with abdominal obesity in males and females. Int J Cancer 2013; 132(9):2192–9.

84. El-Serag HB, Hashmi A, Garcia J, et al. Visceral abdominal obesity measured by CT scan is associated with an increased risk of Barrett's oesophagus: a case-control study. Gut 2014;63(2):220–9.

85. Larsson SC, Wolk A. Obesity and colon and rectal cancer risk: a meta-analysis of prospective studies. Am J Clin Nutr 2007;86(3):556–65.

86. Iwao T, Toyonaga A, Kuboyama S, et al. Effects of omeprazole and lansoprazole on fasting and postprandial serum gastrin and serum pepsinogen A and C. Hepatogastroenterology 1995;42(5):677–82.

87. Abdalla SI, Lao-Sirieix P, Novelli MR, et al. Gastrin-induced cyclooxygenase-2 expression in Barrett's carcinogenesis. Clin Cancer Res 2004;10(14):4784–92.

88. Haigh CR, Attwood SE, Thompson DG, et al. Gastrin induces proliferation in Barrett's metaplasia through activation of the CCK2 receptor. Gastroenterology 2003;124(3):615–25.

89. Ohsawa T, Hirata W, Higichi S. Effects of three H2-receptor antagonists (cimetidine, famotidine, ranitidine) on serum gastrin level. Int J Clin Pharmacol Res 2002;22(2):29–35.

90. Sampliner RE. Practice guidelines on the diagnosis, surveillance, and therapy of Barrett's esophagus. The practice parameters committee of the American College of Gastroenterology. Am J Gastroenterol 1998;93(7):1028–32.

91. Reid BJ, Haggitt RC, Rubin CE, et al. Observer variation in the diagnosis of dysplasia in Barrett's esophagus. Hum Pathol 1988;19(2):166–78.

92. Cameron AJ, Carpenter HA. Barrett's esophagus, high-grade dysplasia, and early adenocarcinoma: a pathological study. Am J Gastroenterol 1997;92(4): 586–91.

93. Reid BJ, Prevo LJ, Galipeau PC, et al. Predictors of progression in Barrett's esophagus II: baseline 17p (p53) loss of heterozygosity identifies a patient subset at increased risk for neoplastic progression. Am J Gastroenterol 2001; 96(10):2839–48.

94. Rygiel AM, van Baal JW, Milano F, et al. Efficient automated assessment of genetic abnormalities detected by fluorescence in situ hybridization on brush cytology in a Barrett esophagus surveillance population. Cancer 2007; 109(10):1980–8.

95. Kerkhof M, Steyerberg EW, Kusters JG, et al. Aneuploidy and high expression of p53 and Ki67 is associated with neoplastic progression in Barrett esophagus. Cancer Biomark 2008;4(1):1–10.

96. Sikkema M, Kerkhof M, Steyerberg EW, et al. Aneuploidy and overexpression of Ki67 and p53 as markers for neoplastic progression in Barrett's esophagus: a case-control study. Am J Gastroenterol 2009;104(11):2673–80.

97. Kastelein F, Biermann K, Steyerberg EW, et al. Aberrant p53 protein expression is associated with an increased risk of neoplastic progression in patients with Barrett's oesophagus. Gut 2013;62(12):1676–83.

98. Sandborn WJ, Hanauer S, Van Assche G, et al. Treating beyond symptoms with a view to improving patient outcomes in inflammatory bowel diseases. J Crohns Colitis 2014;8(9):927–35.

99. Wong DJ, Paulson TG, Prevo LJ, et al. p16(INK4a) lesions are common, early abnormalities that undergo clonal expansion in Barrett's metaplastic epithelium. Cancer Res 2001;61(22):8284–9.
100. Schulmann K, Sterian A, Berki A, et al. Inactivation of p16, RUNX3, and HPP1 occurs early in Barrett's-associated neoplastic progression and predicts progression risk. Oncogene 2005;24(25):4138–48.
101. Prasad GA, Wang KK, Halling KC, et al. Correlation of histology with biomarker status after photodynamic therapy in Barrett esophagus. Cancer 2008;113(3):470–6.
102. Prasad GA, Wang KK, Halling KC, et al. Utility of biomarkers in prediction of response to ablative therapy in Barrett's esophagus. Gastroenterology 2008; 135(2):370–9.
103. Timmer MR, Brankley SM, Gorospe EC, et al. Prediction of response to endoscopic therapy of Barrett's dysplasia by using genetic biomarkers. Gastrointest Endosc 2014;80(6):984–91.
104. Sato F, Jin Z, Schulmann K, et al. Three-tiered risk stratification model to predict progression in Barrett's esophagus using epigenetic and clinical features. PLoS One 2008;3:e1890.
105. Xu E, Gu J, Hawk ET, et al. Genome-wide methylation analysis shows similar patterns in Barrett's esophagus and esophageal adenocarcinoma. Carcinogenesis 2013;34(12):2750–6.
106. Jin Z, Cheng Y, Olaru A, et al. Promoter hypermethylation of CDH13 is a common, early event in human esophageal adenocarcinogenesis and correlates with clinical risk factors. Int J Cancer 2008;123(10):2331–6.
107. Kaz AM, Wong CJ, Luo Y, et al. DNA methylation profiling in Barrett's esophagus and esophageal adenocarcinoma reveals unique methylation signatures and molecular subclasses. Epigenetics 2011;6(12):1403–12.
108. Jin Z, Cheng Y, Gu W, et al. A multicenter, double-blinded validation study of methylation biomarkers for progression prediction in Barrett's esophagus. Cancer Res 2009;69(10):4112–5.
109. Wang JS, Guo M, Montgomery EA, et al. DNA promoter hypermethylation of p16 and APC predicts neoplastic progression in Barrett's esophagus. Am J Gastroenterol 2009;104(9):2153–60.
110. El-Serag HB, Aguirre TV, Davis S, et al. Proton pump inhibitors are associated with reduced incidence of dysplasia in Barrett's esophagus. Am J Gastroenterol 2004;99(10):1877–83.
111. Kastelein F, Spaander MC, Steyerberg EW, et al. Proton pump inhibitors reduce the risk of neoplastic progression in patients with Barrett's esophagus. Clin Gastroenterol Hepatol 2013;11(4):382–8.
112. Hillman LC, Chiragakis L, Shadbolt B, et al. Proton-pump inhibitor therapy and the development of dysplasia in patients with Barrett's oesophagus. Med J Aust 2004;180(8):387–91.
113. Cooper BT, Chapman W, Neumann CS, et al. Continuous treatment of Barrett's oesophagus patients with proton pump inhibitors up to 13 years: observations on regression and cancer incidence. Aliment Pharmacol Ther 2006;23(6):727–33.
114. Hvid-Jensen F, Pedersen L, Funch-Jensen P, et al. Proton pump inhibitor use may not prevent high-grade dysplasia and oesophageal adenocarcinoma in Barrett's oesophagus: a nationwide study of 9883 patients. Aliment Pharmacol Ther 2014;39(9):984–91.
115. Singh S, Garg SK, Singh PP, et al. Acid-suppressive medications and risk of oesophageal adenocarcinoma in patients with Barrett's oesophagus: a systematic review and meta-analysis. Gut 2014;63(8):1229–37.

116. Hong MK, Laskin WB, Herman BE, et al. Expansion of the Ki-67 proliferative compartment correlates with degree of dysplasia in Barrett's esophagus. Cancer 1995;75(2):423–9.

117. Peters FT, Ganesh S, Kuipers EJ, et al. Epithelial cell proliferative activity of Barrett's esophagus: methodology and correlation with traditional cancer risk markers. Dig Dis Sci 1998;43(7):1501–6.

118. Ouatu-Lascar R, Fitzgerald RC, Triadafilopoulos G. Differentiation and proliferation in Barrett's esophagus and the effects of acid suppression. Gastroenterology 1999;117(2):327–35.

119. Peters FT, Ganesh S, Kuipers EJ, et al. Effect of elimination of acid reflux on epithelial cell proliferative activity of Barrett esophagus. Scand J Gastroenterol 2000;35(12):1238–44.

120. Umansky M, Yasui W, Hallak A, et al. Proton pump inhibitors reduce cell cycle abnormalities in Barrett's esophagus. Oncogene 2001;20(55):7987–91.

121. Thanan R, Ma N, Iijima K, et al. Proton pump inhibitors suppress iNOS-dependent DNA damage in Barrett's esophagus by increasing Mn-SOD expression. Biochem Biophys Res Commun 2012;421(2):280–5.

122. Byrne JP, Armstrong GR, Attwood SE. Restoration of the normal squamous lining in Barrett's esophagus by argon beam plasma coagulation. Am J Gastroenterol 1998;93(10):1810–5.

123. Brandt LJ, Blansky RL, Kauvar DR. Repeat laser therapy of recurrent Barrett's epithelium: success with anacidity. Gastrointest Endosc 1995; 41(3):267.

124. Kovacs BJ, Chen YK, Lewis TD, et al. Successful reversal of Barrett's esophagus with multipolar electrocoagulation despite inadequate acid suppression. Gastrointest Endosc 1999;49(5):547–53.

125. Ojima E, Fujimura T, Oyama K, et al. Chemoprevention of esophageal adenocarcinoma in a rat model by ursodeoxycholic acid. Clin Exp Med 2014. [Epub ahead of print].

126. Bozikas A, Marsman WA, Rosmolen WD, et al. The effect of oral administration of ursodeoxycholic acid and high-dose proton pump inhibitors on the histology of Barrett's esophagus. Dis Esophagus 2008;21(4):346–54.

127. Garewal HS, Sampliner RE, Fennerty MB. Chemopreventive studies in Barrett's esophagus: a model premalignant lesion for esophageal adenocarcinoma. J Natl Cancer Inst Monogr 1992;51–4.

128. Sinicrope FA, Broaddus R, Joshi N, et al. Evaluation of difluoromethylornithine for the chemoprevention of Barrett's esophagus and mucosal dysplasia. Cancer Prev Res (Phila) 2011;4(6):829–39.

129. Pollak M. Insulin and insulin-like growth factor signalling in neoplasia. Nat Rev Cancer 2008;8(12):915–28.

130. Towler MC, Hardie DG. AMP-activated protein kinase in metabolic control and insulin signaling. Circ Res 2007;100(3):328–41.

131. Chak A, Buttar NS, Foster NR, et al. Metformin does not reduce markers of cell proliferation in esophageal tissues of patients with Barrett's esophagus. Clin Gastroenterol Hepatol 2015;13(4):665–72.

132. Demierre MF, Higgins PD, Gruber SB, et al. Statins and cancer prevention. Nat Rev Cancer 2005;5(12):930–42.

133. Nguyen DM, Richardson P, El-Serag HB. Medications (NSAIDs, statins, proton pump inhibitors) and the risk of esophageal adenocarcinoma in patients with Barrett's esophagus. Gastroenterology 2010;138(7):2260–6.

134. Kastelein F, Spaander MC, Biermann K, et al. Nonsteroidal anti-inflammatory drugs and statins have chemopreventative effects in patients with Barrett's esophagus. Gastroenterology 2011;141(6):2000–8 [quiz: e13–4].
135. Kantor ED, Onstad L, Blount PL, et al. Use of statin medications and risk of esophageal adenocarcinoma in persons with Barrett's esophagus. Cancer Epidemiol Biomarkers Prev 2012;21(3):456–61.
136. Beales IL, Vardi I, Dearman L. Regular statin and aspirin use in patients with Barrett's oesophagus is associated with a reduced incidence of oesophageal adenocarcinoma. Eur J Gastroenterol Hepatol 2012;24(8):917–23.
137. Nguyen T, Khalaf N, Ramsey D, et al. Statin use is associated with a decreased risk of Barrett's esophagus. Gastroenterology 2014;147(2):314–23.
138. Vinogradova Y, Coupland C, Hippisley-Cox J. Exposure to statins and risk of common cancers: a series of nested case-control studies. BMC Cancer 2011; 11:409.
139. Singh PP, Singh S. Statins are associated with reduced risk of gastric cancer: a systematic review and meta-analysis. Ann Oncol 2013;24(7):1721–30.
140. Brown LM, Devesa SS. Epidemiologic trends in esophageal and gastric cancer in the United States. Surg Oncol Clin N Am 2002;11(2):235–56.
141. Pera M, Manterola C, Vidal O, et al. Epidemiology of esophageal adenocarcinoma. J Surg Oncol 2005;92(3):151–9.
142. Engel LS, Chow WH, Vaughan TL, et al. Population attributable risks of esophageal and gastric cancers. J Natl Cancer Inst 2003;95(18):1404–13.
143. Chow WH, Iot WJ, Vaughan TL, et al. Body mass index and risk of adenocarcinomas of the esophagus and gastric cardia. J Natl Cancer Inst 1998;90(2): 150–5.
144. Lagergren J, Bergström R, Nyrén O. Association between body mass and adenocarcinoma of the esophagus and gastric cardia. Ann Intern Med 1999; 130(11):883–90.
145. Calle EE, Kaaks R. Overweight, obesity and cancer: epidemiological evidence and proposed mechanisms. Nat Rev Cancer 2004;4(8):579–91.
146. Nordenstedt H, El-Serag H. The influence of age, sex, and race on the incidence of esophageal cancer in the United States (1992–2006). Scand J Gastroenterol 2011;46(5):597–602.
147. Steffen A, Schulze MB, Pischon T, et al. Anthropometry and esophageal cancer risk in the European prospective investigation into cancer and nutrition. Cancer Epidemiol Biomarkers Prev 2009;18(7):2079–89.
148. Nelsen EM, Kirihara Y, Takahashi N, et al. Distribution of body fat and its influence on esophageal inflammation and dysplasia in patients with Barrett's esophagus. Clin Gastroenterol Hepatol 2012;10(7):728–34 [quiz: e61–2].
149. Malhi H, Gores GJ, Katzka DA, et al. Mo1898 macrophage related inflammation and phenotype modulation in Barrett's esophagus. Gastroenterology 2013; 144(5):S-688.
150. Mehta SP, Boddy AP, Cook J, et al. Effect of n-3 polyunsaturated fatty acids on Barrett's epithelium in the human lower esophagus. Am J Clin Nutr 2008;87(4): 949–56.
151. Spechler SJ, Lee E, Ahnen D, et al. Long-term outcome of medical and surgical therapies for gastroesophageal reflux disease: follow-up of a randomized controlled trial. JAMA 2001;285(18):2331–8.
152. Wang JS, Varro A, Lightdale CJ, et al. Elevated serum gastrin is associated with a history of advanced neoplasia in Barrett's esophagus. Am J Gastroenterol 2010;105(5):1039–45.

The Effect of Proton Pump Inhibitors on Barrett's Esophagus

Kerry B. Dunbar, MD, PhD*, Rhonda F. Souza, MD,
Stuart J. Spechler, MD

KEYWORDS

- Barrett's esophagus • Proton pump inhibitor • Dysplasia • Esophageal cancer
- Gastroesophageal reflux disease

KEY POINTS

- Gastrointestinal societal guidelines agree that, for patients with Barrett's esophagus, PPIs should be prescribed in whatever dose is necessary to control GERD symptoms and heal reflux esophagitis.
- Routine esophageal pH testing to assess the adequacy of acid suppression with PPIs, and the routine use of high-dose PPIs (beyond what is needed to control GERD), are not recommended by gastrointestinal societies for patients with Barrett's esophagus.
- In Barrett's esophagus, acid reflux can lead to increased cell proliferation, decreased apoptosis, production of reactive oxygen species, DNA damage, and esophageal production of proinflammatory and proproliferative cytokines.
- Although there are no randomized, controlled trials proving that PPI treatment reduces the risk of neoplastic progression in Barrett's esophagus, the bulk of clinical studies published on this issue support a cancer-preventive effect for PPIs.
- The indirect evidence supporting a cancer-protective role for PPIs is strong enough to warrant PPI treatment of virtually all patients with Barrett's esophagus after they have been informed of the potential risks of long-term PPI therapy.

INTRODUCTION

Barrett's esophagus is a major risk factor for the development of esophageal adenocarcinoma, a tumor whose incidence has increased profoundly over the last 40 years in Western countries.[1] The pathogenesis of Barrett's esophagus involves chronic gastroesophageal reflux disease (GERD) wherein the reflux of acid and bile into the

Disclosures: None.
Division of Gastroenterology and Hepatology, Department of Medicine, Dallas VA Medical Center, University of Texas Southwestern Medical Center, 4500 South Lancaster Road, GI Lab – CA-111-B1, Dallas, TX 75231, USA
* Corresponding author.
E-mail address: Kerry.Dunbar@utsouthwestern.edu

esophagus damages the esophageal mucosa and leads to its repair through the process of metaplasia. The specialized intestinal metaplasia of Barrett's esophagus is predisposed to malignancy, and ongoing GERD is likely to contribute to that carcinogenesis. Because chronic GERD plays a role in the pathogenesis of Barrett's metaplasia and in its malignant progression, it makes sense that aggressive treatment of GERD might prevent adenocarcinoma in Barrett's esophagus. The modern medical therapy for GERD is directed primarily at decreasing gastric acid production, and proton pump inhibitors (PPIs), which were introduced into clinical practice in the United States in 1989, are the best medications available for that purpose. This article reviews the effects of PPIs that might impact on the neoplastic progression of Barrett's metaplasia, and the clinical evidence that PPIs may prevent the development of dysplasia and cancer in patients with Barrett's esophagus.

CELLULAR EFFECTS OF ACID REFLUX AND PROTON PUMP INHIBITORS IN BARRETT'S ESOPHAGUS

There are several broad categories of PPI effects that might be expected to protect against carcinogenesis in Barrett's esophagus. First, PPIs heal reflux esophagitis. Chronic inflammation is known to predispose to cancer in several organs, and the elimination of chronic esophageal inflammation by PPIs might protect against malignancy. Next, PPIs decrease esophageal exposure to acid, which can cause cancer-promoting DNA damage and increase proliferation in Barrett's metaplasia. Finally, PPIs can prevent the release of cancer-promoting cytokines by esophageal epithelial cells through mechanisms independent of their acid-suppressive effects. Numerous studies have documented the efficacy of PPIs in healing reflux esophagitis; these data are not reviewed here. Rather, we focus on the latter two mechanisms whereby PPIs might prevent cancer in Barrett's esophagus.

In one study, acid exposure of nondysplastic Barrett's epithelial cells led to the production of reactive oxygen species (ROS) with double-strand breaks in DNA, which can result in genomic instability and carcinogenesis.[2] Those acid-induced DNA double-strand breaks could be prevented by pretreating the Barrett's cells with an ROS scavenger or a compound that inhibited intracellular acidification. These data suggest that refluxed acid can enter Barrett's epithelial cells, leading to the generation of ROS that cause DNA damage. Agents that induce DNA double-strand breaks are considered carcinogens and, thus, PPIs might reduce the risk of cancer by limiting exposure to carcinogenic gastric acid.

Acid also may contribute to cancer by causing increased cellular proliferation in Barrett's esophagus. This has been suggested by studies using Barrett's biopsies maintained in organ culture and using Barrett's biopsies taken before and after acid perfusion of the esophagus.[3,4] Taken together, these studies suggest that acid exposure can cause increased expression of cyclooxygenase-2 and activation of the protein kinase-C and mitogen-activated protein kinase pathways in Barrett's metaplasia, resulting in increased proliferation and decreased apoptosis.

Several clinical studies in patients with Barrett's esophagus have found that protracted treatment with PPIs can cause improvements in markers of proliferation and other potentially beneficial effects. In one study of patients who had biopsies of Barrett's metaplasia taken before and after 6 months of PPI therapy, those patients who achieved normalization of esophageal acid exposure with PPIs showed a significant decrease in proliferation as determined by the biomarker proliferating cell nuclear antigen, unlike the patients who had persistently abnormal esophageal acid exposure despite PPI treatment.[5] Another study compared the proliferative activity in Barrett's mucosal biopsies between patients treated with PPIs and those treated with H_2-receptor antagonists (H_2RAs) for 2 years. Patients treated with H_2RAs showed increased proliferative activity, whereas there was no increase in proliferative activity in patients treated with PPIs.[6]

Patients with Barrett's esophagus often have abnormalities in the expression of certain cell cycle proteins including p16, p21, and cyclins D1 and E in their Barrett's metaplasia. In one study, PPI treatment was associated with fewer abnormalities in mucosal expression of these cell cycle proteins.[7] In another study, tissue samples from patients with Barrett's esophagus were analyzed for levels of iNOS (an oxidant-generating enzyme) and Mn-SOD (an antioxidant enzyme), and DNA damage was measured.[8] In patients who had been treated with PPIs for at least 3 months, iNOS expression was not affected, but Mn-SOD antioxidant levels were higher and DNA damage was reduced. The authors concluded that treatment with PPIs may help trigger the expression of antioxidant genes, potentially reducing oxidative DNA damage.

Gastroesophageal reflux can cause the esophageal mucosa to produce proinflammatory cytokines, such as interleukin (IL)-8, which can increase inflammation and cellular proliferation.[9] In a surgical rat model of reflux esophagitis, for example, increased expression of IL-8 was seen in the esophagus of rats that developed erosive esophagitis. PPIs seem to have anti-inflammatory effects that are independent of their effects on gastric acid suppression, and that might reduce esophageal production of these proinflammatory cytokines. In one study, esophageal squamous cells exposed to acid and bile increased their expression of IL-8 mRNA through effects on nuclear factor-κB and activator protein-1. Treating these cells with omeprazole inhibited IL-8 expression by blocking nuclear translocation of p65, a nuclear factor-κB subunit, and by blocking the binding of activator protein-1 subunits to the IL-8 promoter. This suggests that, in addition to reducing gastric acid production and acid reflux, PPIs also might have beneficial effects in GERD by modulating chemokine expression.[10]

In summary, studies suggest that acid reflux can lead to increased proliferation, decreased apoptosis, production of ROS, and DNA damage in Barrett's metaplasia. Acid reflux also stimulates esophageal production of proinflammatory and proproliferative cytokines. All of these effects might promote cancer development. Through acid-suppressive and acid-independent anti-inflammatory effects, PPIs can prevent or reduce these reflux-induced abnormalities, and thus might protect against carcinogenesis in Barrett's esophagus.

PROTON PUMP INHIBITORS AND CONTROL OF ACID REFLUX IN PATIENTS WITH BARRETT'S ESOPHAGUS

PPIs are highly effective at reducing gastric acid secretion, and they are the mainstay of therapy for GERD. However, one study suggests that almost one-third of patients with GERD taking a PPI once daily continue to have abnormal acid reflux.[11] Patients with long-segment Barrett's esophagus have especially poor antireflux mechanisms and often have more persistent and difficult-to-control acid reflux than patients who have GERD without Barrett's esophagus. Several studies have shown that pathologic acid reflux often persists despite PPI therapy in patients with Barrett's esophagus. One study of patients with long-segment Barrett's esophagus found that 23% had abnormal esophageal acid exposure documented by pH monitoring despite treatment with esomeprazole in high dosage. In these patients, esomeprazole achieved levels of gastric acid suppression similar to those in patients without Barrett's esophagus, but even this reduced amount of gastric acid production resulted in abnormal acid reflux, presumably because antireflux mechanisms were so ineffective in the patients with

Barrett's esophagus.[12] Other studies have shown that control of GERD symptoms with PPI treatment does not guarantee that esophageal acid exposure is controlled.[5,13–15] One of these studies compared the effects of PPIs on acid reflux in patients with Barrett's esophagus and in patients who had GERD without Barrett's esophagus. Despite PPI therapy that controlled GERD symptoms, approximately half of the patients in both groups had abnormal acid reflux documented by esophageal pH monitoring.[14] However, the patients with Barrett's esophagus had higher DeMeester scores than the patients without Barrett's esophagus. These studies suggest that many patients with Barrett's esophagus continue to have abnormal acid reflux despite treatment with PPIs that controls GERD symptoms.

POTENTIAL CARCINOGENIC EFFECTS OF PROTON PUMP INHIBITORS IN BARRETT'S ESOPHAGUS

The studies discussed in the previous sections have suggested plausible mechanisms whereby PPIs might decrease the risk of cancer in Barrett's esophagus. However, PPIs also have effects that conceivably could increase the risk of carcinogenesis, especially PPI effects on serum gastrin levels. Gastrin, which is released from antral G cells in response to meals and other stimuli, causes parietal cells in the gastric body and fundus to secrete acid. This acid stimulates D cells in the antrum to release somatostatin, which then inhibits the further release of gastrin from antral G cells. Thus, in a negative feedback loop, gastrin release stimulates acid secretion, which inhibits further gastrin release. By inhibiting gastric acid secretion, PPIs interrupt this negative feedback loop and cause serum gastrin levels to rise, and gastrin is a growth hormone that can cause proliferation in Barrett's metaplasia. Without gastric acid, furthermore, bacteria can colonize the stomach.[16] These bacteria can deconjugate bile acids, which can injure the esophagus at neutral pH levels, and might convert primary bile acids in the stomach into toxic secondary bile acids, such as deoxycholic acid, which can cause DNA double-strand breaks in Barrett's epithelial cells.[17] Bacteria also can convert dietary nitrates into potentially carcinogenic N-nitroso compounds.[18]

Studies using Barrett's esophageal adenocarcinoma cell lines have found that gastrin activates Janus kinase (JAK2) to trigger STAT3 signaling that stimulates proliferation and also increases levels of several antiapoptotic proteins.[19,20] In addition, gastrin activates the CCK2 receptor, which also increases proliferation and reduces apoptosis in Barrett's metaplasia.[21,22] One retrospective study focused on gastrin levels in patients with GERD, nondysplastic Barrett's metaplasia, low-grade dysplasia, high-grade dysplasia, and adenocarcinoma in Barrett's esophagus who were taking PPIs.[23] Although there were no significant differences in gastrin levels among the patients with dysplasia and adenocarcinoma, the patients with the highest quartile of serum gastrin levels were more likely to have high-grade dysplasia or cancer (odds ratio [OR], 5.46; 95% confidence interval [CI], 1.2–24.8). These studies suggest that gastrin has proproliferative and antiapoptotic effects that could contribute to the neoplastic progression of Barrett's metaplasia.

A prospective randomized trial of low- and high-dose PPI therapy was performed in patients with Barrett's esophagus to address concerns about gastrin and proliferation in Barrett's metaplasia. During a 2-year follow-up period, the investigators followed serum gastrin levels and measured the length of Barrett's metaplasia, with the rationale that PPI-induced elevations of serum gastrin would stimulate the growth of Barrett's tissues. Although serum gastrin levels increased significantly in the study participants, the length of Barrett's metaplasia did not change in either the low- or high-dose PPI groups, suggesting that PPI effects on serum gastrin levels might not have important clinical effects in patients with Barrett's esophagus.[24]

Some epidemiologic studies have found an association between PPI use and esophageal adenocarcinoma, but this association is likely to be the spurious result of a confounding-by-indication bias. Because GERD and Barrett's esophagus are risk factors for esophageal adenocarcinoma, and because PPIs are often prescribed for patients with GERD and Barrett's esophagus, an association between PPIs and esophageal adenocarcinoma might not be caused by the drug, but rather by the underlying conditions for which the PPIs were prescribed. One group explored this issue using the large, general practitioners research database in the United Kingdom.[25] They found that patients who were taking PPIs or H_2RAs for an "esophageal indication," such as GERD, had a significantly increased risk of developing esophageal adenocarcinoma (OR, 5.42; 95% CI, 3.13–9.39), but patients taking those drugs for a "gastroduodenal indication," such as peptic ulcer disease, had no significantly increased risk of adenocarcinoma (OR, 1.74; 95% CI, 0.90–3.34). This is strong evidence of confounding by indication in associating PPI use with esophageal cancer. Furthermore, most studies that have sought an association between PPI use and adenocarcinoma in patients with Barrett's esophagus have found a cancer-protective effect for these agents.

CLINICAL STUDIES ON PROTON PUMP INHIBITORS AND THE RISK OF CANCER IN BARRETT'S ESOPHAGUS

Several studies have documented partial regression of Barrett's metaplasia in some patients on long-term PPI therapy. In one study of nine patients with Barrett's esophagus who had profound suppression of acid reflux on high-dose PPIs and H_2RAs (documented by esophageal pH monitoring), follow-up endoscopy showed a mean decrease in the length of Barrett's metaplasia of 2 cm, accompanied by the frequent development of islands of squamous mucosa in the Barrett's segment.[26] Another study found no regression in the overall length of Barrett's metaplasia in patients on PPIs, but did find an increase in the number of squamous islands the longer PPI therapy was continued.[27] These studies suggest that partial regression of Barrett's metaplasia can occur in some patients with long-term PPI therapy, but they do not establish that this partial regression is clinically important. Although it seems reasonable to assume that a treatment that causes Barrett's metaplasia to regress also should protect against cancer development, no study has demonstrated that partial regression of Barrett's metaplasia is a meaningful surrogate marker for a decreased risk of neoplasia.

Several studies have explored the risk of cancer development in patients with Barrett's esophagus treated with PPIs. In one study of 236 veteran patients with Barrett's esophagus, the cumulative incidence of dysplasia over 10 years was 58% for those who did not take PPIs versus only 21% for the PPI-users.[28] Another study examined pharmacy records of 344 veteran patients with Barrett's esophagus and determined that those who were prescribed PPIs had a significantly reduced risk of developing high-grade dysplasia and cancer, with a hazard ratio (HR) of 0.43 (95% CI, 0.21–0.83).[29] In a study of 540 patients with Barrett's esophagus in the Netherlands, PPI use was associated with a significant reduction in the risk of neoplasia over the 5-year study period, whereas there was no decrease in cancer risk with use of H_2RAs.[30] In this study, PPI use reduced the risk of progression to dysplasia or cancer by 75%, with longer use of PPIs and better adherence associated with a lower risk of neoplastic progression. Additional evidence that PPIs reduce the risk of cancer was provided by a study that examined PPI use after the diagnosis of Barrett's esophagus.

For patients in whom the use of PPIs was delayed for more than 2 years after diagnosis, there was an increased risk for developing low-grade dysplasia (HR, 5.6; 95% CI, 2.0–15.7) and high-grade dysplasia or cancer (HR, 20.9; 95% CI, 2.8–158).[31]

A recent meta-analysis addressed the magnitude of effect of PPIs in reducing cancer risk in patients with Barrett's esophagus.[32] Seven observational studies including 2813 patients with Barrett's esophagus and 317 with esophageal adenocarcinoma were identified. The use of PPIs was associated with a 71% reduction in the risk of high-grade dysplasia and cancer. In addition, longer use (>2–3 years) seemed to provide more protection than shorter-term use.

Although most studies on the issue of PPIs and cancer development in Barrett's esophagus have found a cancer-protective effect for these drugs, there are some contradictory data. For example, a recent, nationwide study of patients with Barrett's esophagus in Denmark examined PPI use and the risk of developing dysplasia and cancer.[33] Among 9883 patients with Barrett's esophagus, 140 developed high-grade dysplasia and/or cancer during a median follow-up period of 10.2 years. Patients who had high adherence to the use of PPIs had a significantly increased relative risk of developing high-grade dysplasia and cancer (relative risk, 3.4; 95% CI, 1.1–10.5), whereas the relative risk was increased, but not significantly, in the low-adherence PPI users (relative risk, 2.2; 95% CI, 0.7–6.7). The authors commented that this association could be caused by confounding by indication, but could also represent a true cancer-promoting effect of PPIs. At this time, there are no published prospective randomized controlled trials proving that PPI treatment reduces the risk of dysplasia and cancer in patients with Barrett's esophagus.

Like PPIs, fundoplication surgery is highly effective at controlling acid reflux in patients with GERD. Unlike PPIs, furthermore, fundoplication can block the reflux of bile acids, which also might contribute to carcinogenesis in Barrett's esophagus. However, high-quality studies of fundoplication have not shown a reduction in risk of cancer for patients with Barrett's esophagus beyond that achieved with PPIs. In one randomized controlled trial comparing fundoplication with medical therapy for GERD, long-term follow-up of 247 patients (10–13 years) showed that there were no statistically significant differences in the development of esophageal adenocarcinoma between patients treated with medical therapy (2.4%) and surgical therapy (1.2%).[34] Several large cohort studies and a meta-analysis examining the risk of cancer in patients with Barrett's esophagus who undergo fundoplication also have not found surgical therapy superior to medical therapy in reducing the development of esophageal adenocarcinoma.[35–37] Thus, antireflux surgery should not be recommended to patients with Barrett's esophagus solely with the rationale that surgery provides better cancer protection than PPI treatment.

The cost-effectiveness of using PPIs for chemoprevention was recently addressed in a study that used a state-transition Markov model to follow a cohort of 50-year-old men with Barrett's esophagus. All patients underwent standard endoscopic surveillance, and the cost-effectiveness of using PPIs for chemoprevention was compared with a strategy of no PPI use for chemoprevention. Chemoprevention with PPIs was found to be cost-effective as long as the PPIs reduced the risk of esophageal cancer by at least 19%.[38]

The American College of Gastroenterology's recent guidelines on the management of GERD recommend maintenance PPI therapy for patients with GERD complications including erosive esophagitis and Barrett's esophagus.[39] The American Gastroenterology Association guidelines on the management of Barrett's esophagus suggest that

PPIs should be used to control reflux symptoms, but that evidence is limited to recommend treatment with PPIs in unusually high doses, or to recommend the use of pH testing to confirm acid suppression as means to prevent cancer in Barrett's esophagus.[40]

The bulk of available evidence supports the use of PPIs for chemoprevention in patients with Barrett's esophagus. This point is moot for patients who require PPI treatment to control their GERD symptoms because those patients are taking PPIs for a clear clinical indication. What remains highly controversial, and largely unaddressed specifically by societal guidelines, is whether PPIs should be prescribed to patients with Barrett's esophagus who have no symptoms or endoscopic signs of GERD, as is common in those with short-segment Barrett's esophagus. We believe that the indirect evidence supporting a cancer-protective role for PPIs is strong enough to warrant conventional-dose PPI treatment of these asymptomatic patients. However, we recommend that patients should share in this decision, and that PPIs should be prescribed in this situation only after patients have been informed of the potential risks of long-term PPI therapy. Patients also should be informed that this approach is not specifically endorsed by medical societies.

THE ROLE OF PROTON PUMP INHIBITORS DURING ENDOSCOPIC ERADICATION THERAPY FOR BARRETT'S ESOPHAGUS

PPIs are used in patients undergoing endoscopic eradication therapy for Barrett's esophagus with the rationale that, after ablation or endoscopic resection of Barrett's metaplasia, control of acid reflux will lead to repair of the eradicated mucosa with squamous epithelium rather than with more Barrett's metaplasia. Several recent studies have addressed risk factors for failure of endoscopic ablation therapy in patients with Barrett's esophagus, focusing on those treated with radiofrequency ablation (RFA). Incomplete healing between RFA treatments, likely caused by persistently abnormal gastroesophageal reflux, is one factor that seems to contribute substantially to an incomplete response to RFA.[41] In one study, patients with Barrett's esophagus on twice-daily PPI therapy were evaluated with esophageal pH/impedance testing before endoscopic eradication therapy with RFA. Patients who had an incomplete response to RFA (defined as persistent Barrett's metaplasia after two RFA sessions) were found to have an increased total number of reflux events, with increased weakly acidic reflux (pH 4–7) and increased nonacid reflux (pH >7).[42] In another study, patients undergoing RFA for Barrett's esophagus underwent pH monitoring while on PPI treatment. Almost one-third of the patients on PPIs were found to have persistent abnormal acid reflux, and persistently elevated esophageal acid exposure (>8% of the study period) was found to be a risk factor for failed endoscopic ablation and persistence of Barrett's metaplasia.[43] These findings suggest that poorly controlled gastroesophageal reflux with abnormal esophageal acid exposure, despite PPI use, may be a contributor to poor response to endoscopic eradication therapy for Barrett's esophagus with RFA.

SUMMARY

PPIs are the mainstay for treatment of GERD. In Barrett's esophagus, authorities agree that PPIs should be used for control of acid reflux symptoms. PPIs also are clearly indicated during endoscopic ablative therapy to allow healing of the ablated Barrett's esophagus with neosquamous epithelium, and adequate acid suppression seems to contribute to the success of ablative therapy. There is also considerable evidence, albeit indirect, that PPIs prevent the neoplastic progression of Barrett's metaplasia.

REFERENCES

1. Pohl H, Sirovich B, Welch HG. Esophageal adenocarcinoma incidence: are we reaching the peak? Cancer Epidemiol Biomarkers Prev 2010;19(6):1468–70.
2. Zhang HY, Hormi-Carver K, Zhang X, et al. In benign Barrett's epithelial cells, acid exposure generates reactive oxygen species that cause DNA double-strand breaks. Cancer Res 2009;69(23):9083–9.
3. Souza RF, Shewmake K, Terada LS, et al. Acid exposure activates the mitogen-activated protein kinase pathways in Barrett's esophagus. Gastroenterology 2002;122(2):299–307.
4. Fitzgerald RC, Omary MB, Triadafilopoulos G. Dynamic effects of acid on Barrett's esophagus. An ex vivo proliferation and differentiation model. J Clin Invest 1996;98(9):2120–8.
5. Ouatu-Lascar R, Fitzgerald RC, Triadafilopoulos G. Differentiation and proliferation in Barrett's esophagus and the effects of acid suppression. Gastroenterology 1999;117(2):327–35.
6. Peters FT, Ganesh S, Kuipers EJ, et al. Effect of elimination of acid reflux on epithelial cell proliferative activity of Barrett esophagus. Scand J Gastroenterol 2000;35(12):1238–44.
7. Umansky M, Yasui W, Hallak A, et al. Proton pump inhibitors reduce cell cycle abnormalities in Barrett's esophagus. Oncogene 2001;20(55):7987–91.
8. Thanan R, Ma N, Iijima K, et al. Proton pump inhibitors suppress iNOS-dependent DNA damage in Barrett's esophagus by increasing Mn-SOD expression. Biochem Biophys Res Commun 2012;421(2):280–5.
9. Souza RF, Huo X, Mittal V, et al. Gastroesophageal reflux might cause esophagitis through a cytokine-mediated mechanism rather than caustic acid injury. Gastroenterology 2009;137(5):1776–84.
10. Huo X, Zhang X, Yu C, et al. In oesophageal squamous cells exposed to acidic bile salt medium, omeprazole inhibits IL-8 expression through effects on nuclear factor-kappaB and activator protein-1. Gut 2014;63(7):1042–52.
11. Charbel S, Khandwala F, Vaezi MF. The role of esophageal pH monitoring in symptomatic patients on PPI therapy. Am J Gastroenterol 2005;100(2):283–9.
12. Spechler SJ, Sharma P, Traxler B, et al. Gastric and esophageal pH in patients with Barrett's esophagus treated with three esomeprazole dosages: a randomized, double-blind, crossover trial. Am J Gastroenterol 2006;101(9):1964–71.
13. Katzka DA, Castell DO. Successful elimination of reflux symptoms does not insure adequate control of acid reflux in patients with Barrett's esophagus. Am J Gastroenterol 1994;89(7):989–91.
14. Gerson LB, Boparai V, Ullah N, et al. Oesophageal and gastric pH profiles in patients with gastro-oesophageal reflux disease and Barrett's oesophagus treated with proton pump inhibitors. Aliment Pharmacol Ther 2004;20(6):637–43.
15. Basu KK, Bale R, West KP, et al. Persistent acid reflux and symptoms in patients with Barrett's oesophagus on proton-pump inhibitor therapy. Eur J Gastroenterol Hepatol 2002;14(11):1187–92.
16. Theisen J, Nehra D, Citron D, et al. Suppression of gastric acid secretion in patients with gastroesophageal reflux disease results in gastric bacterial overgrowth and deconjugation of bile acids. J Gastrointest Surg 2000;4(1):50–4.
17. Peng S, Huo X, Rezaei D, et al. In Barrett's esophagus patients and Barrett's cell lines, ursodeoxycholic acid increases antioxidant expression and prevents DNA damage by bile acids. Am J Physiol Gastrointest Liver Physiol 2014;307(2): G129–39.

18. Williams C, McColl KE. Review article: proton pump inhibitors and bacterial overgrowth. Aliment Pharmacol Ther 2006;23(1):3–10.
19. Beales IL, Ogunwobi OO. Glycine-extended gastrin inhibits apoptosis in Barrett's oesophageal and oesophageal adenocarcinoma cells through JAK2/STAT3 activation. J Mol Endocrinol 2009;42(4):305–18.
20. Ogunwobi OO, Beales IL. Glycine-extended gastrin stimulates proliferation via JAK2- and Akt-dependent NF-kappaB activation in Barrett's oesophageal adenocarcinoma cells. Mol Cell Endocrinol 2008;296(1–2):94–102.
21. Harris JC, Clarke PA, Awan A, et al. An antiapoptotic role for gastrin and the gastrin/CCK-2 receptor in Barrett's esophagus. Cancer Res 2004;64(6):1915–9.
22. Haigh CR, Attwood SE, Thompson DG, et al. Gastrin induces proliferation in Barrett's metaplasia through activation of the CCK2 receptor. Gastroenterology 2003;124(3):615–25.
23. Wang JS, Varro A, Lightdale CJ, et al. Elevated serum gastrin is associated with a history of advanced neoplasia in Barrett's esophagus. Am J Gastroenterol 2010;105(5):1039–45.
24. Obszynska JA, Atherfold PA, Nanji M, et al. Long-term proton pump induced hypergastrinaemia does induce lineage-specific restitution but not clonal expansion in benign Barrett's oesophagus in vivo. Gut 2010;59(2):156–63.
25. Garcia Rodriguez LA, Lagergren J, Lindblad M. Gastric acid suppression and risk of oesophageal and gastric adenocarcinoma: a nested case control study in the UK. Gut 2006;55(11):1538–44.
26. Srinivasan R, Katz PO, Ramakrishnan A, et al. Maximal acid reflux control for Barrett's oesophagus: feasible and effective. Aliment Pharmacol Ther 2001;15(4):519–24.
27. Cooper BT, Chapman W, Neumann CS, et al. Continuous treatment of Barrett's oesophagus patients with proton pump inhibitors up to 13 years: observations on regression and cancer incidence. Aliment Pharmacol Ther 2006;23(6):727–33.
28. El-Serag HB, Aguirre TV, Davis S, et al. Proton pump inhibitors are associated with reduced incidence of dysplasia in Barrett's esophagus. Am J Gastroenterol 2004;99(10):1877–83.
29. Nguyen DM, El-Serag HB, Henderson L, et al. Medication usage and the risk of neoplasia in patients with Barrett's esophagus. Clin Gastroenterol Hepatol 2009;7(12):1299–304.
30. Kastelein F, Spaander MC, Steyerberg EW, et al. Proton pump inhibitors reduce the risk of neoplastic progression in patients with Barrett's esophagus. Clin Gastroenterol Hepatol 2013;11(4):382–8.
31. Hillman LC, Chiragakis L, Shadbolt B, et al. Proton-pump inhibitor therapy and the development of dysplasia in patients with Barrett's oesophagus. Med J Aust 2004;180(8):387–91.
32. Singh S, Garg SK, Singh PP, et al. Acid-suppressive medications and risk of oesophageal adenocarcinoma in patients with Barrett's oesophagus: a systematic review and meta-analysis. Gut 2014;63(8):1229–37.
33. Hvid-Jensen F, Pedersen L, Funch-Jensen P, et al. Proton pump inhibitor use may not prevent high-grade dysplasia and oesophageal adenocarcinoma in Barrett's oesophagus: a nationwide study of 9883 patients. Aliment Pharmacol Ther 2014;39(9):984–91.
34. Spechler SJ, Lee E, Ahnen D, et al. Long-term outcome of medical and surgical therapies for gastroesophageal reflux disease: follow-up of a randomized controlled trial. JAMA 2001;285(18):2331–8.

35. Lagergren J, Ye W, Lagergren P, et al. The risk of esophageal adenocarcinoma after antireflux surgery. Gastroenterology 2010;138(4):1297–301.
36. Corey KE, Schmitz SM, Shaheen NJ. Does a surgical antireflux procedure decrease the incidence of esophageal adenocarcinoma in Barrett's esophagus? A meta-analysis. Am J Gastroenterol 2003;98(11):2390–4.
37. Tran T, Spechler SJ, Richardson P, et al. Fundoplication and the risk of esophageal cancer in gastroesophageal reflux disease: a Veterans Affairs cohort study. Am J Gastroenterol 2005;100(5):1002–8.
38. Sharaiha RZ, Freedberg DE, Abrams JA, et al. Cost-effectiveness of chemoprevention with proton pump inhibitors in Barrett's esophagus. Dig Dis Sci 2014; 59(6):1222–30.
39. Katz PO, Gerson LB, Vela MF. Guidelines for the diagnosis and management of gastroesophageal reflux disease. Am J Gastroenterol 2013;108(3):308–28 [quiz: 329].
40. Spechler SJ, Sharma P, Souza RF, et al. American Gastroenterological Association medical position statement on the management of Barrett's esophagus. Gastroenterology 2011;140(3):1084–91.
41. Bulsiewicz WJ, Kim HP, Dellon ES, et al. Safety and efficacy of endoscopic mucosal therapy with radiofrequency ablation for patients with neoplastic Barrett's esophagus. Clin Gastroenterol Hepatol 2013;11:636–42.
42. Krishnan K, Pandolfino JE, Kahrilas PJ, et al. Increased risk for persistent intestinal metaplasia in patients with Barrett's esophagus and uncontrolled reflux exposure before radiofrequency ablation. Gastroenterology 2012;143(3):576–81.
43. Akiyama J, Marcus SN, Triadafilopoulos G. Effective intra-esophageal acid control is associated with improved radiofrequency ablation outcomes in Barrett's esophagus. Dig Dis Sci 2012;57(10):2625–32.

Cost-Analyses Studies in Barrett's Esophagus
What Is Their Utility?

Lauren B. Gerson, MD, MSc

KEYWORDS

- Cost-effectiveness • Barrett's esophagus • Markov model • Health-state utilities
- Ablation therapy

KEY POINTS

- Cost-effectiveness analyses compare costs associated with administration of therapy for a condition and effectiveness, usually measured in life-years saved or quality-adjusted life years.
- Economic modeling studies in the areas of Barrett's esophagus (BE) have been useful to determine whether current practices of screening and surveillance are cost-effective.
- Key variables in these models include cost of therapy, progression rates from nondysplastic BE to dysplasia and cancer, and efficacy of therapy in eradication of dysplasia and prevention of cancer.
- Modeling studies have demonstrated that screening and surveillance are considered to be cost-effective, particularly for high-risk groups of patients with BE.
- Endoscopic therapy with ablative therapies is considered to be cost-effective for patients with BE and dysplasia.

INTRODUCTION

Any medical therapy rendered is associated with costs, which can include direct costs to patients, hospitals, and/or third-party payers, and indirect costs such as impact on health-related quality of life (HRQL), work productivity, and other measures. Underlying health states and therapies may also be associated with impact on quality of life due to associated symptoms, can impact duration of life expectancy, and in other cases, may affect work productivity and/or quality.

Cost-effectiveness analysis was a concept introduced in the 1990s[1] as a means to evaluate costs and effectiveness of different medical therapies. Costs are typically estimated based on third-party payers or Medicare rates for medications and

Disclosure Statement: Dr L.B. Gerson receives grant support from CDx Diagnotics, Inc.
California Pacific Medical Center, 2340 Clay Street, 6th Floor, San Francisco, CA 94115, USA
E-mail address: GersonL@sutterhealth.org

procedures performed. Effectiveness measures can include impact on life expectancy, calculated from the US Life Tables based on patient age, or quality-adjusted life years (QALYs) adjusted by number of life years remaining. All costs and health state utility values are discounted, typically by 3% per year. Scores from generalized or disease-specific instruments cannot be used in the calculation; rather cost-effectiveness analyses require utility values, numbers representing health-quality of life states between 0 and 100. To obtain utilities, either the time-tradeoff or the standard gamble (SG) exercises can be used. Although traditionally paper probability wheels were used, most studies now use computer programs to interview patients. First, the life expectancy of the patient is calculated based on current US Life Tables. In the time-tradeoff exercise, patients are asked how much of their remaining life they would like to trade to rid themselves of their current disorder or health state. The amount traded can range from months to years and is calculated by the formula:

$$\frac{\text{Number of life years remaining} - \text{number of years traded}}{\text{Life years remaining}}$$

which generates a number between 0 and 1, where 0 represents the state of death, and a score of 1, a state of perfect health.

In the SG exercise, patients are invited to engage in a gamble exercise wherein they are told there is a cure for their underlying disorder, but the treatment is associated with a small risk of death. The patient is asked to determine the risk of death that would be acceptable to achieve a cure. In both of these exercises, a "ping-pong" strategy is used whereby patients are initially presented with large values of risk or life years to trade alternating with very small values, and this value is adjusted until the patient decides on a final value.

In the setting of Barrett's esophagus (BE) cost-effectiveness analysis, health-state utility values that might be of interest include those included with the symptoms of gastroesophageal reflux disease (GERD) in patients with BE, risks of cancer associated with states of dysplasia, symptoms associated with cancer, and symptoms that might develop after esophagectomy. Values that have been derived from the literature and have been used in the cost-effectiveness studies to be discussed are shown in **Table 1**. Based on the presence of GERD symptoms, patients with BE did not show lower quality of life scores compared with patients with GERD in one study.[2] When patients with BE were asked theoretically to imagine they had BE in association with a dysplastic state and were educated about associated risks of cancer, lower HRQL values were obtained. Of note is that values obtained using SG techniques are typically higher compared with time tradeoff techniques (TTO) because patients are less willing to undergo therapies with a certain percentage risk of death compared to a trade where they are able to give away a certain amount of time in order to eliminate a certain condition or health state.

Creation of a Decision Model

The first decision in the creation of a cost-effectiveness model is the duration of the model, based on the available literature. In situations where there are only short-term data available, such as, for example, duration of an endoscopic therapy for GERD, a model can be created in a fixed time period to reflect the available data regarding treatment duration. If patients progress in the model from one state to another without the possibility of transitioning back to the original state, then a standard decision tree can be created. If, however, the patient can transition between

Table 1
Health-state utility values for patients with gastroesophageal reflux disease and Barrett's esophagus

Author, Year	Utility Exercise	Patients	Findings
Gerson et al,[2] 2005	TTO and SG	220 GERD 40 (25%) BE	TTO 0.94 on medications and 0.90 off PPI SG 0.94 for both TTO for BE 0.92 on medications and 0.90 off PPI
Hur et al,[22] 2006	SG	20 patients BE	NDBE = 0.95; Postesophagectomy for HGD with dysphagia = 0.92; Post-PDT for HGD with recurrence uncertainty = 0.93; Post-PDT for HGD with recurrence uncertainty and dysphagia = 0.91; Intensive endoscopic surveillance for HGD = 0.9
Gerson et al,[23] 2007	TTO	60 patient BE 40 patients GERD	NDBE = 0.91 LGD = 0.85 HGD = 0.77 Esophageal cancer = 0.67

Abbreviations: HGD, high grade dysplasia; LGD, low grade dysplasia; NDBE, nondysplastic Barrett's esophagus; PDT, photodynamic therapy; PPI, proton pump inhibitor; SG, standard gamble; TTO, time trade-off.
Data from Refs.[2,22,23]

different states of the model until death occurs, a Markov process should be used (**Fig. 1**). These models can be created using standard programs including Excel, or commercially available programs for modeling (for example, TreeAge Software, Boston, MA, USA). To create the model, the investigator needs to be able to input the duration of each cycle (which could range from a month to several years), the probability of being in each health state, probabilities for transitioning to different health states, costs associated with each treatment rendered, and utility values for each health state. The end result is a calculation of total costs and utility values for each treatment arm of the model.

A base case for each model is required and usually involves a typical patient with a condition (in the case of BE, a 50-year-old Caucasian man with chronic GERD) with the baseline being absence of treatment or screening. In this arm, the probabilities for the development of dysplasia and/or cancer are calculated based on natural history information. If the comparator treatment is both less expensive and more effective compared with the baseline arm, it is stated to "dominate" the other strategies, and a cost-effectiveness ratio is not calculated. If, on the other hand, the comparator treatment is more expensive but also more effective, then an incremental cost-effectiveness ratio (ICER) is calculated using the following formula:

$$ICER = \frac{\text{Cost therapy} - \text{Cost baseline treatment}}{\text{QALY therapy} - \text{QALY baseline treatment}}$$

and is expressed as dollars per QALY in a cost-utility analysis, or life-years saved if life expectancy is used for a cost-effectiveness analysis. A treatment is deemed to be acceptable from a societal point of view if the ICER is roughly less than $50,000 per QALY.

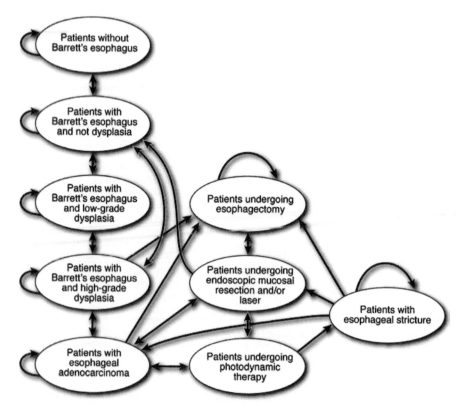

Fig. 1. The Markov model showing possible transitions between health states. Patients continue to cycle between states until death occurs. Circular arrows represent states where patients can stay permanently. (*From* Gerson L, Lin OS. Cost-benefit analysis of capsule endoscopy compared with standard upper endoscopy for the detection of Barrett's esophagus. Clin Gastroenterol Hepatol 2007;5:320; with permission.)

Methods for This Analysis

To perform the analysis of the literature for this article, a search was performed using PubMed/Medline from 2000 to 2014 using the following search terms, including "Cost-Benefit Analysis," "Barrett's esophagus," "Markov chains," "esophageal cancer," "chemoprevention," "aspirin," "proton pump inhibitor therapy," and "quality-adjusted life years." Only articles performing an analysis using US dollars and either QALY or life-years gained were included in this analysis.

Studies Assessing Cost-Effectiveness of Screening and Surveillance for Barrett's Esophagus

As shown in **Table 2**, there have been 7 cost-effectiveness studies assessing whether screening and surveillance of BE are cost-effective. The method of screening included standard sedated upper endoscopy (EGD) in 3 studies,[3–5] unsedated transnasal endoscopy (uTNE) in one study,[6] esophageal capsule endoscopy (ECE) in 2 studies,[7,8] and use of a Cytosponge in a recent analysis.[9]

In the first study by Sonnenberg and colleagues,[5] the authors compared surveillance of nondysplastic BE (NDBE) with upper endoscopy every 2 years to no screening and found that this practice was cost-effective with an ICER of $17K per life-year saved. Patients with high-grade dysplasia (HGD) were modeled to undergo esophagectomy. Costs included $644 for EGD, $21K for esophagectomy, and $44K for cancer care. Surveillance became less cost-effective if the decrement in HRQL increased after esophagectomy or when the efficacy of screening in reducing the incidence of adenocarcinoma decreased. With sensitivity analyses, the ICER of surveillance ranged from $5000 to $85,000 per life-year saved.

Inadomi and colleagues[4] published a model focusing on surveillance in high-risk BE groups in the *Annals of Internal Medicine* in 2003. In this study, the authors used a Markov model for a base-case patient who was a 50-year-old Caucasian man with chronic GERD. The authors compared 2 strategies to no surveillance: the first involved identification of BE followed by surveillance only if dysplasia was detected; in the second arm, identification of BE was followed by surveillance for nondysplastic as well as dysplastic BE. The authors modeled that the presence of HGD would increase surveillance to every 3 months, and that esophagectomy would be performed in the presence of cancer. QALYs were used with health-state utility values estimated from TTO values obtained from experts. QALY values after esophagectomy were available from patients. Based on data from the Health Care Financing Administration, costs for EGD were estimated at $830, esophagectomy at $19,000, and care of cancer $34,000. The authors found that compared with no surveillance, screening with surveillance of dysplastic BE only was cost-effective with an ICER of $10,440 per QALY, but that surveillance of NDBE was not cost-effective compared with surveillance only of dysplastic cases. It should be noted, however, that surveillance of NDBE would be considered to be cost-effective, if compared with the strategy of no screening or surveillance. However, because the primary aim of the model was to examine the cost-effectiveness of surveillance of dysplasia compared with no screening or surveillance, the arm examining surveillance of NDBE was not cost-effective because of the very small to no change in QALY values between arms. The model was most sensitive to progression rates for HGD to cancer and the prevalence of BE.

A subsequent model by Gerson and colleagues[3] in 2004 examined the cost-effectiveness of screening and surveillance for patients with BE. Surveillance intervals occurred according to the current society guidelines, including every 3 years for NDBE, every 1 year for LGD, and every 3 months for HGD. Patients found to have cancer who were not surgical candidates could undergo endoscopic mucosal resection for nodular disease, or photodynamic therapy (PDT) for flat disease. Costs included $810 for EGD, $15,500 for esophagectomy, $6100 for PDT, $10,700 for chemotherapy, and $5700 for radiation therapy. The ICER for screening and surveillance was $12K/life-year gained but exceeded $100K if the prevalence of BE decreased to 1%. Overall, these 3 models demonstrated that surveillance of BE is cost-effective depending on the prevalence of BE and the progression rates to cancer. If, however, most cancers are found on the initial screening examination, then subsequent surveillance may not be cost-effective. The addition of endoscopic therapy prolongs survival and renders surveillance more cost-effective.

Unsedated transnasal endoscopy (uTNE) has demonstrated excellent sensitivity and specificity as a screening tool for BE with lower associated patient costs and indirect costs, such as time lost from work. A 2003 cost-utility analysis compared screening with uTNE to sedated EGD and no screening. The costs for uTNE and EGD based on Medicare reimbursement rates were $97 and $506, respectively. The authors assumed a 95% sensitivity and specificity for uTNE in the detection of BE. Compared with no screening and assuming a BE prevalence of 3%, the ICER of

Table 2
Cost-effectiveness studies of screening and surveillance for Barrett's esophagus

Author, Year	Patient Population/ Screening Modality	Model Design	Results	Key Model Parameters
Sonnenberg et al,[5] 2002	100,000 subjects 60-y-old with BE	Markov model Surveillance with EGD every 2 y Esophagectomy for HGD	ICER $17K/life-saved for screening	BE to cancer 0.5% 20% survive postesophagectomy Life-years saved
Inadomi et al,[4] 2003	50-y-old Caucasian men with chronic GERD undergoing sedated EGD	Markov model Surveillance only if dysplasia present Esophagectomy for HGD or cancer	ICER $10K/QALY for screen + surveillance dysplasia ICER $596K/QALY surveillance all BE every 5 y compared with surveillance for dysplasia	BE prevalence 10% Prevalent cancer in BE 6.7% BE to cancer 0.5% Quality-adjusted life-years with TTO based on expert opinion Esophagectomy only for cancer
Gerson et al,[3] 2004	50-y-old Caucasian men with chronic GERD undergoing sedated EGD	Markov model Surveillance according to guidelines Esophagectomy for HGD Endoscopic therapy for nonsurgical candidates	ICER for screening of $12K/ life-year gained	BE prevalence 10% BE to cancer 0.5% Prevalent cancer 0.8% Outcome: life-years saved
Nietert et al,[6] 2003	50-y-old man with chronic GERD	Markov model	Compared with no screening uTE: $56K/QALY EGD: $87K/QALY Screening with uTE compared with EGD: $709K/QALY	Outcome: QALY BE prevalence 3% BE to EAC 0.5% per year Sensitivity and specificity of uTNE: 95%

Study	Population	Model	Results	Assumptions
Rubenstein et al,[7] 2007	50-y-old Caucasian men with chronic GERD	Markov model Screening with EGD or ECE followed by EGD compared with no screening	EGD compared with no screening ICER $11K/QALY ECE less effective and more expensive compared with EGD	Outcome: QALY BE prevalence: 10% BE to EAC: 0.5% ECE sensitivity: 85% EGD sensitivity: 100%
Gerson & Lin,[8] 2007	50 y-old men with chronic GERD	Markov model Screening with EGD or ECE followed by EGD compared with no screening	Compared with no screening, ICER for EGD $5K/LY ECE arm more expensive and less effective	Outcome: life-years saved BE prevalence: 10% BE to EAC: 0.5% Sensitivity of ECE: 70% Sensitivity of EGD: 85%
Benaglia et al,[9] 2013	50 y-old man with chronic GERD	Microsimulation model Cytosponge or EGD compared with no screening Endotherapy (RFA + EMR) and esophagectomy modeled to treat HGD or EAC	Cytosponge screening compared with no screening with ICER $16K/QALY EGD more expensive and less effective	Outcome: QALY BE prevalence: 8% BE to EAC: 0.15% Cytosponge participation: 45% EGD participation: 23% EGD sensitivity and specificity: 100% Cytosponge sensitivity 73% and specificity 94%

Data from Refs.[3-9]

uTNE was $56K/QALY. The ICER estimates were very sensitive to the prevalence of esophageal adenocarcinoma (EAC). If 1% of BE patients developed EAC per year, the ICERs for uTNE and EGD decreased to $15K/QALY and $25/QALY, respectively. The no screening strategy dominated when the EAC incidence decreased to 0.25%/y. In addition, if the cost of uTNE exceeded $330, then the EGD strategy became the most cost-effective. The QALY value used for most of these models for patients after esophagectomy was 0.97, based on a prior work by Provenzale and colleagues[10] published in abstract form interviewing patients with TTO. The authors noted that if this value decreased to 0.90, then both screening arms would no longer be cost-effective with ICERs exceeding $150K/QALY, and at a value of 0.86, the no screening arm would dominate.

Esophageal capsule endoscopy (ECE) was introduced in 2004 as a noninvasive means of imaging the esophagogastric junction (EGJ).[11] By capturing 14 frames per second compared with 2 frames per second with conventional small bowel capsule endoscopy, the hope was to successfully image the EGJ with the patient in the supine position after ingestion to slow down esophageal transit. A meta-analysis published in 2009 based on 9 studies and 618 patients demonstrated sensitivity and specificity of 78% and 90% for ECE in the diagnosis of BE using EGD as the gold standard.[12]

Two cost-effectiveness studies were published to determine whether usage of ECE would be cost-effective as a screening modality. In the first study by Rubenstein and colleagues,[7] the authors included costs for EGD with biopsy of $830 and ECE of $740 based on 2005 Medicare reimbursement rates. Compared with EGD, which was assumed to have an accuracy of 100% for the diagnosis of BE, the sensitivity of ECE was modeled to be 85%. Compared with the no screening strategy where patients lived an average of 23 additional years after the enrollment age of 50 and accrued an average of 16.47 QALYs with average costs of $102, the patients in the EGD arm accrued costs of $2304 with an average of 16.66 QALYs resulting in an ICER of $11K per QALY gained compared with no screening. The esophageal capsule arm had costs of $2348, was associated with 16.64 QALYs, and was therefore dominated (more costly and less effective) by the standard EGD arm.

In the second study comparing ECE to standard EGD by Gerson and Lin,[8] a similar Markov model was constructed comparing no screening with ECE followed by EGD if BE was suspected, or standard EGD. Using weighted probabilities of sensitivities for ECE from recent clinical trials, the sensitivity of ECE was 70% and the sensitivity of EGD was 85% based on clinical trial data. It was assumed that there would be poor visualization of the EGJ in 50% of the cases, which would lead to an EGD examination. Costs used included $785 for ECE and $179 for EGD with biopsy. Assuming a theoretic cohort of 10,000 patients with GERD, the initial EGD cost was $1988 and was associated with 18.54 life-years compared with $2392 and 18.36 life-years for the ECE arm and $901 and 18.30 life-years for the no screening arm. The ICER of screening with EGD compared with the no screening arm was $4530 per life-year gained and again dominated the ECE arm, which was more expensive and less effective. Since the publication of these 2 cost-effectiveness analyses, there have not been further advances in esophageal capsule technology to warrant updates in cost-effectiveness analyses for this technology.

A recent cost analysis examined the potential of a Cytosponge for BE screening. As described by the authors, the Cytosponge is an ingestible gelatin capsule containing a compressed mesh attached to a string; once swallowed, the capsule is dissolved and the sponge is released at the level of the EGJ. The cytology specimen is then collected and analysis is performed with immunostaining for trefoil factor 3, a diagnostic marker of BE.[9] For patients with BE segments 1 cm or larger, the Cytosponge has a sensitivity of 73% and specificity of 94% for BE.[13] Patients found to have NDBE underwent surveillance every 3 months and LGD every 6 months. HGD or esophageal cancer was treated with either endotherapy (radiofrequency ablation [RFA] with or without endoscopic mucosal resection [EMR]) or esophagectomy. Costs in the model included $152 for the Cytosponge and $786 for endoscopy with biopsy. The ICER for usage of the Cytosponge was $16K/QALY; Cytosponge screening followed by treatment of patients with dysplasia or intramucosal cancer (IMC) cost an additional $240 with a mean gain of 0.015 QALYs. Compared with no screening, the EGD arm cost $299 and was associated with 0.013 QALYs with an ICER of $22K/QALY. Therefore, the Cytosponge arm was less costly and more effective compared with standard EGD.

Chemoprevention in Barrett's Esophagus

There were 3 published studies examining the potential role of chemopreventive agents including aspirin (ASA),[14] statins plus aspirin,[15] and proton pump inhibitor (PPI) therapy.[16]

In the first study published in 2004, Hur and colleagues[14] constructed a Markov model to compare ASA usage, endoscopic surveillance with biopsies, both therapies, or neither therapy. The authors modeled risk of stroke and gastrointestinal (GI) bleeding associated with daily ASA therapy. The costs were $1 for daily ASA usage per month and $830 for EGD with biopsy. Base-case results (**Table 3**) demonstrated that ASA was less expensive and more effective compared with no therapy. ASA plus endoscopic therapy was also cost-effective. The benefits of ASA continued down to an effectiveness for cancer prevention of 10%.

The second study by Choi and colleagues[15] examined the impact of ASA, statins, or both in addition to endoscopic surveillance in the reduction of EAC in patients with BE. The authors modeled reductions from BE to EAC of 53% for ASA, 54% for statins, and 78% for combination therapy in addition to complication risks associated with these medications. Costs included $930 for EGD with biopsy, $19/y for ASA, and $872/y for statins. When progression of BE to EAC was 0.33%/y or less, the combination therapy was not preferred over the ASA arm. The authors concluded that ASA therapy was the most cost-effective, but that statins could be considered in patients unable or unwilling to take ASA therapy.

A 2014 cost-effectiveness study examined the role of PPIs as chemopreventive agents for patients with BE.[16] A recent meta-analysis demonstrated a 71% reduction in the risk of HGD and/or EAC in PPI users with BE based on data from 7 studies in 2813 patients (odds ratio 0.3, 95% confidence interval 0.1–0.8).[17] In this Markov model, the authors assumed a 50% reduction in EAC with PPI usage and included potential complications of hip fracture and *Clostridium difficile* infection in PPI users compared with nonusers. Compared with endoscopic surveillance without PPI therapy, usage of PPI cost $23K per patient and was associated with 0.32 QALYs resulting in an ICER of $12K/QALY. The PPI arm resulted in 2.3 EAC cases compared with 6 in the non-PPI arm. The authors found that the ICER would remain less than $50K/QALY if PPI therapy was associated with at least a 19% reduction in EAC progression.

Cost-Effectiveness of Endoscopic Therapy for Dysplastic Barrett's Esophagus

Several studies have been published examining the role of endoscopic therapy compared with esophagectomy and/or surveillance for patients with BE and HGD (**Table 4**). In the first study by Hur and colleagues,[18] the authors compared the cost-effectiveness of photodynamic therapy (PDT) with esophagectomy or surveillance for patients with BE and HGD. The cost of PDT was $9K compared with $23K for esophagectomy and $830 for EGD with biopsy. Overall, PDT was more expensive

Table 3
Studies assessing chemoprevention in Barrett's esophagus

Author, Year	Chemopreventive Agent	Model Design	Results	Key Model Parameters
Hur et al,[14] 2004	325 mg ASA daily	Markov model 55-y-old man with BE. Compared no therapy to daily ASA, endoscopic surveillance alone or both ASA + endoscopy	• ASA therapy arm was dominant (cost $2900 less and more effective 0.19 QALYs) than no therapy • Endoscopic therapy $118K per QALY • ASA + EGD $49K/QALY • EGD alone $203K/QALY compared with ASA alone	• Outcome: QALY • ASA associated with reduction esophageal cancer 50% • False positive and negative rates for histology incorporated • Incorporated costs associated with stroke and GI bleeding • BE to EAC: 0.5%
Choi et al,[15] 2014	Statins/ASA	Markov model 50-y-old with BE Surveillance with EGD or surveillance with EGD plus ASA 325 mg daily or EGD plus statin daily or EGD plus ASA + statin	ASA strategy dominated EGD alone ($6900 less and 0.167 QALYs). ICER of $38K/QALY for statin + EGD and $16K/QALY for statin + ASA + EGD	Outcome: QALY ASA 53% reduction in EAC Statins 54% reduction in EAC ASA + statin 78% reduction in EAC Complications for ASA and statins included
Sharaiha et al,[16] 2014	PPI	Markov model 50-y-old white men with BE PPI + EGD Endotherapy and esophagectomy for HGD and/or cancer	ICER for PPI $12K/QALY compared with no PPI	Outcome: QALY BE to EAC 0.5% PPI therapy 50% reduction in EAC risk

Abbreviations: APC, argon plasma coagulation; ASA, aspirin; EAC, esophageal adenocarcinoma; EGD, upper endoscopy; HGD, high grade dysplasia; ICER, incremental cost-effectiveness ratio; IM, intestinal metaplasia; LGD, low grade dysplasia; MPEC, multipolar electrocoagulation; NDBE, non-dysplastic Barrett's esophagus; PDT, photodynamic therapy; PPI, proton pump inhibitor; QALY, quality-adjusted life year; RFA, radiofrequency ablation.
Data from Refs.[14–16]

Table 4
Studies assessing cost-effectiveness of endoscopic therapy for dysplasia

Author, Year	Endoscopic Therapy	Model Design	Results	Key Model Parameters
Hur et al,[18] 2003	PDT	Markov model 50-y-old man with BE and HGD Options esophagectomy for HGD and operative candidates vs palliative care compared with PDT therapy	ICER $12K/QALY for PDT compared with surveillance ICER $3K/QALY comparing PDT with esophagectomy	HGD to EAC progression rates 15% first year, 10% subsequent years PDT success 43% HGD recurrence 11%
Shaheen et al,[19] 2004	PDT	Markov model 50 y-old man with BE and HGD No therapy vs EGD vs PDT vs esophagectomy	ICER $26K/QALY for PDT compared with no therapy. All other arms less expensive but less effective	Outcome: QALY BE to EAC: 0.5% PDT success 88% HGD PDT success 40% all BE HGD to EAC 2.5%
Inadomi et al,[20] 2009	RFA, APC, MPEC, PDF	Markov model 50 y-old patients with BE with or without dysplasia who would be candidates for endoscopic therapy or surgery	Compared with no surveillance, ICER for RFA $5839/QALY for HGD, and ICER for PDT $32K/QALY For LGD and NDBE, ablation without surveillance most cost-effective	Outcome: QALY ND to EAC 0.5% HGD to EAC 5.5% PDT success BE 60%; dysplasia 58% RFA success 82%, dysplasia 64% APC success 65%, dysplasia 62% MPEC success 75%
Hur et al,[21] 2012	RFA	Markov model 50 y-old men with NDBE, LGD, or HGD	RFA dominant strategy for HGD compared with surgery Initial RFA cost-effective for LGD with ICER $18K/QALY RFA for NDBE ICER $118K	Outcome: QALY HGD to EAC 2.4% Efficacy RFA for ablation of IM 74% for HGD, 81% for LGD, and 70% for NDBE; Efficacy of RFA for ablation of dysplasia 81% for HGD and 91% for LGD

Data from Refs.[18–21]

but also more effective than esophagectomy and surveillance; PDT cost $48K compared with $41K for esophagectomy and $28K for EGD but was associated with 11.6 QALYs compared with 9.44 for esophagectomy and 10 for EGD. The overall ICER was $12K/QALY for PDT compared with surveillance and $3K/QALY comparing PDT with esophagectomy. In sensitivity analyses, surveillance was preferred over esophagectomy in most cases, except for patients over the age of 65 years.

In the second study by Shaheen and colleagues,[19] the authors compared no surveillance with strategies of esophagectomy, ablation with PDT, or surveillance with upper endoscopy for 50-year-old men with BE and HGD. Costs in the mode included $20K for PDT, $830 for EGD with biopsy, and $19K for esophagectomy. Compared with all of the other arms, PDT was more expensive (cost of $42K compared with $35K for EGD, $35K for esophagectomy, and $750 for no therapy) but was also most effective, resulting in an ICER of $26K/QALY. The cost of PDT had to be less than $15K for the cost of PDT to be less than the standard EGD arm.

In a study published in *Gastroenterology* in 2009, Inadomi and colleagues[20] compared strategies for treatment of HGD, LGD, and NDBE, including no endoscopic surveillance; endoscopic surveillance with ablation for incident dysplasia; immediate ablation followed by endoscopic surveillance in all patients or only for to patients in whom metaplasia persisted; and esophagectomy. Modalities included for ablation were PDT, RFA, and multipolar electrocoagulation (MPEC).

For patients with HGD, no surveillance cost $1859 per person and was associated with 12.4 discounted QALYs compared with $21K and 15.67 QALYs for RFA, and $35K and 15.67 QALYs for PDT. The other strategies were less effective. The calculated ICERs were $5839/QALY for RFA and $32,588 for PDT for treatment of HGD. For LGD, ablation without subsequent surveillance was the most cost-effective with an ICER of $11,147/QALY, and for NDBE this strategy was associated with an ICER of $16,286/QALY. The results were sensitive to the amounts of residual dysplasia postablation.

The most recent study by Hur and colleagues[21] in 2012 examined the cost-effectiveness of radiofrequency ablation (RFA) for NDBE, LGD, and HGD patients compared with a strategy of surveillance and esophagectomy for cancer. Costs for procedures included $930 for EGD with biopsy, $6400 for RFA, and $26K for esophagectomy. RFA was both less expensive and more effective ($46K and 16.7 QALYs) compared with surveillance and surgery ($71K and 16.04 QALYs) for patients with HGD. For patients with LGD (confirmed by a gastrointestinal pathologist and stable: present on 2 examinations 6 months apart), an initial approach of RFA was associated with an ICER of $18K/QALY compared with the other strategies of surveillance and surgery for cancer, or surveillance and RFA for HGD. For patients with NDBE, RFA was not cost-effective when the progression of NDBE to cancer was 0.5% per year, with an ICER of $118K/QALY.

SUMMARY

Approximately 10% to 15% of the chronic GERD population is at risk for the development of BE, particularly in the setting of other risk factors, including male gender, Caucasian race, age more than 50, and central obesity. The risk of cancer progression for patients with NDBE has been estimated to be approximately 0.2% to 0.5% per year. Given these low progression rates and the high cost of endoscopic surveillance, cost-effectiveness analyses in this area are useful to determine appropriate resource allocation. Although surveillance of NDBE appears to be cost-effective to no surveillance if performed at appropriate intervals and if endoscopic therapy can be offered for patients with dysplasia, newer techniques including uTNE and usage of a Cytosponge may confer additional advantages by lowering costs without loss of efficacy. The current generations of ECE do not appear to be cost-effective means for screening. Usage of ASA, statins, and PPI therapy may be useful to prevent progression of BE to EAC, depending on the risk of potential side effects associated with therapy. Endoscopic therapy for patients with dysplastic BE appear to be cost-effective compared with esophagectomy, particularly the usage of PDT and RFA. For patients with NDBE, however, RFA does not appear to be a cost-effective approach given the low rate of progression to EAC.

REFERENCES

1. Russell LB, Gold MR, Siegel JE, et al. The role of cost-effectiveness analysis in health and medicine. Panel on Cost-Effectiveness in Health and Medicine. JAMA 1996;276:1172–7.
2. Gerson LB, Ullah N, Hastie T, et al. Patient-derived health state utilities for gastroesophageal reflux disease. Am J Gastroenterol 2005;100:524–33.
3. Gerson LB, Groeneveld PW, Triadafilopoulos G. Cost-effectiveness model of endoscopic screening and surveillance in patients with gastroesophageal reflux disease. Clin Gastroenterol Hepatol 2004;2:868–79.
4. Inadomi JM, Sampliner R, Lagergren J, et al. Screening and surveillance for Barrett esophagus in high-risk groups: a cost-utility analysis. Ann Intern Med 2003; 138:176–86.
5. Sonnenberg A, Soni A, Sampliner RE. Medical decision analysis of endoscopic surveillance of Barrett's oesophagus to prevent oesophageal adenocarcinoma. Aliment Pharmacol Ther 2002;16:41–50.
6. Nietert PJ, Silverstein MD, Mokhashi MS, et al. Cost-effectiveness of screening a population with chronic gastroesophageal reflux. Gastrointest Endosc 2003;57: 311–8.
7. Rubenstein JH, Inadomi JM, Brill JV, et al. Cost utility of screening for Barrett's esophagus with esophageal capsule endoscopy versus conventional upper endoscopy. Clin Gastroenterol Hepatol 2007;5:312–8.
8. Gerson L, Lin OS. Cost-benefit analysis of capsule endoscopy compared with standard upper endoscopy for the detection of Barrett's esophagus. Clin Gastroenterol Hepatol 2007;5:319–25.
9. Benaglia T, Sharples LD, Fitzgerald RC, et al. Health benefits and cost effectiveness of endoscopic and nonendoscopic cytosponge screening for Barrett's esophagus. Gastroenterology 2013;144:62–73.e6.
10. Provenzale D, Kemp JA, Arora S, et al. A guide for surveillance of patients with Barrett's esophagus. Am J Gastroenterol 1994;89:670–80.
11. Koslowsky B, Jacob H, Eliakim R, et al. PillCam ESO in esophageal studies: improved diagnostic yield of 14 frames per second (fps) compared with 4 fps. Endoscopy 2006;38:27–30.
12. Bhardwaj A, Hollenbeak CS, Pooran N, et al. A meta-analysis of the diagnostic accuracy of esophageal capsule endoscopy for Barrett's esophagus in patients with gastroesophageal reflux disease. Am J Gastroenterol 2009;104:1533–9.
13. Kadri SR, Lao-Sirieix P, O'Donovan M, et al. Acceptability and accuracy of a non-endoscopic screening test for Barrett's oesophagus in primary care: cohort study. BMJ 2010;341:c4372.
14. Hur C, Nishioka NS, Gazelle GS. Cost-effectiveness of aspirin chemoprevention for Barrett's esophagus. J Natl Cancer Inst 2004;96:316–25.

15. Choi SE, Perzan KE, Tramontano AC, et al. Statins and aspirin for chemoprevention in Barrett's esophagus: results of a cost-effectiveness analysis. Cancer Prev Res (Phila) 2014;7:341–50.
16. Sharaiha RZ, Freedberg DE, Abrams JA, et al. Cost-effectiveness of chemoprevention with proton pump inhibitors in Barrett's esophagus. Dig Dis Sci 2014;59: 1222–30.
17. Singh S, Garg SK, Singh PP, et al. Acid-suppressive medications and risk of oesophageal adenocarcinoma in patients with Barrett's oesophagus: a systematic review and meta-analysis. Gut 2014;63:1229–37.
18. Hur C, Nishioka NS, Gazelle GS. Cost-effectiveness of photodynamic therapy for treatment of Barrett's esophagus with high grade dysplasia. Dig Dis Sci 2003;48: 1273–83.
19. Shaheen NJ, Inadomi JM, Overholt BF, et al. What is the best management strategy for high grade dysplasia in Barrett's oesophagus? A cost effectiveness analysis. Gut 2004;53:1736–44.
20. Inadomi JM, Somoouk M, Madanick RD, et al. A cost-utility analysis of ablative therapy for Barrett's esophagus. Gastroenterology 2009;136:2101–14.e1–6.
21. Hur C, Choi SE, Rubenstein JH, et al. The cost effectiveness of radiofrequency ablation for Barrett's esophagus. Gastroenterology 2012;143:567–75.
22. Hur C, Wittenberg E, Nishioka NS, et al. Quality of life in patients with various Barrett's esophagus associated health states. Health Qual Life Outcomes 2006;4:45.
23. Gerson LB, Ullah N, Hastie T, et al. Does cancer risk affect health-related quality of life in patients with Barrett's esophagus? Gastrointest Endosc 2007; 65:16–25.

Advanced Imaging in Barrett's Esophagus

V. Raman Muthusamy, MD[a],*, Stephen Kim, MD[a], Michael B. Wallace, MD[b]

KEYWORDS

- Barrett's esophagus • Imaging • Chromoendoscopy • Narrow-band imaging
- Autofluorescence imaging • Confocal laser endomicroscopy

KEY POINTS

- A careful endoscopic examination using high-resolution white light endoscopy (HR-WLE) is the current standard in the evaluation of Barrett's esophagus (BE).
- Advances in imaging technology have led to promising new endoscopic tools that may improve the detection of BE and early neoplasia.
- The optimal combination of wide-field surveillance and focal high-resolution imaging for BE has yet to be determined.

INTRODUCTION

BE is estimated to be present in up to 5.6% of the US population and is the precursor lesion for esophageal adenocarcinoma, which has a poor 5-year survival rate of 17%.[1,2] Surveillance endoscopy is now the primary management approach for BE, with 4-quadrant biopsies being obtained every 1 to 2 cm at designated intervals in an attempt to identify dysplasia and early neoplasia. The goal of this approach is to treat patients with identified dysplastic or neoplastic lesions with endoscopic eradication therapies in lieu of surgery or chemoradiation, which is used for patients presenting with more advanced cancers. However, standard protocol biopsies have been associated with a miss rate of up to 57% for dysplastic/neoplastic lesions in patients with BE.[3] Thus, a variety of methods to optimize the imaging of BE have been developed to improve the efficiency and diagnostic yield of surveillance endoscopy in detecting early neoplasia (**Table 1**). These techniques use changes that occur at macroscopic, microscopic, and subcellular levels in early neoplasia and are the focus of this article.

[a] Division of Digestive Diseases, David Geffen School of Medicine at UCLA, 200 UCLA Medical Plaza, Room 330-37, Los Angeles, CA 90095, USA; [b] Division of Gastroenterology and Hepatology, Mayo School of Medicine, 4500 San Pablo Road, Jacksonville, FL 32224, USA
* Corresponding author.
E-mail address: raman@mednet.ucla.edu

Gastroenterol Clin N Am 44 (2015) 439–458
http://dx.doi.org/10.1016/j.gtc.2015.02.012
0889-8553/15/$ – see front matter © 2015 Elsevier Inc. All rights reserved.

gastro.theclinics.com

Table 1 Optical technologies for Barrett's esophagus		
Technology	**Advantages**	**Disadvantages**
Standard WLE	Wide-field imaging, widely available, no contrast	Limited sensitivity and specificity
High resolution WLE	Wide-field imaging, improved image quality, no contrast	Cost of upgrading entire endoscopy system
Dye-based chromoendoscopy	Wide-field imaging, mucosal enhancement	Time consuming, tedious, requires contrast, contrast may be harmful
Optical chromoendoscopy	Wide-field imaging, mucosal enhancement, no contrast	Unclear if there is added benefit to high-resolution WLE alone
AFI	Wide-field imaging, high sensitivity	High false-positive rate
CLE	In vivo histology, probe can be used in any endoscope	Near-field imaging, expensive, requires fluorescein, interpretation of imaging
OCT	In vivo assessment of tissue architecture, no contrast; ability for subsurface imaging	Near-field imaging, early in development
HRME	In vivo histology, can be used in any endoscope	Near-field imaging, requires contrast, not commercially available
Endocytoscopy	In vivo histology, probe can be used in any therapeutic endoscope	Near-field imaging, expensive, requires contrast agents, labor-intensive, not commercially available

Abbreviations: AFI, autofluorescence imaging; CLE, confocal laser endomicroscopy; HRME, high-resolution microendoscopy; OCT, optical coherence topography; WLE, white light endoscopy.

HIGH-DEFINITION WHITE LIGHT EXAMINATION

BE is a diagnosis made based on endoscopic visualization and histologic confirmation. Careful inspection of the esophageal mucosa on upper endoscopy is essential in the detection and surveillance of BE. Consequently, the quality of endoscopic imaging has diagnostic implications on the gastroenterologist's ability to detect and identify intestinal metaplasia, dysplasia, and even early neoplasia.

The quality of endoscopic visualization depends on image resolution and magnification. Resolution refers to the amount of detail within an image and is a function of the pixel density. As the number of pixels increases, the resolution correspondingly improves, providing sharper, more defined, and more detailed images. Standard definition (SD) endoscopes are equipped with charge-coupled device (CCD) chips, which can produce images with up to 400,000 pixels that are then displayed on a traditional display in a 4:3 (width:height) aspect ratio. Technologic advances now enable smaller CCD chips that are capable of producing images with much higher resolution. High-definition or high-resolution endoscopes can capture images with more than 800,000 to 2.1 million pixels that can be displayed on monitors with a 16:9 aspect ratio (**Fig. 1**).[4] The superior imaging quality of the high-resolution endoscopes is 2- to 5-fold better than SD white light endoscopy (WLE), enabling improved visualization of the mucosal surface in BE.

The other essential component of endoscopic visualization is image magnification. Standard endoscopes are designed to magnify the video image by 30 to 35 times.

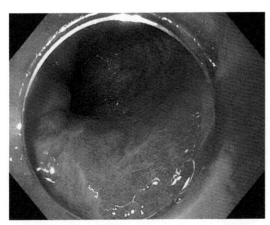

Fig. 1. Barrett's esophagus as seen with high-resolution white light endoscopy.

Many endoscopes may also have a built-in 1.5× to 2× digital zoom, an electronic zoom that brings the center of the image closer without improvement in resolution. This feature should not be confused with specially designed high-definition magnification endoscopes that can optically magnify images by 70 to 140 times their normal size, 2 to 4 times the capability of the standard endoscope. High-resolution magnification endoscopes provide detailed imaging of the mucosal patterns while maintaining image resolution.[4] These highly specialized endoscopes have been studied, primarily in combination with chromoendoscopy, with regards to their ability to enhance the visualization of the mucosal pit patterns and microvasculature morphology of BE.

Expert opinion recommends that HR-WLE should be the minimum standard in the evaluation of patients with BE.[5] However, in their consensus statement, the investigators acknowledge that there is limited high-quality evidence to support this recommendation. At present, there are no randomized studies that directly compare high-resolution to standard WLE in the management of BE. However, the notion that higher resolution may be more sensitive for detecting early neoplastic changes in BE may be inferred from several studies in which standard WLE has been compared with HR-WLE with chromoendoscopy.[6–8] In a prospective, blinded, tandem endoscopy study, patients with BE with known dysplasia underwent SD endoscopy followed by HR-WLE with narrow band imaging (NBI; Olympus, Center Valley, PA, USA) by 2 different endoscopists. HR-WLE with NBI was superior to SD endoscopy in identifying patients with dysplasia as well as detecting higher grades of dysplasia.[6] The study design makes it difficult to determine if the improved detection of early neoplastic changes can be attributed to the HR-WLE, mucosal enhancement with NBI, or the combination of the 2 modalities. Subsequent studies suggest that most of the benefit is derived from the HR-WLE alone and that the added value of using either dye-based or optical chromoendoscopy is uncertain. In a prospective, randomized, crossover study comparing HR-WLE with either indigo carmine chromoendoscopy or NBI, HR-WLE was able to successfully identify subtle dysplastic and early neoplastic changes in BE in 11 of 14 patients (79%). Targeted biopsies using indigo carmine and NBI had limited added benefit to high-resolution endoscopy alone (79% for both procedures, $P = 1$).[7] Another study comparing HR-WLE still images of dysplastic BE with and without indigo carmine, acetic acid, and NBI found that these additional imaging techniques did not improve the identification of early neoplasia compared with the HR-WLE alone (diagnostic yields: HR-WLE alone, 86%; indigo carmine, 70%; acetic acid, 83%; and NBI, 84%).[8] Although direct head-to-head comparison studies are limited, HR-WLE seems to be more sensitive than standard WLE in the detection of BE and its associated early neoplasia.

The role of high-resolution magnification endoscopy alone in BE is unclear. The high-power magnification capability of these scopes is an adjunct usually used in concert with chromoendoscopy (dye based and optical) to closely visualize the mucosal and microvascular patterns of BE. The first use of magnification endoscopy in BE was described in 1994 in which Lugol solution and indigo carmine were used to identify a villiform surface mucosal pattern, which correlated with histologic intestinal metaplasia.[9] Subsequent studies have similarly used indigo carmine or methylene blue with high-magnification endoscopy for identification of BE and surveillance of dysplasia and neoplasia.[10–12] NBI has also been combined with high-resolution magnification endoscopy in the management of BE. A meta-analysis has shown that NBI with magnification can accurately diagnose high-grade dysplasia (HGD) in BE.[13] One small study required 5 expert endoscopists to examine images of BE taken with high-resolution magnification white light and NBI to predict final histopathology. NBI with magnification was superior to high-resolution magnification alone in identifying both nondysplastic BE and HGD in this cohort.[14] Further studies are necessary before any specific conclusions can be made about the role of high-resolution magnification endoscopy in BE.

In summary, despite the limited evidence, it seems reasonable that HR-WLE should be the minimum standard in the initial evaluation and subsequent surveillance of BE. The additional benefit of adding magnification to HR-WLE is uncertain, as this modality has only been studied in conjunction with chromoendoscopy.

DYE-BASED CHROMOENDOSCOPY

Dye-based chromoendoscopy is a wide-field diagnostic imaging tool in which a dye or chemical solution is sprayed onto the gastrointestinal mucosa to enhance visualization of the subtle mucosal and microvascular patterns. In many studies, dye-based chromoendoscopy is often used in combination with high-resolution magnification endoscopes to image the mucosa in exquisite detail. Various stains have proved to be useful in the evaluation of BE by highlighting features of intestinal metaplasia, dysplasia, and early neoplasia that may not be readily apparent with WLE (**Fig. 2**). The different types of dyes used in BE as chromoendoscopy agents include methylene blue, indigo carmine, and acetic acid, each with its own unique properties to facilitate detection of mucosal abnormalities (**Table 2**).

Spraying catheters are typically used to apply the dye in a fine mist covering the esophageal mucosa. The staining dye solution should be sprayed evenly to provide a consistent light coating on the mucosal surface. Excessive spraying can lead to pooling of the dye solution in dependent areas, making the underlying mucosa difficult to interpret. In such instances, any excess dye should be washed away to provide better visualization.

Methylene blue is a vital stain that is preferentially absorbed by intestinal and colonic epithelium.[15] Hence, the intestinal metaplasia of BE stands out from the background of normal squamous epithelium. Methylene blue chromoendoscopy is generally preceded by applying 10% N-acetylcysteine to clean the surface mucosa, followed by spraying 0.5% methylene blue onto the mucosa, waiting 2 to 3 minutes to allow absorption, and subsequently irrigating with water. The methylene blue staining begins to highlight absorptive mucosa within 2 to 3 minutes and wears off after 20 minutes.

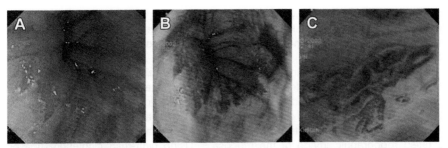

Fig. 2. Barrett's esophagus as seen with (A) high-resolution white light endoscopy and (B, C) methylene blue dye-based chromoendoscopy. (*From* Kiesslich R, Neurath MF. Magnifying chromoendoscopy for the detection of premalignant gastrointestinal lesions. Best Pract Res Clin Gastroenterol 2006;20:68; with permission.)

In BE, the intestinal metaplasia preferentially absorbs the dye, transitioning from the typical salmon-colored mucosa to mucosa with a dark blue hue with a regular, homogeneous pattern. Irregular, heterogeneous staining of the mucosa with varying dark and light blue discoloration can be a cause of concern for dysplastic BE. Initial studies found methylene blue to be an effective tool in targeting intestinal metaplasia and dysplasia, but subsequent studies have had equivocal results.[10,16–19] A meta-analysis ultimately concluded that chromoendoscopy using methylene blue provided no benefit over standard 4-quadrant biopsies in detecting intestinal metaplasia and dysplasia in patients with BE.[20] In addition, in a cohort of patients undergoing surveillance for BE, methylene blue was found to induce oxidative damage to DNA when photosensitized with white light.[21] Although the clinical significance of this finding is unclear, the potential to accelerate carcinogenesis in a well-recognized premalignant

Table 2
Dye-based chromoendoscopy agents in Barrett's esophagus

Chromoendoscopy Agent	Type of Dye	What Does It Stain?	What Does It Not Stain?	Barrett's Esophagus	Early Neoplasia
Methylene blue	Vital stain	Intestinal mucosa	Squamous epithelium	Regular, homogenous, dark blue colored mucosa	Irregular, heterogenous, varying dark and light blue colored mucosa
Indigo carmine	Contrast dye	Not absorbed; pools in mucosal grooves and crevices	Does not stain mucosa	Villiform pattern with tortuous, thick villi	Distortion and irregularity of cerebriform and villous pattern
Acetic acid	Colorless stain	Enhances mucosal surface and vascular patterns	All mucosa stained	Fine villiform appearance with regular shape and arrangement	Irregular surface pattern, increased vascularity

condition has understandably raised concerns regarding the safety profile of methylene blue in BE. Given the lack of clinical efficacy, the time-consuming spray protocol, and the potential risks of methylene blue chromoendoscopy, this technique is no longer popular.

Chromoendoscopy using indigo carmine may be useful in the evaluation of BE and its associated high-risk lesions. Indigo carmine was used in the first successful demonstration of dye-based chromoendoscopy in the evaluation of BE.[9] Indigo carmine is unique in that the dye is not absorbed by the epithelium. Rather, the solution settles between the pits and grooves of the surface epithelium, providing a detailed topographic image of the mucosa.[15] Using high-resolution magnification endoscopy with indigo carmine, targeted biopsies of ridged and villous-appearing mucosa accurately identified intestinal metaplasia in 57 of 62 patients (97%), whereas irregular and distorted mucosa was associated with HGD in 6 of 6 patients (100%).[11] In a subsequent prospective multicenter study of 56 patients with BE, targeted biopsies using high-resolution magnification endoscopy in conjunction with indigo carmine proved to have high sensitivity (83%) and specificity (88%) for HGD while taking less time than performing standard random biopsies.[22]

Acetic acid is a colorless dye and reacts with the epithelium to enhance the surface mucosal pattern.[15] A 1.5% to 3% acetic acid solution is sprayed onto the mucosa, causing whitish discoloration of the epithelium, and examined under high-resolution magnification endoscopy. Close inspection of the surface pit pattern in areas of suspected BE can distinguish normal esophagus from intestinal metaplasia and neoplasia, with a high correlation with final histology ($r = 0.98$).[23] Although no randomized studies have been performed to date, acetic acid has been shown to significantly improve the detection of neoplasia as compared with WLE with routine random biopsies.[23,24]

For a variety of reasons, dye-based chromoendoscopy has not gained widespread clinical use, including a perception that the technique is time consuming and tedious, the concurrent need for high-magnification endoscopy, and concerns regarding the potential to cause bodily harm to the patient. In addition, no standardized classification criteria have been established for dye-based chromoendoscopy, leading to wide variability in sensitivity and specificity.[10,11,16–20,22–24]

In summary, dye-based chromoendoscopy seems to have a limited role in the evaluation of patients with suspected or established BE. This technique has been largely supplanted by optical chromoendoscopy because of the ease and safety of this method.

OPTICAL CHROMOENDOSCOPY

Optical chromoendoscopy is a wide-field diagnostic tool that uses light filters and computer processing technology within the endoscope to enhance visualization of the esophageal mucosa. The principle is similar to that of traditional dye-based chromoendoscopy but without the unwieldy process of spraying and instilling dyes. There are 3 commercially available forms of optical chromoendoscopy as designed by each of the major endoscope manufacturers incorporated into the endoscopes. NBI filters white light into 2 specific wavelengths, 415 nm and 540 nm, that are strongly absorbed by hemoglobin. The filtered light serves to highlight both superficial veins and capillaries along the surface, as well as deeper blood vessels within the mucosa. Fujinon intelligent color enhancement (FICE; Fujinon, Inc, Wayne, NJ, USA) and I-Scan (Pentax Medical, Montvale, NJ, USA) use proprietary postimage acquisition processing technology to modify the white light image and create an enhanced view of the esophageal mucosa. Among these 3 modalities, NBI is most commonly used and has been studied more rigorously than FICE or I-Scan. The few studies that have evaluated FICE and I-SCAN were used in conjunction with acetic acid chromoendoscopy.[25,26] Therefore, NBI is the focus of the following discussion.

BE and HGD have characteristic findings on optical chromoendoscopy that are readily recognizable by the abnormal vascular and mucosal patterns.[27] Intestinal metaplasia has a flat, villous-appearing mucosal pattern with long branching vessels, whereas HGD is described as having disrupted mucosa with irregular blood vessels (**Fig. 3**). NBI has consistently been shown to detect intestinal metaplasia and HGD with a high degree of accuracy when correlated with histology.[27–30] No formal classification of mucosal and vascular patterns have been standardized or validated, which has likely limited the routine clinical use of optical chromoendoscopy in evaluating patients with BE.

Studies comparing NBI to WLE in detecting dysplasia have had equivocal results (**Table 3**). In a prospective tandem study, NBI was superior to SD WLE as NBI was able to detect more patients with dysplasia and higher grades of dysplasia.[6] However, NBI was unable to improve the diagnostic yield of HGD or early neoplasia when compared with HR-WLE alone.[8,31] In the most comprehensive study comparing NBI with HR-WLE, an international, randomized controlled crossover trial found that NBI with targeted biopsies had the same detection rate of intestinal metaplasia as HR-WLE with standard protocol biopsies, detecting a higher proportion of dysplasia (30% vs 21%, $P = .01$) using fewer biopsies per patient (3.6 vs 7.6, $P<.0001$).[32] A meta-analysis of 8 studies found favorable test characteristics of NBI in the diagnosis of HGD (sensitivity 96%, specificity 94%) and BE (sensitivity 95%, specificity 65%).[13] Evidence suggests that NBI may increase the diagnostic yield of targeted biopsies of early neoplasia in BE and may be useful as an adjunctive tool to HR-WLE.

Optical chromoendoscopy has also been shown to be comparable to dye-based chromoendoscopy in the assessment of Barrett's epithelium. In 2 head-to-head studies, acetic acid and I-Scan had similar results in diagnosing intestinal metaplasia (57% vs 66%, $P = .075$)[26] and indigo carmine and NBI were also found to be comparable in detecting HGD and early neoplasia (93% vs 86%, $P = 1$).[7] Given their similar clinical efficacy, optical chromoendoscopy offers several practical advantages over traditional dye-based chromoendoscopy, including ease of use, uniformity of the mucosal distribution, and likely shorter procedure times, all without any potential additional risk to the patient.

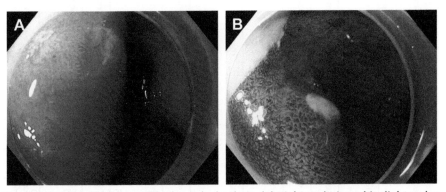

Fig. 3. Barrett's esophagus with high-grade dysplasia. (*A*) High-resolution white light endoscopy shows nodular mucosa with a cerebriform villous architecture. (*B*) Narrow band imaging enhances the abnormal mucosal pattern and microvasculature.

Table 3
Studies evaluating efficacy of narrow band imaging in Barrett's esophagus

Study	Study Design	Patients, n	Lesions, n	Histologic Reference Standard	Results
Sharma et al, 2013	Crossover trial	123	977	BE, dysplasia	BE: NBI equivalent to WLE Dysplasia: NBI detected more dysplasia than WLE (P = .01)
Wolfsen et al, 2008	RCT (tandem)	65	—	BE, dysplasia	NBI detected more dysplasia than WLE (57% vs 43% patients)
Singh et al, 2009	Cross-sectional	109	1021	BE, HGD	NBI grading correlated with histology in 903 of 1021 lesions (87.9%)
Curvers et al, 2008	Cross-sectional	84	165	HGD	NBI used to decrease the false-positive rate of autofluorescence in detecting HGD from 81% to 26%
Sharma et al, 2006	Cross-sectional	51	204	BE, HGD	BE: NBI detects with sensitivity 93.5%, specificity 86.7%, PPV 94.7% HGD: NBI detects with sensitivity 100%, specificity 98.7%, PPV 95.3%
Goda et al, 2007	Cross-sectional	58	217	BE, carcinoma	6 adenocarcinoma sites had irregular mucosal and capillary patterns on NBI
Anagnostopoulos et al, 2007	Cross-sectional	50	344	BE, HGD	BE: NBI detects with sensitivity 100%, specificity 78.8%, PPV 93.5%, NPV 100% HGD: NBI detects with sensitivity 90%, specificity 100%, PPV 99.2%, NPV 100%
Kara et al, 2006	Cross-sectional	63	161	BE, HGD	HGD: NBI detects with sensitivity 94%, specificity 76%, PPV 64%, NPV 98%
Kara et al, 2006	Cross-sectional	20	47	HGD	NBI used to decrease the false-positive rate of autofluorescence in detecting HGD from 40% to 10%

Abbreviations: NPV, negative predictive value; PPV, positive predictive value; RCT, randomized controlled trial.
Data from Refs.[6,14,27–32,69]

For these reasons, optical chromoendoscopy has developed an important role in the evaluation of BE and detection of early neoplasia. Although the magnitude of the additional benefit of optical chromoendoscopy over HR-WLE is still debated, it remains an easy and effective tool in targeting high-risk lesions arising in a background of BE.

AUTOFLUORESCENCE IMAGING

Similar to chromoendoscopy, autofluorescence imaging (AFI) is a wide-field technique that allows the assessment of a large area of tissue with the aim of identifying foci of neoplastic change by identifying alterations in endogenous esophageal fluorophores that develop when neoplastic change occurs. The primary fluorophores in the esophageal epithelium include mitochondrial reduced nicotinamide adenine dinucleotide (NADH) and flavin adenine dinucleotide (FAD), the levels of which increase when dysplasia develops. This technique uses the excitation of these fluorophores (NADH to UV wavelengths of 330–370 nm and FAD to green excitation wavelengths of 510–550 nm) and requires no exogenous contrast.[33] Regions that are "positive" are typically violet or purple, whereas "negative" regions on AFI are green (**Fig. 4**). AFI

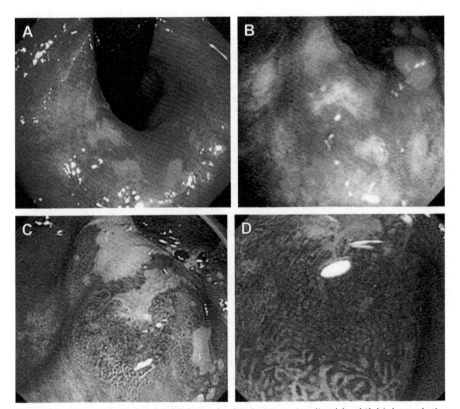

Fig. 4. Barrett's esophagus with high-grade dysplasia as visualized by (*A*) high-resolution white light endoscopy, (*B*) autofluorescence, (*C*) narrow band imaging, and (*D*) narrow band imaging with near focus. (*From* Shahid MW, Wallace MB. Endoscopic imaging for the detection of esophageal dysplasia and carcinoma. Gastrointest Endosc Clin N Am 2010;20:15; with permission.)

has been used in conjunction with NBI and HR-WLE, and this combination of imaging has been dubbed trimodal imaging.[34]

The data regarding the utility of AFI in BE have generally been disappointing. The overall accuracy of identifying dysplasia in a single-center study of 74 images from 63 patients was modest (69%–76%) and was better when AFI and HR-WLE images were combined (75%–85%).[35] The rates of interobserver agreement for AFI positive lesions were fair to moderate using AFI images alone. An assessment of 5 studies (including 2 randomized trials) totaling 371 patients using first-, second-, and third-generation AFI imaging found that the incremental benefit of AFI over standard WLE with random biopsies in detecting HGD or intramucosal cancer was only 2% (5 of 211).[36] Similarly, AFI identified 6 intramucosal cancers that were not identified by the standard surveillance protocol, for an impact on the choice of therapy of 2% (6 of 371).

In addition to its minimal effect on clinical management, AFI has been beset by rates of false positivity of up to 70%, and these rates have remained unacceptably high even after assessing AFI positive regions with HR-WLE and NBI.[34] In an attempt to improve the specificity of AFI, a study combined the use of AFI with biomarker analysis of tissue obtained from areas identified by AFI as positive.[37] This study identified aneuploidy, p53, and cyclin A immunohistochemistry as having the strongest association with dysplasia. When using this 3-biomarker panel, AFI had a sensitivity of 95.8% and a specificity of 88.6% for detecting HGD/esophageal cancer, which was comparable with the results achieved by a standard biopsy protocol. In addition, this combination of techniques was associated with a 4.5-fold reduction in the number of biopsies obtained. In summary, although AFI has many theoretic advantages, it has produced disappointing results to date because of the high rates of false positivity and the minimal incremental benefit in detecting dysplasia over standard endoscopic imaging combined with random biopsies. Future work combining this technique with biomarker analysis may define a role for AFI in the endoscopic evaluation of BE.

CONFOCAL LASER ENDOMICROSCOPY

Confocal laser endomicroscopy (CLE) is an emerging near-field technology that allows real-time in vivo histologic visualization of the gastrointestinal tract during endoscopy. There are 2 CLE systems used in BE. CLE imaging can be performed using a specially equipped endoscope that incorporates the confocal laser endomicroscope (eCLE, Pentax Medical, Montvale, NJ, USA) or via a probe that can be inserted through the working channel of a standard endoscope (pCLE, Mauna Kea Technologies, Paris, France). At the time of this publication, only the pCLE system is commercially available. Following application of a fluorescent agent, an argon blue laser light (488 nm wavelength) is used to illuminate and detect fluorescent light reflected from the mucosa. The laser is placed directly in contact with the mucosa to allow histologic examination along a single plane of cells. The reconstructed image of the mucosa is magnified more than 1000-fold, providing real-time optical microscopy. The 2 CLE systems have slightly different specifications, although both are capable of generating high-resolution endomicroscopy images. The eCLE provides a larger field of view (475 × 475 μm) with an image depth that can vary from the surface to 250 μm. However, the image resolution is limited by a slower acquisition speed of 0.8 to 1.6 images per second. The pCLE has a smaller 240-μm field of view with a tighter range of depth between 55 and 65 μm, but its rapid image acquisition speed of 12 frames per second allows generation of video-quality imaging. CLE requires the use of a fluorescing agent to enhance the underlying mucosa. Although several topical solutions have been tried,[38,39] intravenous fluorescein has emerged as the preferred fluorescent agent.

Patients should be informed that the fluorescein may temporarily cause their skin and urine to become yellow to orange for up to 24 hours following the procedure. Fortunately, the safety of intravenous fluorescein (typically 3–5 mL of a 10% solution) in CLE has been well demonstrated in a multicenter study including more than 2200 CLE procedures in which no major adverse effects were recorded.[40]

Although there were initial concerns regarding the endoscopist's ability to interpret real-time histology, CLE imaging of neoplasia has been shown to be easy to learn with a high degree of accuracy and reliability.[41] In addition, a consensus among CLE users established the Miami classification, a standardized system to diagnose and differentiate between BE, HGD, and adenocarcinoma.[42] An example of pCLE imaging of BE with HGD is shown in **Fig. 5**.

With the ability to obtain optical biopsies, CLE provides a means of identifying and diagnosing BE and dysplasia in real time during upper endoscopy. The potential value of CLE in the management of BE was first demonstrated in 2006 in a small study of 63 patients. In vivo imaging with CLE was able to predict BE and associated neoplasia with a sensitivity of 98.1% and 92.9% and a specificity of 94.1% and 98.4%, respectively.[43] Subsequent studies have repeatedly shown that a strategy of CLE with targeted mucosal biopsies of dysplastic lesions improves the diagnostic yield for dysplastic BE when compared with the standard 4-quadrant, random biopsy protocol (**Table 4**).[44–47] In an international multicenter study, 101 patients with known BE were examined with HR-WLE, NBI, and CLE before sampling biopsies. HR-WLE in combination with CLE significantly improved the detection of neoplasia in patients with BE compared with HR-WLE alone.[46] A subsequent multicenter trial of 192 patients undergoing surveillance of BE were randomized to either HR-WLE with standard random biopsies or HR-WLE with CLE with targeted biopsies. The implementation of CLE during surveillance increased the sensitivity for detecting neoplasia from 40% to 96% ($P<.001$) without significant reduction in specificity. CLE also improved procedural efficiency by tripling the diagnostic yield (22% vs 6%, $P = .002$) while requiring only a fifth of the number of biopsies. The impact of real-time, in vivo histology with CLE ultimately altered the treatment plan in 36% of patients.[47]

Despite the growing body of evidence in support of CLE, there remain several important limitations. CLE is capable of imaging only a small field of mucosa, leaving

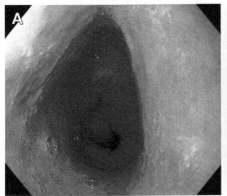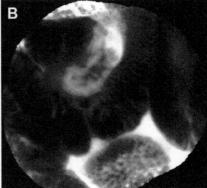

Fig. 5. Barrett's esophagus with high-grade dysplasia. (*A*) High-resolution white light endoscopy shows irregularity of the surface mucosa in the 3-o'clock position without obvious evidence of nodularity or ulceration. (*B*) Confocal laser endomicroscopy reveals a saw-toothed epithelial surface, no apparent goblet cells, and enlarged, irregular-appearing columnar cells consistent with dysplastic Barrett's esophagus.

Table 4
Studies evaluating efficacy of confocal laser endomicroscopy in Barrett's esophagus

Study	Type of CLE	Study Design	Patients, n	Lesions, n	Histologic Reference Standard	Results
Canto et al, 2014	eCLE	RCT	192	1371	BE, dysplasia	eCLE with targeted biopsies tripled the diagnostic yield for neoplasia compared with WLE with random biopsies (22% vs 6% $P = .002$)
Bertani et al, 2013	pCLE	Prospective cohort	100	635	BE, dysplasia	pCLE detected dysplasia at a higher rate than WLE ($P = .04$)
Wallace et al, 2011	pCLE	RCT	164	458	Residual BE after treatment	No difference between pCLE and high-resolution WLE in detecting residual Barrett's esophagus of neoplasia after treatment
Sharma et al, 2011	pCLE	RCT (tandem)	101	874	HGD, carcinoma	High-definition WLE with pCLE improved sensitivity and specificity for detecting HGD and adenocarcinoma as compared with high-definition WLE alone ($P = .002$)
Bajbouj et al, 2010	pCLE	Prospective cohort	68	670	HGD, carcinoma	pCLE had poor PPV (46%) and sensitivity (18%) for detecting Barrett's neoplasia
Pohl et al, 2007	pCLE	Prospective cohort	38	296	HGD, carcinoma	pCLE has high NPV (98.8%) for HGD and adenocarcinoma, but sensitivity remains low (75%)
Dunbar et al, 2008	eCLE	Crossover study	39	—	BE, HGD, carcinoma	eCLE had a higher mean diagnostic yield for HGD or carcinoma as compared with WLE with random biopsies (33.7% vs 17.2%, $P = .01$)
Kiesslich et al, 2006	eCLE	Prospective cohort	63	156	BE, dysplasia	eCLE predicted BE and associated neoplasia with high sensitivity (98.1%, 92.9%) and high specificity (94.1%, 98.4%), respectively

Abbreviations: NPV, negative predictive value; PPV, positive predictive value; RCT, randomized controlled trial.
Data from Refs.[42–47,67,70]

the possibility of sampling error. This limitation was illustrated in a randomized, double-blind, controlled crossover trial of 39 patients with BE in which HGD was missed in 2 patients randomized to CLE but later detected using standard WLE with random biopsies.[45] Even when suspicious neoplastic lesions are identified on CLE, performing a targeted biopsy of the mucosa at the exact site visualized by CLE can be technically challenging. Thus, the obtained biopsy specimen may not necessarily correlate with sites seen on CLE imaging. Lastly, the studies evaluating the efficacy of CLE have all been performed at academic centers in the hands of expert endoscopists involving high-risk patient populations. The effectiveness of CLE in the community setting is unclear, and the adoption of this new technology may prove to be impractical for the practicing gastroenterologist with limited resources to obtain the device, limited time to obtain proper training to perform the technique and interpret the images, and a patient population with a reduced incidence of dysplastic BE.[48]

Nevertheless, CLE remains a promising advanced imaging technology in the diagnosis and surveillance of dysplastic BE. Future advances that enable more rapid visualization of the entire Barrett's segment and more readily distinguish neoplastic lesions from normal mucosa may allow for better surveillance. The development of fluorescent-labeled probes specific to neoplastic Barrett's mucosa is already beginning to expand the molecular imaging capabilities of CLE.[49]

OPTICAL COHERENCE TOMOGRAPHY

Optical coherence tomography (OCT) uses endogenous variations in the time it takes light to be reflected from surface and subsurface structures to generate image contrast of the wall of the gastrointestinal tract in a manner analogous to ultrasound imaging. However, unlike ultrasound imaging, OCT uses light rather than sound. The obtained high-resolution images are comparable with those obtained from a low-power microscope but do not allow for cellular imaging. OCT offers a higher spatial resolution (1–15 μm) but lower depth of penetration than endosonography.[50] Application of OCT in the gastrointestinal tract dates back 15 years, with initial technologies using conventional time-domain OCT. More recently, frequency domain OCT has been developed to provide faster real-time imaging with a higher resolution.[50] A system based on frequency-domain OCT (volumetric laser endomicroscopy [VLE]; Ninepoint Medical, Cambridge, MA, USA) has been developed and is commercially available. It provides a resolution of 10 μm and an imaging depth down to 3 mm. The device scans a 6-cm length of esophagus over a period of 90 seconds. Newer iterations of this device are being developed that will incorporate laser marking to accurately sample abnormalities seen on imaging.[51]

Several early studies assessed the utility of OCT in detecting dysplasia.[52–54] One prospective study of 33 patients found a sensitivity of 68% and a specificity of 82% for dysplasia,[55] whereas another developed a scoring system for OCT that had a sensitivity of 83% and a specificity of 75% for HGD/intramucosal cancer.[56] More recently, OCT, particularly with the VLE device, has been used to assess for subsquamous intestinal metaplasia or buried glands in patients before and after ablation therapy **(Fig. 6)**.[56,57] OCT found such glands in 63% of such patients who had achieved complete endoscopic eradication of their BE.[58] VLE seems to have great potential in assessing the esophagus before planned endoscopic ablation for predictors of prolonged or failed ablation, such as Barrett's epithelium thickness and the number of subepithelial, or buried, glands present.[59] It may also have utility in the surveillance of patients postendoscopic ablation to assess for buried glands, and this information may potentially be used to stratify surveillance intervals. However, further studies are

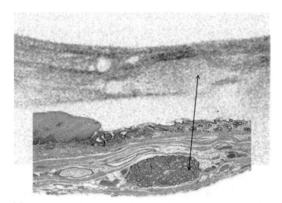

Fig. 6. VLE image of resected Barrett's esophagus with demonstration of subepithelial, or buried, high-grade dysplasia. The *arrow* shows the corresponding VLE image (above) with the ex vivo histologic findings (below).

needed to correlate OCT images to actual pathologic findings and to assess the ability to accurately sample the regions being visualized.

EMERGING TECHNOLOGIES

High-resolution microendoscopy (HRME) was first described in 2007 and uses a slender and flexible fiberoptic probe that has 30,000 optical fibers, is 3 m long, and has a diameter of 1 mm so it can pass through the accessory channel of a standard endoscope.[60] This probe is connected to a combined light source and camera, and the resultant images are processed by a laptop or tablet-based processor. It requires the use of a topical contrast agent, typically proflavine at a 0.01% concentration. Similar to CLE, images are obtained by placing the tip of the probe in contact with the mucosa, with each optical fiber acting as an individual pixel of the image. A 455-nm blue light–emitting diode illuminates and excites the previously administered fluorophore. The resulting emitted light is collected by the probe and transmitted through the computer to a digital camera, allowing real-time mucosal imaging. HRME provides a 1000× magnification, allowing for subcellular resolution (4.4 mm). The field of view is approximately 720 mm. The probe is small and portable and can be reused about 60 to 75 times, and current prototypes have been built for less than $3500.[61]

An initial study showed the feasibility of HRME to assess ex vivo endoscopic mucosal resection (EMR) specimens in patients with a prior diagnosis of BE with HGD or adenocarcinoma.[62] One study compared 20 gastroenterologists with no prior microendoscopic experience to 3 endoscopists who had performed greater than 50 HRME cases in assessing HRME images.[63] The overall sensitivity and specificity for HRME to identify either HGD or cancer was 90% and 82%, respectively. No significant differences in accuracy were noted between experts and novices, with a moderate interrater reliability (kappa 0.56 [0.54–0.58]). An ongoing in vivo study is prospectively comparing standard high-definition WLE with or without HRME in patients with BE, with subjects undergoing both targeted and random optical biopsies with HRME.[64] Initial results show improved sensitivity with WLE/HRME (100% vs 50%), with comparable specificities (94.9% vs 96.3%) for each group. The diagnostic yield was higher when HRME was used (37.5%–1.71%), and HRME could reduce the number of biopsies taken by 92.2%, with 70.8% of patients not requiring any biopsies at all.

Limitations of HRME include its use of a currently investigational contrast agent (proflavine), an inability to assess below the mucosa, and the need for direct mucosal contact to obtain imaging. Despite these limitations, preliminary data suggest potential for this low-cost, near-field technique to be used in the endoscopic surveillance of BE, particularly if paired with a red-flag technology that could select specific regions of interest within a large mucosal field.

Endocytoscopy (EC) produces detailed images of a thin superficial layer of tissue located within a thicker sample using the principles of light microscopy and requires a light source and image processors. EC uses a high-power lens with a fixed focus objective that provides ultrahigh-magnification (up to 1000×) images of surface morphology, allowing for cellular resolution. Similar to CLE, EC comes as a probe-based system or one that is incorporated into the endoscope (Olympus Medical Systems Co., Tokyo, Japan) and requires direct tissue contact. Neither EC device is currently available commercially. The probe is 3.2 mm in diameter, measures 380 cm in length, and is available at 2 levels of magnification.[65] The lower magnification device (XEC 300 Endocytoscope) has a 450× magnification, 30 μm depth of penetration, and a 300 μm × 300 μm field of view. In contrast, the higher-magnification device (XEC 120 Endocytoscope) enables 1125× magnification and 120 μm × 120 μm field of view. Given the 3.2 mm diameter of the probes, they must be used in therapeutic endoscopes, which provide a channel large enough to accommodate them. The integrated EC device is available in upper (103 cm long, XGIF-Q260EC1) and lower endoscopes (133 cm long, XCF-Q260EC1), each with a magnification of 580×, 30 μm depth of penetration, and a 400 μm × 400 μm field of view.

EC uses vital staining to enhance cellular imaging. The mucosa is aggressively washed, and a mucolytic agent (10% N-acetylcysteine) is usually administered. Methylene blue (1%) applied for 60 seconds has typically been used in the esophagus.[66] Typically, 2 to 3 layers of cells can be observed, with nuclei able to be seen at low power and nucleoli able to be visualized at high power. In nondysplastic BE, the cell density is low with uniform nuclei arranged radially to form regular glands and crypts. In cancer, the organization of the crypts and glands is destroyed with increased cell density and pleomorphic nuclei.[65] Although initial studies in BE yielded disappointing results,[67] more recent studies in ex vivo BE EMR specimens have suggested this technique may be associated with an acceptable diagnostic accuracy and excellent interobserver agreement.[68]

SUMMARY

During the past 2 decades, endoscopic imaging has been substantially enhanced through advances in endoscope optics, chromoendoscopy (both dye based and optical), and the introduction of novel technologies such as CLE that allow for cellular and subcellular imaging. Numerous additional technologies such as HRME and EC are in the early stages of assessment. However, although conceptually attractive, clinical studies have failed to show a clear benefit of these methods over a careful high-quality endoscopic examination coupled with random endoscopic biopsies obtained in a 4-quadrant manner every 1 to 2 cm. In the future, a combination of a sensitive broad-field or red-flag technology and a highly specific near-field technique (ideally with the capability of subsurface imaging) to confirm the presence of neoplastic change may be used. The theoretic benefits of such an approach could include improving the diagnostic yield for dysplasia/cancer, the ability to more appropriately select endoscopic eradication therapies in real time, reducing the number of surveillance biopsies taken, and increasing surveillance intervals. Such benefits could offset the costs associated with the utilization of these technologies. However, until that time, current efforts are best spent in ensuring that a careful endoscopic examination is performed, all identified mucosal abnormalities are resected, and the currently recommended surveillance biopsy protocol is adhered to.

REFERENCES

1. Hayeck TJ, Kong CY, Spechler SJ, et al. The prevalence of Barrett's esophagus in the US: estimates from a simulation model confirmed by SEER data. Dis Esophagus 2010;23:451–7.
2. Rustgi AK, El-Serag HB. Esophageal carcinoma. N Engl J Med 2014;371: 2499–509.
3. Vieth M, Ell C, Gossner L, et al. Histological analysis of endoscopic resection specimens from 326 patients with Barrett's esophagus and early neoplasia. Endoscopy 2004;36:776–81.
4. ASGE Technology Committee, Chand B, Conway JD, et al. High-resolution and high-magnification endoscopes. Gastrointest Endosc 2009;69(3 Pt 1):399–407.
5. Bennett C, Vakil N, Bergman J, et al. Consensus statements for management of Barrett's dysplasia and early-stage esophageal adenocarcinoma, based on a Delphi process. Gastroenterology 2012;143:336–46.
6. Wolfsen HC, Crook JE, Krishna M, et al. Prospective, controlled tandem endoscopy study of narrow band imaging for dysplasia detection in Barrett's esophagus. Gastroenterology 2008;135:24–31.
7. Kara MA, Peters FP, Rosmolen WD, et al. High-resolution endoscopy plus chromoendoscopy or narrow-band imaging in Barrett's esophagus: a prospective randomized crossover study. Endoscopy 2005;37:929–36.
8. Curvers W, Baak L, Kiesslich R, et al. Chromoendoscopy and narrow-band imaging compared with high-resolution magnification endoscopy in Barrett's esophagus. Gastroenterology 2008;134:670–9.
9. Stevens PD, Lightdale CJ, Green PH, et al. Combined magnification endoscopy with chromoendoscopy for the evaluation of Barrett's esophagus. Gastrointest Endosc 1994;40:747–9.
10. Sharma P, Topalovski M, Mayo MS, et al. Methylene blue chromoendoscopy for detection of short-segment Barrett's esophagus. Gastrointest Endosc 2001;54:289–93.
11. Sharma P, Weston AP, Topalovski M, et al. Magnification chromoendoscopy for the detection of intestinal metaplasia and dysplasia in Barrett's oesophagus. Gut 2003;52:24–7.
12. Ham NS, Jang JY, Ryu SW, et al. Magnifying endoscopy for the diagnosis of specialized intestinal metaplasia in short-segment Barrett's esophagus. World J Gastroenterol 2013;19:7089–96.
13. Mannath J, Subramanian V, Hawkey CJ, et al. Narrow band imaging for characterization of high grade dysplasia and specialized intestinal metaplasia in Barrett's esophagus: a meta-analysis. Endoscopy 2010;42:351–9.
14. Singh R, Karageorgiou H, Owen V, et al. Comparison of high-resolution magnification narrow-band imaging and white-light endoscopy in the prediction of histology in Barrett's oesophagus. Scand J Gastroenterol 2009;44:85–92.
15. Trivedi PJ, Braden B. Indications, stains and techniques in chromoendoscopy. QJM 2013;106:117–31.
16. Canto MI, Setrakian S, Willis JE, et al. Methylene blue-directed biopsies improve detection of intestinal metaplasia and dysplasia in Barrett's esophagus. Gastrointest Endosc 2000;51:560–8.

17. Gossner L, Pech O, May A, et al. Comparison of methylene blue-directed biopsies and four-quadrant biopsies in the detection of high-grade intraepithelial neoplasia and early cancer in Barrett's oesophagus. Dig Liver Dis 2006;38:724–9.

18. Wo JM, Ray MB, Mayfield-Stokes S, et al. Comparison of methylene blue-directed biopsies and conventional biopsies in the detection of intestinal metaplasia and dysplasia in Barrett's esophagus: a preliminary study. Gastrointest Endosc 2001;54:294–301.

19. Lim CH, Rotimi O, Dexter SP, et al. Randomized crossover study that used methylene blue or random 4-quadrant biopsy for the diagnosis of dysplasia in Barrett's esophagus. Gastrointest Endosc 2006;64:195–9.

20. Ngamruengphong S, Sharma VK, Das A. Diagnostic yield of methylene blue chromoendoscopy for detecting specialized intestinal metaplasia and dysplasia in Barrett's esophagus: a meta-analysis. Gastrointest Endosc 2009;69:1021–8.

21. Olliver JR, Wild CP, Sahay P, et al. Chromoendoscopy with methylene blue and associated DNA damage in Barrett's oesophagus. Lancet 2003;362:373–4.

22. Sharma P, Marcon N, Wani S, et al. Non-biopsy detection of intestinal metaplasia and dysplasia in Barrett's esophagus: a prospective multicenter study. Endoscopy 2006;38:1206–12.

23. Longcroft-Wheaton G, Duku M, Mead R, et al. Acetic acid spray is an effective tool for the endoscopic detection of neoplasia in patients with Barrett's esophagus. Clin Gastroenterol Hepatol 2010;8:843–7.

24. Tholoor S, Bhattacharyya R, Tsagkournis O, et al. Acetic acid chromoendoscopy in Barrett's esophagus surveillance is superior to the standardized random biopsy protocol: results from a large cohort study (with video). Gastrointest Endosc 2014;80:417–24.

25. Camus M, Coriat R, Leblanc S, et al. Helpfulness of the combination of acetic acid and FICE in the detection of Barrett's epithelium and Barrett's associated neoplasias. World J Gastroenterol 2012;18:1921–5.

26. Hoffman A, Korczynski O, Tresch A, et al. Acetic acid compared with I-scan imaging for detecting Barrett's esophagus: a randomized, comparative trial. Gastrointest Endosc 2014;79:46–54.

27. Kara MA, Ennahachi M, Fockens P, et al. Detection and classification of the mucosal and vascular patterns (mucosal morphology) in Barrett's esophagus by using narrow band imaging. Gastrointest Endosc 2006;64:155–66.

28. Kara MA, Peters FP, Fockens P, et al. Endoscopic video-autofluorescence imaging followed by narrow band imaging for detecting early neoplasia in Barrett's esophagus. Gastrointest Endosc 2006;64:176–85.

29. Sharma P, Bansal A, Mathur S, et al. The utility of a novel narrow band imaging endoscopy system in patients with Barrett's esophagus. Gastrointest Endosc 2006;64:167–75.

30. Anagnostopoulos GK, Pick B, Cunliffe R, et al. Barrett's esophagus specialist clinic: what difference can it make? Dis Esophagus 2006;19:84–7.

31. Curvers WL, Bohmer CJ, Mallant-Hent RC, et al. Mucosal morphology in Barrett's esophagus: interobserver agreement and role of narrow band imaging. Endoscopy 2008;40:799–805.

32. Sharma P, Hawes RH, Bansal A, et al. Standard endoscopy with random biopsies versus narrow band imaging targeted biopsies in Barrett's oesophagus: a prospective, international, randomised controlled trial. Gut 2013;62:15–21.

33. Thekkek N, Anandasabapathy S, Richards-Kortum R. Optical molecular imaging for detection of Barrett's-associated neoplasia. World J Gastroenterol 2011;17: 53–62.

34. Curvers WL, Alvarez Herrero L, Wallace MB, et al. Endoscopic tri-modal imaging is more effective than standard endoscopy in identifying early-stage neoplasia in Barrett's esophagus. Gastroenterology 2010;139:1106–14.

35. Mannath J, Subramanian V, Telakis E, et al. An inter-observer agreement study of autofluorescence endoscopy in Barrett's esophagus among expert and non-expert endoscopists. Dig Dis Sci 2013;58:465–70.

36. Boerwinkel DF, Holz JA, Kara MA, et al. Effects of autofluorescence imaging on detection and treatment of early neoplasia in patients with Barrett's esophagus. Clin Gastroenterol Hepatol 2014;12:774–81.

37. di Pietro M, Boerwinkel DF, Shariff MK, et al. The combination of autofluorescence endoscopy and molecular biomarkers is a novel diagnostic tool for dysplasia in Barrett's oesophagus. Gut 2015;64:49–56.

38. Goetz M, Toermer T, Vieth M, et al. Simultaneous confocal laser endomicroscopy and chromoendoscopy with topical cresyl violet. Gastrointest Endosc 2009;70: 959–68.

39. Hoffman A, Goetz M, Vieth M, et al. Confocal laser endomicroscopy: technical status and current indications. Endoscopy 2006;38:1275–83.

40. Wallace MB, Meining A, Canto M, et al. The safety of intravenous fluorescein for confocal laser endomicroscopy in the gastrointestinal tract. Aliment Pharmacol Ther 2010;31:548–52.

41. Wallace MB, Sharma P, Lightdale C, et al. Preliminary accuracy and interobserver agreement for the detection of intraepithelial neoplasia in Barrett's esophagus with probe-based confocal laser endomicroscopy. Gastrointest Endosc 2010; 72:19–24.

42. Wallace MB, Lauwers GY, Chen Y, et al. Miami classification for probe-based confocal laser endomicroscopy. Endoscopy 2011;43:882–91.

43. Kiesslich R, Gossner L, Goetz M, et al. In vivo histology of Barrett's esophagus and associated neoplasia by confocal laser endomicroscopy. Clin Gastroenterol Hepatol 2006;4:979–87.

44. Bajbouj M, Vieth M, Rosch T, et al. Probe-based confocal laser endomicroscopy compared with standard four-quadrant biopsy for evaluation of neoplasia in Barrett's esophagus. Endoscopy 2010;42(6):435–40.

45. Dunbar KB, Okolo P 3rd, Montgomery E, et al. Confocal laser endomicroscopy in Barrett's esophagus and endoscopically inapparent Barrett's neoplasia: a prospective, randomized, double-blind, controlled, crossover trial. Gastrointest Endosc 2009;70:645–54.

46. Sharma P, Meining AR, Coron E, et al. Real-time increased detection of neoplastic tissue in Barrett's esophagus with probe-based confocal laser endomicroscopy: final results of an international multicenter, prospective, randomized, controlled trial. Gastrointest Endosc 2011;74:465–72.

47. Canto MI, Anandasabapathy S, Brugge W, et al, Confocal Endomicroscopy for Barrett's Esophagus or Confocal Endomicroscopy for Barrett's Esophagus Trial Group. In vivo endomicroscopy improves detection of Barrett's esophagus-related neoplasia: a multicenter international randomized controlled trial (with video). Gastrointest Endosc 2014;79:211–21.

48. Berzosa M, Wallace MB. Surveillance of Barrett's esophagus: why biopsy if you can endomicroscopy. Gastrointest Endosc 2014;79:222–3.

49. Sturm MB, Piraka C, Elmunzer BJ, et al. In vivo molecular imaging of Barrett's esophagus with confocal laser endomicroscopy. Gastroenterology 2013;145:56–8.

50. ASGE Technology Committee. Enhanced imaging in the GI tract: spectroscopy and optical coherence tomography. Gastrointest Endosc 2013;78:568–73.

51. Suter MJ, Gora MJ, Lauwers GY, et al. Esophageal-guided biopsy with volumetric laser endomicroscopy and laser cautery marking: a pilot clinical study. Gastrointest Endosc 2014;79:886–96.

52. Evans JA, Poneros JM, Bouma BE, et al. Optical coherence tomography to identify intramucosal carcinoma and high-grade dysplasia in Barrett's esophagus. Clin Gastroenterol Hepatol 2006;4:38–43.

53. Chen Y, Aguirre AD, Hsiung PL, et al. Ultrahigh resolution optical coherence tomography of Barrett's esophagus: preliminary descriptive clinical study correlating images with histology. Endoscopy 2007;39:599–605.

54. Zuccaro G, Gladkova N, Vargo J, et al. Optical coherence tomography of the esophagus and proximal stomach in health and disease. Am J Gastroenterol 2001;96:2633–9.

55. Isenberg G, Sivak MV Jr, Chak A, et al. Accuracy of endoscopic optical coherence tomography in the detection of dysplasia in Barrett's esophagus: a prospective, double-blinded study. Gastrointest Endosc 2005;62:825–31.

56. Cobb MJ, Hwang JH, Upton MP, et al. Imaging of subsquamous Barrett's epithelium with ultrahigh-resolution optical coherence tomography: a histologic correlation study. Gastrointest Endosc 2010;71:223–30.

57. Adler DC, Zhou C, Tsai TH, et al. Three-dimensional optical coherence tomography of Barrett's esophagus and buried glands beneath neosquamous epithelium following radiofrequency ablation. Endoscopy 2009;41:773–6.

58. Zhou C, Tsai TH, Lee HC, et al. Characterization of buried glands before and after radiofrequency ablation by using 3-dimensional optical coherence tomography (with videos). Gastrointest Endosc 2012;76:32–40.

59. Tsai TH, Zhou C, Tao YK, et al. Structural markers observed with endoscopic 3-dimensional optical coherence tomography correlating with Barrett's esophagus radiofrequency ablation treatment response (with videos). Gastrointest Endosc 2012;76:1104–12.

60. Muldoon TJ, Pierce MC, Nida DL, et al. Subcellular-resolution molecular imaging within living tissue by fiber microendoscopy. Opt Express 2007;15:16413–23.

61. Louie JS, Richards-Kortum R, Anandasabapathy S. Applications and advancements in the use of high-resolution microendoscopy for detection of gastrointestinal neoplasia. Clin Gastroenterol Hepatol 2014;12:1789–92.

62. Muldoon TJ, Anandasabapathy S, Maru D, et al. High-resolution imaging in Barrett's esophagus: a novel, low-cost endoscopic microscope. Gastrointest Endosc 2008;68:737–44.

63. Vila PM, Kingsley MJ, Polydorides AD, et al. Accuracy and interrater reliability for the diagnosis of Barrett's neoplasia among users of a novel, portable high-resolution microendoscope. Dis Esophagus 2014;27:55–62.

64. Lee M, Parikh N, Polydorides AD, et al. Diagnostic yield and clinical impact of a low-cost microendoscope in the early diagnosis of Barrett's associated neoplasia: a prospective, single-center randomized controlled trial. Gastroenterology 2014;146:S522.

65. Singh R, Chen Yi Mei SL, Tam W, et al. Real-time histology with the endocytoscope. World J Gastroenterol 2010;16:5016–9.

66. Kodashima S, Fujishiro M, Takubo K, et al. Ex-vivo study of high-magnification chromoendoscopy in the gastrointestinal tract to determine the optimal staining conditions for endocytoscopy. Endoscopy 2006;38:1115–21.

67. Pohl H, Koch M, Khalifa A, et al. Evaluation of endocytoscopy in the surveillance of patients with Barrett's esophagus. Endoscopy 2007;39:492–6.

68. Tomizawa Y, Iyer PG, Wongkeesong LM, et al. Assessment of the diagnostic performance and interobserver variability of endocytoscopy in Barrett's esophagus: a pilot ex-vivo study. World J Gastroenterol 2013;19:8652–8.

69. Goda K, Tajiri H, Ikegami M, et al. Usefulness of magnifying endoscopy with narrow band imaging for the detection of specialized intestinal metaplasia in columnar-lined esophagus and Barrett's adenocarcinoma. Gastrointest Endosc 2007;65(1):36–46.

70. Bertani H, Frazzoni M, Dabizzi E, et al. Improved detection of incident dysplasia by probe-based confocal laser endomicroscopy in a Barrett's esophagus surveillance program. Dig Dis Sci 2013;58(1):188–93.

Surgical Management of Barrett's Esophagus

Christian G. Peyre, MD, Thomas J. Watson, MD*

KEYWORDS

- Barrett's esophagus • Antireflux surgery • Esophagectomy • Nissen fundoplication
- Intramucosal adenocarcinoma

KEY POINTS

- Antireflux surgery is a safe and effective treatment option to control gastroesophageal reflux disease in patients with Barrett's esophagus.
- Antireflux surgery prevents reflux of acid and nonacid gastric content, and can induce regression in some cases of Barrett's metaplasia or dysplasia.
- Antireflux has not been proved to be superior to medical therapy in preventing the progression of Barrett's esophagus to esophageal adenocarcinoma.
- Esophagectomy has been supplanted by endoscopic therapies as the ideal treatment option for most patients with high-grade dysplasia or focal intramucosal adenocarcinoma.
- Esophagectomy may be the preferred treatment option in a minority of select cases with multifocal dysplasia, high-risk tumor characteristics, an esophagus otherwise not worth salvaging, or because of patient preference.

INTRODUCTION

Gastroesophageal reflux disease (GERD) is the major risk factor for the development of Barrett's esophagus (BE) and esophageal adenocarcinoma (EAC).[1,2] The treatment of BE is focused primarily on controlling reflux, most commonly with antisecretory medication to abolish gastric acid production.[3] In patients with dysplastic BE or early esophageal neoplasia, endoscopic therapies, including various forms of ablation and resection, have become the primary treatment options to eradicate the pathologic mucosa.[4] Adjunctive medical or surgical antireflux therapies are necessary to control ongoing reflux, in an effort to reduce the recurrence of esophageal metaplasia, dysplasia, or neoplasia.

Although medical therapy is the most commonly used treatment modality for BE, antireflux surgery is a safe and effective alternative and should be considered in all

Disclosure: The authors have no disclosures.
Division of Thoracic and Foregut Surgery, Department of Surgery, University of Rochester School of Medicine and Dentistry, University of Rochester Medical Center, 601 Elmwood Avenue, Box Surgery, Rochester, NY 14642, USA
* Corresponding author.
E-mail address: Thomas_watson@urmc.rochester.edu

Gastroenterol Clin N Am 44 (2015) 459–471
http://dx.doi.org/10.1016/j.gtc.2015.02.013
0889-8553/15/$ – see front matter © 2015 Elsevier Inc. All rights reserved.

Box 1
Relative indications for esophagectomy in patients with high-grade dysplasia or intramucosal adenocarcinoma

- Tumor characteristics with a significant risk of lymph node metastasis
  - Poorly differentiated tumors
  - Positive deep margin after endoscopic resection
  - Lymphovascular invasion
  - Invasion beyond the muscularis mucosa
- Dysplastic or neoplastic Barrett's esophagus, which is difficult to eradicate
  - Ultra-long segment Barrett's esophagus
  - Diffusely nodular esophagus with multifocal high-grade dysplasia or intramucosal adenocarcinoma
  - Long or large intramucosal adenocarcinomas
- Failed eradication of disease following endoscopic therapy
- Patient unwilling or unable to comply with the required repeat endoscopies and long-term surveillance
- Esophagus not worth salvage
  - Recalcitrant stricture
  - End-stage motility disorder

---

patients to control underlying GERD. In select cases, such as individuals with end-stage esophageal motility disorders, recalcitrant strictures, or long-segment BE (LSBE) with multifocal high-grade dysplasia (HGD) or intra-mucosal adenocarcinoma (IMC), esophagectomy should be considered in the treatment paradigm (**Box 1**).

This article reviews the role of antireflux surgery in the management of nondysplastic and dysplastic BE, and highlights the evolution of esophagectomy in the treatment of patients with HGD or early esophageal neoplasia.

GOALS OF THERAPY FOR BARRETT'S ESOPHAGUS

Although most patients treated for GERD without BE can be managed successfully with medical therapy alone, those patients identified with BE are at increased risk for the development of EAC and may require a more intense treatment regimen.[5] Such patients should (1) undergo a detailed endoscopic examination, with multiple biopsies per established protocols, to rule out dysplasia or early neoplasia; (2) be treated aggressively for reflux to prevent further mucosal injury; and (3) be enrolled in an ongoing endoscopic surveillance program for early detection of progression of disease. The ideal treatment of BE should control troublesome reflux symptoms, result in healing of mucosal injury, induce regression of Barrett's epithelium to normal squamous mucosa, and prevent progression of BE to EAC, all with few side effects.

LIMITATIONS OF MEDICAL THERAPY IN PATIENTS WITH BARRETT'S ESOPHAGUS

Long-term, continuous control of reflux is critical in patients with BE to allow healing of the esophageal mucosa and to prevent progression of disease. Patients with GERD and BE compared with those without BE, however, have increased amounts of acid and bile reflux, and a higher prevalence of incompetent lower esophageal sphincters, hiatal hernias, and impaired esophageal motility.[6,7] Consequently, control of GERD in patients with BE is much more challenging than in patients with GERD without BE.[8,9]

Although the primary treatment end point in patients with GERD is symptom control, it has been shown in patients with BE that control of reflux symptoms does not equate to control of gastric pH or esophageal acid exposure.[10,11] Greater than 50% of patients with BE have pathologic levels of esophageal acid exposure despite relief of symptoms.[12] To maintain tight control of acid production, strict adherence to daily, and often twice daily, proton pump inhibitor (PPI) is necessary, making patient compliance a challenge. Additionally, antisecretory medications are directed at abolishment of acid production alone; they are ineffective at controlling the reflux of biliopancreatic substrates and nonacid gastric contents (eg, pepsin) that can contribute to ongoing mucosal injury.[13,14]

BENEFITS OF ANTIREFLUX SURGERY

Antireflux surgery is a safe and effective alternative to medical therapy for patients with BE. Surgery corrects an incompetent lower esophageal sphincter and concomitant hiatal hernia, preventing the reflux of acid, bile, and other nonacid substrates. Complete reflux control can lead to healing and regression of Barrett's mucosa, and may reduce the risk of progression to cancer. Surgery also eliminates the concern for patient compliance with medical therapy, and may reduce the cost of treatment compared with life-long antisecretory therapy.[15]

Approach to Antireflux Surgery for Barrett's Esophagus

Beginning with Rudolph Nissen's transabdominal open "gastroplication," first described in 1956 and modified for laparoscopy by Dallemagne in 1991, modern antireflux surgery has undergone a tremendous evolution over the past half century.[16] Surgery can be accomplished via open transabdominal or transthoracic approaches, but laparoscopic fundoplication has become the gold standard for surgical management of GERD because of decreased morbidity, quicker recovery, improved cosmesis, and superior patient satisfaction over open surgery. Most patients with GERD are candidates for laparoscopic antireflux surgery, although in a select group open surgery may be required because of extensive abdominal adhesions from previous surgery or other patient factors.

The technique of constructing the fundoplication has also evolved over time. The original fundic wrap described by Nissen was approximately 6 cm long and was associated with significant postoperative dysphagia.[17] The modern Nissen technique consists of a short (1.5–2 cm) floppy wrap over a large (56–60F catheter) bougie, affording excellent reflux control but with a lower risk of postoperative dysphagia.[18,19] If esophageal motility is significantly impaired, a partial fundoplication may be better suited than a 360-degree Nissen wrap to prevent dysphagia. The efficacy of a partial fundoplication in patients with BE is questionable, however, with some studies suggesting decreased long-term control of reflux compared with a complete Nissen fundoplication.[20,21] Other less used surgical techniques have been described as well, including near-total or subtotal gastrectomy with Roux-en-y reconstruction, or duodenal switch with biliopancreatic diversion. Perioperative risks and long-term gastrointestinal side effects may be increased with these more complex operations, and the data are less robust to support such interventions.[22] As a result, this discussion focuses on the results of fundoplication.

Outcomes of Antireflux Surgery in Patients with Barrett's Esophagus

Success following antireflux surgery can be assessed in several different domains.[23] Primary end points include symptom relief, normalization of esophageal acid exposure, prevention of dysplasia or neoplasia, and regression of metaplasia or dysplasia. Most data are derived from cohort analyses from high-volume esophageal surgery centers, although there are limited publications comparing medical and surgical therapies.

Safety of antireflux surgery for Barrett's esophagus

Laparoscopic antireflux surgery is safe with low morbidity and mortality. A recent review of the American College of Surgeons National Surgical Quality Improvement Program database, examining more than 7500 laparoscopic antireflux surgeries performed across the United States, revealed the 30-day operative mortality to be only 0.3%, and morbidity 3.8%.[24] As expected, mortality increased with age, but was only 0.8% for patients older than 70 years.

Control of gastroesophageal reflux disease symptoms

The primary focus of the treatment of GERD is the control of troublesome symptoms, most commonly "typical" heartburn and regurgitation. Studies assessing short-term outcomes of laparoscopic Nissen fundoplication (LNF) have revealed excellent control of such typical GERD symptoms. In one study looking at 100 consecutive patients treated with LNF, including 37 patients with BE, 87% of patients considered themselves "cured" and another 11% had significantly improved symptoms at a median follow-up of 2 years.[19]

When focusing on patients with BE treated with antireflux surgery, similar results for the control of symptoms have been seen. In a cohort of 85 patients followed for a median of 5 years, 77% of patients considered themselves "cured," and an additional 22% had significant improvement of symptoms, following antireflux surgery.[25] Similarly, a series of 59 patients followed for a median of 59 months revealed that 90% of patients undergoing antireflux surgery had no or only minor postoperative symptoms.[26] "Minor" symptoms were defined as not interfering with quality of life or requiring medication. A third study of 215 patients followed for a median of 8 years after antireflux surgery demonstrated that 86% of patients had control of heartburn and regurgitation.[27] As these studies demonstrate, laparoscopic antireflux surgery results in excellent control of GERD symptoms in most patients with BE.

Control of esophageal acid exposure: postoperative pH monitoring

Antireflux surgery has been shown to control the reflux of gastric acid into the esophagus, and to normalize esophageal acid exposure, in most patients treated for GERD.[28] Because patients with BE represent a challenging patient population with severe reflux disease, control of esophageal acid exposure may not be as effective as in patients with GERD without BE. In a study of 53 patients with BE examined with preoperative and postoperative esophageal pH monitoring (at a median follow-up of 40 months after surgery), a significant reduction in distal esophageal acid exposure as measured by percent time pH less than 4 was seen (27.9% vs 4.0%; $P<.001$).[23] However, abnormal distal esophageal acid exposure postoperatively was found in 14 of 53 (26%) patients. Similarly, an analysis by Hofstetter and colleagues[25] of 21 patients studied with esophageal pH monitoring before and after antireflux surgery revealed that 4 of 21 (19%) patients had abnormal postoperative distal esophageal acid exposure. All four patients with a positive postoperative pH test had recurrent clinical symptoms of GERD. Although most patients undergoing antireflux surgery for BE can expect excellent reflux control, the lack of universal control of pathologic esophageal acid exposure reinforces the need for ongoing monitoring of patients with BE after antireflux surgery.

Control of histologic mucosal changes

The fate of the metaplastic or dysplastic Barrett's epithelium may be the most important end point in assessing the results of antireflux surgery in patients with BE. Because esophageal pH monitoring has shown that approximately 20% to 25% of patients may suffer from recurrent reflux, the potential for progression of metaplasia exists. In a study of 77 consecutive patients with BE treated with antireflux surgery (61 undergoing Nissen fundoplication), histologic regression occurred in 28 (36%) patients and 8 (10%) had progression at a median follow-up of 50 months.[29] The cohort included 17 of 25 patients with low-grade dysplasia (LGD) who regressed to BE without dysplasia, and 11 patients with nondysplastic BE who had no further intestinal metaplasia on follow-up. Of the eight patients who progressed, three went from nondysplastic BE to LGD and five from LGD to HGD. No esophageal cancers developed. The authors noted that patients with short-segment BE (SSBE) were more likely than those with LSBE to undergo histologic regression (58% vs 28%; $P<.0016$), with a median time to regression of 18.5 months. Progression occurred only in patients with LSBE.

Similarly, a study of 58 consecutive patients treated with antireflux surgery and followed for a median of 59 months showed complete regression of BE in eight (14%), regression of LGD to BE without dysplasia in six of eight (75%), and only four (7%) with progression of disease (two from BE without dysplasia to LGD, and two to EAC discovered at 4 and 7 years after surgery).[26] All four patients with progression had abnormal postoperative esophageal pH monitoring.

Another study assessed 109 consecutive patients treated with antireflux surgery for BE, 90 of whom returned for continued endoscopic surveillance.[23] At a median follow-up of 30 months, 30 (33%) patients had complete regression of BE, and only three (3.3%) had progression. Regression occurred only in patients with SSBE (30 of 54; 55%) and in no patients with LSBE. Progression included one patient with preoperative indefinite dysplasia who developed LGD, and two patients with BE with LGD who developed HGD (at 4 years) and EAC (at 10 months).

Antireflux surgery versus medical therapy

To determine whether antireflux surgery is superior to medical therapy in the management of BE, several comparative studies, including small, randomized controlled trials and meta-analyses, have been undertaken.

In a cohort study by Oberg and colleagues,[30] 140 patients with BE without dysplasia were followed for a median of 5.8 years (945 patient-years) with surveillance endoscopies every 1 to 2 years. Only those patients whose two initial surveillance endoscopies were without dysplasia were included to assess for progression of disease. Forty-six patients were treated with antireflux surgery (43 Nissen fundoplications), eight with H_2 blockers (early patients in the cohort), and 85 with PPIs (60% single-daily dose, 40% twice-daily dose). The treatment strategy was at the discretion of the physician. Progression developed in 46 patients (33%) during the course of follow-up, including 39 patients to LGD, four to HGD, and three to EAC. No patients in the surgical arm developed HGD or EAC, and patients treated with antireflux surgery were 2.3 times less likely to develop LGD compared with the patients treated with medical therapy.

A study by Attwood and colleagues[31] included a subgroup analysis of patients enrolled in the LOTUS trial, a European, multicenter, randomized, controlled trial that compared laparoscopic antireflux surgery with dose-escalating esomeprazole therapy. Of the 554 patients enrolled in the main study, 60 had BE without dysplasia, including 32 treated with LNF. All patients underwent pH monitoring at baseline and at 6 months after initiation of therapy. Those patients with BE treated with surgery had a significant reduction in esophageal acid exposure compared with patients treated with medical therapy (median percentage exposure time, 13.2% → 0.4% vs 7.4% → 4.9%; P = .002). Despite the differences in pH testing, symptomatic outcomes assessed at 3 years of follow-up were similar, and treatment failures were uncommon in either treatment arm (three medical, one surgical). Histologic follow-up was not reported.

In a study by Parrilla and colleagues,[32] 101 patients with BE were randomized to open Nissen fundoplication (N = 58) versus twice-daily PPI therapy (N = 43) and followed annually. The mean follow-up was 5 years. The success of each treatment was similar, with 91% of patients in each arm of the study having a "good" or "excellent" symptomatic outcome. Objective physiologic testing, including esophageal pH and bile (Bilitec) monitoring, was performed. Surgical therapy was significantly more effective than medical therapy at controlling esophageal acid and bile exposure. There was no significant difference in the histologic changes seen in patients in each arm. No patients in either arm had resolution of BE. In the medical arm, two patients had regression of LGD to no dysplasia but eight patients (20%) developed dysplasia, including one with HGD and one with EAC. In the surgical arm, five patients had regression of LGD, but three patients (6%) had progression during follow-up, including one to HGD and one to EAC.

Two meta-analyses have assessed the impact of medical and surgical therapy in patients with BE on the development of EAC. Chang and colleagues[33] reviewed 25 articles that had at least 1 year endoscopic follow-up after initiation of therapy. The analysis pooled the results of 996 patients treated with antireflux surgery and 700 patients treated with medical therapy, and followed for 3711 and 2939 patients-years, respectively. The surgical analysis included patients undergoing either partial or complete (Nissen) fundoplication. The incidence of EAC was significantly lower in surgically treated patients (2.8 vs 6.3 cases per 1000 patient years; P = .034). The authors noted, however, that this difference was predominantly driven by uncontrolled case-series, suggesting a publication bias. When only controlled studies were considered, the difference between surgical and medical therapy was no longer significant (4.8 vs 6.5 cases per 1000 patient-years; P = .32). The authors also examined the risk of regression and progression of BE. The probability of regression was significantly higher in surgically treated patients (15.4% vs 1.9%; P = .004). When the analysis was limited to controlled studies, the probability of regression remained significantly higher in surgical patients (6.4% vs 0.5%; P = .024). The probability of progression of disease was similar between both groups (2.9% vs 6.8%; P = .054). The authors concluded that, whereas the data suggest antireflux surgery promotes regression of BE better than medical therapy, antireflux surgery is not better at preventing the development of EAC.

A meta-analysis by Corey and colleagues[34] yielded similar results with respect to EAC risk. The authors analyzed 34 publications with a cumulative 4678 patient-years of follow-up in surgical patients, and 4906 patient-years of follow-up in medically treated patients. The incidence of EAC was similar in both groups (3.8 vs 5.3 cancers per 1000 patient-years; P = .29, respectively). The difference between the two therapies was even smaller (3.8 vs 4.3 cancers per 1000 patient-years; P = .33) when the analysis limited the medically therapy arm to studies published in the preceding 5 years to eliminate patients for whom PPI therapy was not the primary medical treatment. The authors concluded that the incidence of EAC in patients with BE was low, and that antireflux surgery did not prevent cancer development better than medical therapy. Both meta-analyses concluded that antireflux surgery should not be recommended as an "antineoplastic" therapy.

EVOLUTION IN THERAPY FOR BARRETT'S ESOPHAGUS WITH EARLY NEOPLASIA

The link between GERD, BE, and EAC has been well established.[1,2] Esophageal cancer is a highly lethal disease of which relatively few are cured. Data from the American Cancer Society predict an overall 5-year survival of only 17% for patients diagnosed with esophageal carcinoma in 2014.[35] Similar to other gastrointestinal malignancies, cancer of the esophagus is usually asymptomatic in its early stages. As a consequence, most symptomatic patients present with advanced, often incurable disease. Fortunately, growing enthusiasm for endoscopic surveillance of patients with BE has led to increased detection of patients with early esophageal neoplasia who can be treated with the expectation of cure. This fact should not be lost in the pessimism surrounding the treatment of more advanced EAC. Given the anticipated long-term survival for patients with early esophageal malignancy, quality of life considerations become important in deciding on a management strategy that avoids morbidity while still ensuring eradication of disease.

The introduction of new endoscopic technologies that have improved the ability to treat mucosal disease has resulted in a revolution in the standard of care for the treatment of early neoplasia in the setting of BE. Although only a few years ago the recommended therapy for cases of BE with HGD or IMC was esophagectomy, assuming a medically suitable patient and the availability of an expert surgical team, the treatment paradigm has shifted such that most cases now are treated endoscopically. Guidelines recently proposed by the American Gastroenterological Association recommend endoscopic mucosal resection (EMR) and ablation as the procedures of choice for BE with HGD in most patients.[3] Because of the widespread adoption of these effective and low-risk endoscopic therapies, many individuals who previously would have been referred for surgery are now spared from esophageal resection.

ESOPHAGECTOMY FOR EARLY ESOPHAGEAL NEOPLASIA

For decades, esophagectomy was the standard of care for BE with HGD or IMC. As a result, the indications, surgical techniques, perioperative outcomes, cure rates, and long-term quality of life relative to esophageal resection and reconstruction have been extensively studied and elucidated. With the recent, rapid changes in treatment toward endoscopic therapy for early esophageal neoplasia, the physician must be mindful of this surgical experience so as to have a basis against which endoscopic alternatives should be compared. In the course of therapy for early neoplasia, the treating physician runs the risk of being overaggressive, recommending esophagectomy when less invasive endoscopic therapies would have been appropriate. Alternatively, the physician may be underaggressive, continuing on a course of endoscopic treatment when it should have been abandoned, leading to the development of incurable, locoregionally advanced, or systemic disease from what started as a readily curable disease process.

The rationale for esophageal resection in cases of BE with HGD has been based on two factors: occult invasive carcinoma has been found in a significant proportion of esophagectomy specimens in patients undergoing resection for HGD, averaging approximately 37% in multiple large surgical series[36]; and invasive cancer may arise within dysplastic BE over the short to medium term if the esophagus is left in situ.

Esophagectomy, therefore, is curative and prophylactic relative to the treatment of invasive disease. Of course, the ability to eliminate pathologic mucosa by surgical extirpation must be weighed against the invasiveness of the procedure and its implications with regards to perioperative morbidity, mortality, recovery time, and long-term impact on quality of life. Thus, esophagectomy in this circumstance may rightly be considered "radical prophylaxis" for a microscopic disease process.[37]

Esophagectomy has traditionally been considered to be a morbid operation. Large population-based studies have shown a significant mortality rate when esophagectomy is performed for cancer. In a report from 2003 describing the experience in US Veterans Administration hospitals from 1991 to 2000, 30-day postoperative mortality in 1777 esophagectomies performed in 109 facilities was 9.8%.[38] Most operations were performed in low-volume institutions, because only 1.6 esophagectomies were done per year in the average facility. Similarly, a publication from 2007 used the Nationwide Inpatient Sample to assess esophagectomy outcomes in 17,395 patients over the years 1999 to 2003.[39] Overall mortality after esophagectomy was 8.7%, with high-volume centers obtaining significantly lower rates compared with low-volume institutions. In specialty centers, contemporary data derived from the United States and Europe show far better rates of perioperative mortality following esophagectomy for cancer, in the range of 2% to 5%.[40–43] Unfortunately, these data are commonly quoted by gastroenterologists and surgeons when discussing esophagectomy as an alternative for BE with HGD or IMC.

Of greater relevance, however, are data specific to outcomes when esophagectomy is performed for early neoplasia. A literature review published in 2007 detailed the reported experience with esophagectomy for HGD over the 20-year period from 1987 to 2007.[36] In 22 studies covering 530 patients, the overall perioperative mortality was 0.94%, representing only five total deaths in the literature, and roughly one-tenth the mortality rate quoted previously for all cases of esophagectomy for cancer.

The morbidity and mortality associated with esophagectomy fortunately have improved over recent decades, a trend that is likely to continue. When operating for early disease with a low potential for lymph node metastasis and high expectation for cure, the surgeon should consider operative approaches, such as transhiatal esophagectomy,[40] minimally invasive esophagectomy,[44] or vagal-sparing esophagectomy,[45] which avoid some of the morbidity and negative impact on long-term alimentary function associated with more aggressive procedures.

Based on these data verifying the safety and efficacy of endoscopic resection and ablation for early esophageal neoplasia, including BE with HGD and IMC, an endoscopic treatment paradigm seems appropriate for most cases. Esophagectomy will continue to have a role in select circumstances, such as the following:

1. When tumor characteristics (eg, large or poorly differentiated tumors, presence of lymphovascular invasion, positive deep margin on EMR specimen, or invasion beyond the muscularis mucosa) impart a significant risk of lymph node metastases[46]
2. When the patient prefers surgery, or is unwilling or unable to comply with the rigorous, often prolonged requirements of serial endoscopic treatments and subsequent surveillance
3. In cases that are difficult to eradicate with ablation, such as ultra-long segments of BE, a diffusely nodular esophagus with multifocal HGD or IMC, or long intramucosal tumors
4. When attempts at ablation have failed
5. When the esophagus is otherwise not worth salvaging (eg, recalcitrant stricture or end-stage motility disorder)

STUDIES COMPARING ESOPHAGECTOMY AND ENDOSCOPIC THERAPIES FOR EARLY ESOPHAGEAL NEOPLASIA

Three retrospectively reviewed case series have compared surgical and endoscopic treatment of BE with HGD or esophageal IMC. The first report, from the Mayo Clinic group published in 2009, compared outcomes in 178 patients with IMC treated between 1998 and 2007.[47] Endoscopic therapy was undertaken in 132 patients (74%) and 46 patients (26%) underwent an initial esophagectomy. Endoscopic therapy consisted of EMR alone in 75 (57%) and a combination of EMR with photodynamic therapy in 57 (43%). At a mean follow-up of 43 months in the endoscopic cohort, 24 patients (18.2%) experienced persistent or recurrent cancer, nine requiring esophagectomy, one undergoing chemoradiation, and 14 being treated with repeat EMR. The overall mortality during the follow-up interval was 17%. For the cohort undergoing an initial esophagectomy, the mean follow-up was 64 months and the overall mortality was 20%. The survival was thought to be comparable between the two groups.

The second report, from 2011, described the experience at the University of Southern California.[48] Their cohort consisted of 101 patients with either HGD or IMC, 40 treated via endoscopy and 61 undergoing esophagectomy. The endoscopic treatment group underwent a total of 109 EMRs and 70 ablation sessions. The median number of endoscopic interventions per patient was three. The metachronous neoplasia rate was 20%, with three patients (7.5%) subsequently requiring esophagectomy for endoscopic treatment failure. Comparing endoscopic and surgical therapy, the former was associated with lower morbidity (0% vs 39%), although similar overall (94% in both groups) and disease-free survival at 3 years.

A third report assessed outcomes at two high-volume specialty centers in Germany between 1996 and 2009.[49] Seventy-six patients who underwent EMR and argon plasma coagulation in Wiesbaden were compared with 38 patients who underwent transthoracic esophagectomy with two-field lymphadenectomy for IMC at the University of Cologne. The groups were matched for age, gender, depth of invasion, and differentiation. Similar to the prior studies, endoscopic treatment was associated with equivalent cure rates compared with esophagectomy, but with lower morbidity and no mortality.

The esophageal surgeon must be well-versed in the indications for endoscopic resective and ablative therapies so that they are appropriately applied. Before any treatment decisions are made, the patient should be evaluated and counseled by an experienced endoscopist and an esophageal surgeon on the available management options, including the pros and cons of each. The best treatment decision for a given patient depends on patient factors, such as their desires, their comorbidities, the specifics of their disease, the salvageability of their esophagus, physician expertise, and local or regional institutional resources.

SUMMARY

The management of BE and underlying GERD is a challenge for the treating physician or surgeon. The patient and their physician must enter into a long-term relationship to chronically manage these related diseases, with treatment aimed at controlling troublesome GERD symptoms while monitoring for potential progression of BE toward malignancy. The clinician must be well versed in medical, endoscopic, and surgical alternatives to therapy. Fortunately, few patients with BE ever progress to EAC.

Antireflux surgery is a safe and effective treatment option for patients with BE. Most patients can expect long-lasting relief of symptoms, control of esophageal acid and bile exposure, and stabilization or regression of the metaplastic esophageal epithelium. Although there are reasonable data to suggest that antireflux surgery induces regression of BE better than medical therapy, especially in patients with SSBE, surgery has not been shown to be better than medical therapy at reducing the incidence of progression to EAC. As with medical therapy, a small proportion of patients may experience recurrent GERD after antireflux surgery, leaving them at risk not only for recurrent symptoms but, more importantly for progression to dysplasia or neoplasia. As a result, continued surveillance with serial endoscopies is mandatory, and a full evaluation to assess possible breakdown of the fundoplication should be performed in patients with recurrent symptoms.

In patients with dysplastic BE or IMC, endoscopic therapies including ablation and mucosal resection have become the standard of care and have supplanted esophagectomy as the preferred treatment options in most cases. These endoscopic therapies are associated with rates of lower morbidity and mortality, and improved long-term quality of life, compared with esophageal resection without compromising survival. Select patients, however, still may be best treated with esophagectomy. In the hands of experienced esophageal surgeons, esophagectomy for HGD or IMC can be done with low mortality, acceptable morbidity, and good long-term alimentary function and quality of life.

REFERENCES

1. Lagergren J, Bergstrom R, Lindgren A, et al. Symptomatic gastroesophageal reflux as a risk factor for esophageal adenocarcinoma. N Engl J Med 1999;340(11): 825–31.
2. Spechler SJ. Barrett esophagus and risk of esophageal cancer: a clinical review. JAMA 2013;310(6):627–36.
3. American Gastroenterological Association, Spechler SJ, Sharma P, et al. American Gastroenterological Association medical position statement on the management of Barrett's esophagus. Gastroenterology 2011;140(3):1084–91.
4. Spechler SJ, Sharma P, Souza RF, et al, American Gastroenterological Association. American Gastroenterological Association technical review on the management of Barrett's esophagus. Gastroenterology 2011;140(3):e18–52 [quiz: e13].
5. Spechler SJ, Souza RF. Barrett's esophagus. N Engl J Med 2014;371(9): 836–45.
6. Cameron AJ. Barrett's esophagus: prevalence and size of hiatal hernia. Am J Gastroenterol 1999;94(8):2054–9.
7. Avidan B, Sonnenberg A, Schnell TG, et al. Hiatal hernia size, Barrett's length, and severity of acid reflux are all risk factors for esophageal adenocarcinoma. Am J Gastroenterol 2002;97(8):1930–6.
8. Kahrilas PJ. Review article: is stringent control of gastric pH useful and practical in GERD? Aliment Pharmacol Ther 2004;20(Suppl 5):89–94 [discussion: 95–6].
9. Gerson LB, Boparai V, Ullah N, et al. Oesophageal and gastric pH profiles in patients with gastro-oesophageal reflux disease and Barrett's oesophagus treated with proton pump inhibitors. Aliment Pharmacol Ther 2004;20(6):637–43.
10. Katzka DA, Castell DO. Successful elimination of reflux symptoms does not insure adequate control of acid reflux in patients with Barrett's esophagus. Am J Gastroenterol 1994;89(7):989–91.
11. Yeh RW, Gerson LB, Triadafilopoulos G. Efficacy of esomeprazole in controlling reflux symptoms, intraesophageal, and intragastric pH in patients with Barrett's esophagus. Dis Esophagus 2003;16(3):193–8.

12. Milkes D, Gerson LB, Triadafilopoulos G. Complete elimination of reflux symptoms does not guarantee normalization of intraesophageal and intragastric pH in patients with gastroesophageal reflux disease (GERD). Am J Gastroenterol 2004;99(6):991–6.
13. Vela MF, Camacho-Lobato L, Srinivasan R, et al. Simultaneous intraesophageal impedance and pH measurement of acid and nonacid gastroesophageal reflux: effect of omeprazole. Gastroenterology 2001;120(7):1599–606.
14. Kauer WK, Peters JH, DeMeester TR, et al. Mixed reflux of gastric and duodenal juices is more harmful to the esophagus than gastric juice alone. The need for surgical therapy re-emphasized. Ann Surg 1995;222(4):525–31 [discussion: 531–3].
15. Thijssen AS, Broeders IA, de Wit GA, et al. Cost-effectiveness of proton pump inhibitors versus laparoscopic Nissen fundoplication for patients with gastroesophageal reflux disease: a systematic review of the literature. Surg Endosc 2011; 25(10):3127–34.
16. Stylopoulos N, Rattner DW. The history of hiatal hernia surgery: from Bowditch to laparoscopy. Ann Surg 2005;241(1):185–93.
17. Nissen R. Gastropexy as the lone procedure in the surgical repair of hiatus hernia. Am J Surg 1956;92(3):389–92.
18. DeMeester TR, Bonavina L, Albertucci M. Nissen fundoplication for gastroesophageal reflux disease. Evaluation of primary repair in 100 consecutive patients. Ann Surg 1986;204(1):9–20.
19. Peters JH, DeMeester TR, Crookes P, et al. The treatment of gastroesophageal reflux disease with laparoscopic Nissen fundoplication: prospective evaluation of 100 patients with "typical" symptoms. Ann Surg 1998;228(1):40–50.
20. Farrell TM, Archer SB, Galloway KD, et al. Heartburn is more likely to recur after Toupet fundoplication than Nissen fundoplication. Am Surg 2000;66(3):229–36 [discussion: 236–7].
21. Horvath KD, Jobe BA, Herron DM, et al. Laparoscopic Toupet fundoplication is an inadequate procedure for patients with severe reflux disease. J Gastrointest Surg 1999;3(6):583–91.
22. Csendes A. Surgical treatment of Barrett's esophagus: 1980–2003. World J Surg 2004;28(3):225–31.
23. Oelschlager BK, Barreca M, Chang L, et al. Clinical and pathologic response of Barrett's esophagus to laparoscopic antireflux surgery. Ann Surg 2003;238(4): 458–64 [discussion: 464–6].
24. Niebisch S, Fleming FJ, Galey KM, et al. Perioperative risk of laparoscopic fundoplication: safer than previously reported-analysis of the American College of Surgeons National Surgical Quality Improvement Program 2005 to 2009. J Am Coll Surg 2012;215(1):61–8 [discussion: 68–9].
25. Hofstetter WL, Peters JH, DeMeester TR, et al. Long-term outcome of antireflux surgery in patients with Barrett's esophagus. Ann Surg 2001;234(4):532–8 [discussion: 538–9].
26. O'Riordan JM, Byrne PJ, Ravi N, et al. Long-term clinical and pathologic response of Barrett's esophagus after antireflux surgery. Am J Surg 2004; 188(1):27–33.
27. Morrow E, Bushyhead D, Wassenaar E, et al. The impact of laparoscopic anti-reflux surgery in patients with Barrett's esophagus. Surg Endosc 2014;28(12):3279–84.
28. DeMeester TR, Johnson LF. Evaluation of the Nissen antireflux procedure by esophageal manometry and twenty-four hour pH monitoring. Am J Surg 1975; 129(1):94–100.

29. Gurski RR, Peters JH, Hagen JA, et al. Barrett's esophagus can and does regress after antireflux surgery: a study of prevalence and predictive features. J Am Coll Surg 2003;196(5):706–12 [discussion: 712–3].

30. Oberg S, Wenner J, Johansson J, et al. Barrett esophagus: risk factors for progression to dysplasia and adenocarcinoma. Ann Surg 2005;242(1):49–54.

31. Attwood SE, Lundell L, Hatlebakk JG, et al. Medical or surgical management of GERD patients with Barrett's esophagus: the LOTUS trial 3-year experience. J Gastrointest Surg 2008;12(10):1646–54 [discussion: 1654–5].

32. Parrilla P, Martinez de Haro LF, Ortiz A, et al. Long-term results of a randomized prospective study comparing medical and surgical treatment of Barrett's esophagus. Ann Surg 2003;237(3):291–8.

33. Chang EY, Morris CD, Seltman AK, et al. The effect of antireflux surgery on esophageal carcinogenesis in patients with Barrett esophagus: a systematic review. Ann Surg 2007;246(1):11–21.

34. Corey KE, Schmitz SM, Shaheen NJ. Does a surgical antireflux procedure decrease the incidence of esophageal adenocarcinoma in Barrett's esophagus? A meta-analysis. Am J Gastroenterol 2003;98(11):2390–4.

35. Siegel R, Ma J, Zou Z, et al. Cancer statistics, 2014. CA Cancer J Clin 2014;64(1):9–29.

36. Williams VA, Watson TJ, Herbella FA, et al. Esophagectomy for high grade dysplasia is safe, curative, and results in good alimentary outcome. J Gastrointest Surg 2007;11(12):1589–97.

37. Barr H. Ablative mucosectomy is the procedure of choice to prevent Barrett's cancer. Gut 2003;52(1):14–5.

38. Bailey SH, Bull DA, Harpole DH, et al. Outcomes after esophagectomy: a ten-year prospective cohort. Ann Thorac Surg 2003;75(1):217–22 [discussion: 222].

39. Connors RC, Reuben BC, Neumayer LA, et al. Comparing outcomes after transthoracic and transhiatal esophagectomy: a 5-year prospective cohort of 17,395 patients. J Am Coll Surg 2007;205(6):735–40.

40. Orringer MB, Marshall B, Chang AC, et al. Two thousand transhiatal esophagectomies: changing trends, lessons learned. Ann Surg 2007;246(3):363–72 [discussion: 372–4].

41. Portale G, Hagen JA, Peters JH, et al. Modern 5-year survival of resectable esophageal adenocarcinoma: single institution experience with 263 patients. J Am Coll Surg 2006;202:588–96.

42. Swanson SJ, Batirel HF, Bueno R, et al. Transthoracic esophagectomy with radical mediastinal and abdominal lymph node dissection and cervical esophagogastrostomy for esophageal carcinoma. Ann Thorac Surg 2001;72:1918–25.

43. Hulscher JB, Tijssen JG, Obertorp H, et al. Transthoracic versus transhiatal resection for carcinoma of the esophagus: a meta-analysis. Ann Thorac Surg 2001;72:306–13.

44. Fernando HC, Luketich JD, Buenaventura PO, et al. Outcomes of minimally invasive esophagectomy (MIE) for high-grade dysplasia of the esophagus. Eur J Cardiothorac Surg 2002;22(1):1–6.

45. Peyre CG, DeMeester SR, Rizzetto C, et al. Vagal-sparing esophagectomy: the ideal operation for intramucosal adenocarcinoma and barrett with high-grade dysplasia. Ann Surg 2007;246(4):665–71.

46. Lee L, Ronellenfitsch U, Hofstetter WL, et al. Predicting lymph node metastases in early esophageal adenocarcinoma using a simple scoring system. J Am Coll Surg 2013;217(2):191–9.

47. Prasad GA, Wu TT, Wigle DA, et al. Endoscopic and surgical treatment of mucosal (T1a) esophageal adenocarcinoma in Barrett's esophagus. Gastroenterology 2009;137(3):815–23.
48. Zehetner J, DeMeester SR, Hagen JA, et al. Endoscopic resection and ablation versus esophagectomy for high-grade dysplasia and intramucosal adenocarcinoma. J Thorac Cardiovasc Surg 2011;141(1):39–47.
49. Pech O, Bollschweiler E, Manner H, et al. Comparison between endoscopic and surgical resection of mucosal esophageal adenocarcinoma in Barrett's esophagus at two high-volume centers. Ann Surg 2011;254(1):67–72.

Genetic and Epigenetic Alterations in Barrett's Esophagus and Esophageal Adenocarcinoma

 CrossMark

Andrew M. Kaz, MD[a,b,c], William M. Grady, MD[b,c,*],
Matthew D. Stachler, MD, PhD[d], Adam J. Bass, MD[e]

KEYWORDS

- Barrett's esophagus • Esophageal adenocarcinoma • Cancer genomics • LOH
- Aneuploidy • Genomic instability • DNA methylation

KEY POINTS

- Genetic and epigenetic alterations play a central role in the formation of Barrett's esophagus (BE) and esophageal adenocarcinoma (EAC).
- Global epigenetic alterations occur early in the BE to EAC sequence.
- Genomic analysis of EAC and BE has revealed a set of commonly altered genes that are likely drivers of cancer formation in the esophagus.
- There is considerable genetic and epigenetic heterogeneity in BE and EAC.

INTRODUCTION

Esophageal cancer can be separated into 2 major histotypes, esophageal adenocarcinoma (EAC) and esophageal squamous cell carcinoma, and is the eighth most

Disclosure Statement: The authors all report that they have no significant disclosures to make. Grant Support: Support for this work was provided by National Institutes of Health (NIH) National Cancer Institute (NCI) RO1CA115513, P30CA15704, UO1CA152756, U54CA143862, and P01CA077852 (W. M. Grady) and PO1CA098101 (A. J. Bass); and a Burroughs Wellcome Fund Translational Research Award for Clinician Scientist (W. M. Grady).
[a] R&D Department, VA Puget Sound Health Care System, 1660 South Columbian Way, S-111-Gastro, Seattle, WA 98109, USA; [b] Clinical Research Division, Fred Hutchinson Cancer Research Center, 1100 Fairview Avenue North, Seattle, WA, USA; [c] Department of Internal Medicine, University of Washington School of Medicine, 1959 NE Pacific Street, Seattle, WA 98195, USA; [d] Department of Pathology, Brigham & Women's Hospital, Harvard Medical School, 75 Francis Street, Boston, MA 02115, USA; [e] Department of Medical Oncology, Dana-Farber Cancer Institute, 450 Brookline Avenue, Boston, MA 02215, USA
* Corresponding author. Fred Hutchinson Cancer Research Center, 1100 Fairview Avenue North, D4-100, Seattle, WA 98109.
E-mail address: wgrady@fhcrc.org

Gastroenterol Clin N Am 44 (2015) 473–489
http://dx.doi.org/10.1016/j.gtc.2015.02.015
0889-8553/15/$ – see front matter © 2015 Elsevier Inc. All rights reserved.

common cancer worldwide.[1] The incidence of EAC has been rising more rapidly than any other type of solid cancer in the United States for the past several decades, possibly secondary to the increasing prevalence of risk factors, such as obesity.[2] EAC is a particularly lethal cancer, with 5-year survival rates of less than 20%.[3]

EAC develops from Barrett's esophagus (BE), intestinal metaplasia of the lower esophagus, which can then progress through low-grade dysplasia and high-grade dysplasia (HGD) to intramucosal carcinoma and then invasive carcinoma.[4] Several concurrent histologic and molecular changes have been described for BE and EAC.[5–8] The molecular changes observed include structural genomic alterations (amplifications and deletions, translocations), DNA sequence alterations (eg, missense mutations), and epigenetic modifications, primarily in the form of DNA hypermethylation and hypomethylation of CpG dinucleotides.

In light of the increased risk of EAC in those with BE, individuals diagnosed with BE are advised to undergo periodic endoscopic surveillance with biopsies of the affected segment to detect early histologic changes (ie, the presence of dysplasia) thought to confer risk for EAC development. However, because the overall risk of progression to EAC is minimal, a challenge when managing individuals with BE is to balance the risks and costs of endoscopic surveillance with the potential benefit of early identification or prevention of cancer. Assays for molecular alterations in BE samples might ultimately complement histologic, demographic, and/or endoscopic data and provide a more accurate prediction of an individual's risk for dysplasia or cancer. This article summarizes the current understanding of genetic and epigenetic alterations that underpin the development of BE, dysplastic BE, and EAC, with an emphasis on global alterations observed in BE and EAC.

GENETIC ALTERATIONS IN BARRETT'S ESOPHAGUS, BARRETT'S ESOPHAGUS WITH DYSPLASIA, AND ESOPHAGEAL ADENOCARCINOMA
Somatic Genomic Alterations in Barrett's Esophagus

The progression of BE to EAC provides a unique system to characterize the process by which a carcinoma emerges from its precursor state. Genomic studies of BE have revealed that it is not simply a metaplastic tissue; it also harbors frequent somatic alterations. The analysis of the process of BE progression has been greatly enhanced by dramatic improvements in genomic technologies, including tools to examine genetic mutations as well as larger structural alterations in cancer (and precancer) genomes.

Early studies of BE identified frequent loss of heterozygosity (LOH) at 17p, 5q, 9p, and 13q.[9,10] The 17p and 9p harbor the tumor suppressors TP53 and CDKN2A, respectively, and studies have revealed frequent LOH through mutation (TP53 and CKN2A) or promoter methylation (CDKN2A). Galipeau and colleagues[11] analyzed a series of esophageal biopsies from patients with BE and HGD without invasive EAC, finding patients commonly develop 9p LOH before the onset of 17p LOH. A 17p LOH was associated with genomic doubling to a 4N state, consistent with the impact of p53 loss upon genomic instability. When multiple biopsies from a single patient and time point were analyzed, 9p LOH was identified frequently in a greater percentage of the overall area of BE. These data contributed to the development of a popular model, where CDKN2A loss is thought to be an initiating event in BE progression, whereas TP53 alterations are later events, associated with neoplastic progression and aneuploidy.

Beyond aneuploidy, BE progression has been associated with increasing clonal diversity.[8] Indeed, the presence of genomically distinct clones in the field of BE has been proposed by some researchers, with data suggesting the potential for certain clones to become dominant over time, that is, a 'clonal sweep.'[8,12,13]

One limitation of studies of populations with BE is that the vast majority of patients with BE do not progress to cancer, making the contribution of specific genomic alterations to the process of carcinogenesis less certain. More recent prospectively established collections have permitted researchers to study differences in structural genomic profiles in BE patients who did or did not progress to cancer. Li and colleagues[14] studied serial BE biopsies using high-density single nucleotide polymorphism arrays. They identified chromosomal instability, genome doubling, and an increase in genetic diversity in BE samples taken within 48 months of EAC diagnosis compared with BE samples from nonprogressors. Interestingly, whereas the genomes in nonprogressors were relatively stable with fewer copy number changes, 9p (*CDKN2A*) loss was still identified. These results were consistent with the model of aneuploidy being associated with neoplastic progression, but were novel in demonstrating that aneuploidy was acquired just before the diagnosis of cancer.

The advent of next-generation massively parallel sequencing technologies has enabled systematic studies of the coding mutations in BE. Agrawal and colleagues[15] performed whole exome sequencing on a set of EAC samples, including 2 cases of EAC with adjacent BE. They were able to identify the majority of mutations found in EAC in the paired BE tissue, confirming that EAC emerges from BE and showing that many coding mutations are already present in BE, including mutations in the tumor suppressor *TP53*. Through sequencing of multiple biopsy samples of BE and EAC from the same patient, Streppel and colleagues[16] identified loss of the tumor suppressor *ARID1A* in both BE and EAC. In a larger cohort of patients, this group identified loss of *ARID1A* in 4.9%, 14.3%, 16.0%, and 12.2% of BE, BE with low-grade dysplasia, BE with HGD, and EAC, respectively. In addition, by immunohistochemical staining, they identified abnormal nuclear accumulation of P53 in 34.1% of nondysplastic BE samples.

The most comprehensive, large-scale sequencing study in BE samples to date analyzed 26 genes (selected because they are commonly mutated in EAC) in a collection of nondysplastic BE, BE with HGD, and EAC samples.[17] A striking result of this study was that, with the exception of *TP53* and *SMAD4*, the other genes did not show differential mutation rates between BE and EAC, even for bona fide tumor suppressors such as *CDKN2A* and *ARID1A*. Although only 2.5% of nondysplastic BE contained a mutation in *TP53*, 70% of cases of HGD and EAC were *TP53* mutant. Nondysplastic BE samples were chosen because they showed no signs of progression; thus, it is notable that they contained tumor suppressor inactivation. Because most of these patients likely never progress to cancer, it will be important to determine whether mutations in genes such as *ARID1A* in BE are markers for increased progression risk.

Somatic Genomic Alterations in Esophageal Adenocarcinoma

Modern genomics tools are being applied widely to the study of cancers, including EAC. The earliest efforts used genome-wide array platforms for copy number analysis and found a wide range of copy number disruptions in EAC. Nancarrow and colleagues[18] identified frequent copy number alterations including homozygous deletions at putative fragile sites in the genome at genes such as *FHIT* and *WWOX*. Goh and colleagues[19] used comparative genomic hybridization to confine regions of amplification to targets that included known oncogenes, such as *MYC* and *EGFR*. Their results also suggested that patients with highly aneuploid tumors have a poorer prognosis. However, other studies have not validated the relationship between aneuploidy and survival.[20,21]

The resolution of array platforms has recently improved, as have the statistical tools with which to analyze copy number data to identify significantly recurrent alterations.[22] Comparisons across tumor types have also shown that copy number patterns in EAC are strikingly similar to those in gastric cancers.[22,23] The copy number study with the largest number of samples to date evaluated 186 EACs in conjunction with a large set of gastric and colorectal cancers.[23] A key finding from this group was that the predilection for recurrent genomic amplifications was an important feature distinguishing EAC (and gastric cancer) from lower intestinal tumors. Rates of genomic deletion, by contrast, were not highly divergent between upper and lower gastrointestinal cancers. Statistical analysis demonstrated that amplifications were highly recurrent at the loci of a number of established oncogenes involved with cell signaling (EGFR, ERBB2, KRAS, MET, FGFR2), the cell cycle (CCND1, CDK6 and CCNE1), and transcription factors (MYC, GATA4 and GATA6). Alterations in some of these oncogenes, including CDK6 and GATA6, were validated in other studies.[24,25] Many recurrent deletions were at loci of putative fragile site genes; thus, their pathologic significance is unclear. As in studies of BE, these data were consistent with a model where aneuploidy and oncogene activation seem to be important precursors for progression to cancer. Similarly, other analyses of these data established that whole-genome doubling is a prominent feature of EAC.[18,19,26] Newer sequencing technologies that have now been used to characterize EAC have demonstrated relatively high somatic mutation rates compared with most other epithelial cancers.[15,17,26–28] Agrawal and colleagues[15] were the first to publish data focusing on exome sequencing of esophageal cancer. They demonstrated the occurrence of common TP53 mutations and the absence of Notch family mutations in esophageal squamous cell cancers. Dulak and colleagues[27] performed whole exome sequencing on 149 EACs, along with whole genome sequencing of 15 of these EACs (Fig. 1). Canonical oncogene mutations in genes such as KRAS and PIK3CA were uncommon, whereas evidence of oncogene amplification was frequent. By contrast, there were widespread mutations affecting tumor suppressor genes, including TP53 and CDKN2A and chromatin-modifying enzymes including ARID1A, SMARCA4, and PBRM1. Novel recurrent mutations, including those involving TLR4 and ELMO1, were also noted, but their pathologic significance remains unclear.

Utilizing this large-scale sequencing, Dulak and colleagues were also able to evaluate mutation patterns, and found a predilection for A to C transversions at AA dinucleotides. The etiology of these mutations is unknown, but it has been hypothesized to be linked to bile acid exposure and the induction of oxidative DNA damage. This novel mutation signature was also observed in whole genome sequencing of esophageal cancers by other groups.[17,28] The Nones group also performed additional structural analysis of whole genome data, finding that EACs commonly emerge after catastrophic genomic disruptive events termed chromotripsis. These recent genomic studies are consistent with the earlier BE studies in suggesting the significant role of acquisition of aneuploidy in the transition to EAC.

Alterations in MicroRNA Expression in Barrett's Esophagus and Esophageal Adenocarcinoma

MicroRNAs (miRNAs) are small noncoding RNA molecules that can interact with other RNA molecules, resulting in posttranscriptional regulation of gene expression and gene silencing.[29] Although most of the data regarding the role of miRNAs in esophageal cancer pertains to squamous cell carcinoma, there is evidence that miR-21 and miR-375 play a functional role in BE and EAC. Several studies have demonstrated that miR-21 is upregulated in BE and EAC compared with the normal esophagus. Feber

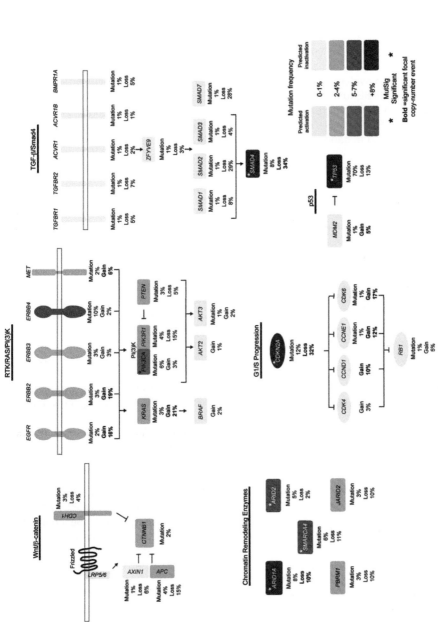

Fig. 1. Genetic alterations and affected pathways in esophageal adenocarcinoma identified by whole exome sequencing. Percentages represent the number of alterations across the cohort. Predicted gain-of-function alterations are represented in red and loss-of-function alterations are shown in blue. The darker the shade, the more frequently the gene is mutated. (*From* Dulak AM, Stojanov P, Peng S, et al. Exome and whole-genome sequencing of esophageal adenocarcinoma identifies recurrent driver events and mutational complexity. Nat Genet 2013;45(5):483; with permission.)

and colleagues[30] showed that miRNA expression profiles distinguished normal esophagus from EAC, and that *miR-21* expression was 3- to 5-fold greater in EAC compared with normal epithelia. Meanwhile, another study that utilized microarray-based technology found 34 differentially expressed miRNAs between normal squamous epithelium and BE/EACs, although the miRNA profile did not reliably distinguish BE from EAC.[31] In a validation cohort, the 5 miRNAs chosen for validation with quantitative reverse transcriptase polymerase chain reaction, including *miR-21*, were successfully able to discriminate normal esophagus from BE/EAC.

There is also evidence that differential expression of miRNAs is associated with the progression of BE to EAC. Revilla-Nuin and colleagues[32] recently identified 23 miR-NAs involved in BE progression using miRNA sequencing analysis, finding 4 miRNAs (*miR-192*, *miR-194*, *miR-196a*, and *miR-196b*) had higher expression in BE patients who progressed to cancer compared with those who did not progress.

EPIGENETIC ALTERATIONS IN BARRETT'S ESOPHAGUS, BARRETT'S ESOPHAGUS WITH DYSPLASIA, AND ESOPHAGEAL ADENOCARCINOMA

Epigenetics broadly refers to heritable and stable alterations in gene expression that are not mediated by changes in the DNA sequence. Since the discovery of DNA hypomethylation in colorectal cancer in 1982, epigenetic research has revealed an epigenetic landscape consisting of a complex array of epigenetic regulatory mechanisms that control gene expression in both cancer[33,34] and normal tissue, where it plays a crucial role in embryonic development, imprinting, and tissue differentiation.[35] The epigenetic landscape largely impacts the condensation state of the chromatin, determining whether the DNA is accessible to transcription factors and other proteins that control gene transcription.[35] The epigenetic mechanisms currently believed to play a role in cancer include (1) DNA methylation of cytosine bases in CG-rich sequences, called CpG islands, (2) posttranslational modifications of histones, proteins that form the nucleosomes, which regulate packaging of DNA in chromatin, (3) miRNAs and noncoding RNAs, and (4) nucleosome positioning.[35] In this review, we focus on aberrant DNA methylation because it is the most extensively studied epigenetic mechanism in BE and EAC. A number of excellent publications focusing on other classes of epigenetic alterations, such as histone modifications, have been written recently, and the interested reader is directed to those reviews.[36–39]

DNA Methylation: An Overview

DNA methylation refers to the enzymatic addition of a methyl group to the 5-carbon position of the nucleotide cytosine by DNA methyltransferases (DNMT1, DNMT3a, or DNMT3b) to produce 5-methylcytosine, a normal base in DNA.[40] Generally, the favored substrate for the DNMTs is the CG dinucleotide sequence, which has been termed CpG. The majority of CpGs are methylated in mammalian cells with unmethylated CpGs being typically present only in regions of DNA called CpG islands, genomic regions 200 to 500 bases in length with greater than 50% GC (guanine-cytosine) content and a ratio of observed-to-expected CpGs of greater than 0.6.[41] CpG islands overlap the promoter region of 60% to 70% of genes and tend to be protected from methylation; however, they can become aberrantly methylated in cancer. CpG methylation can lead to transcriptional inactivation via multiple mechanisms, including directly inhibiting cis-binding elements, including the following transcription factors: AP-2, CREB, E2F, CBF, and NF-KB.[42–46] Although this aberrant methylation is correlated traditionally with silencing of gene expression, it seems that decreased gene expression is characteristic of only a subset of methylated genes in most cancers.[47,48]

The methylation that occurs in CpG sites outside of promoter regions, termed gene body methylation, paradoxically has been correlated with transcriptional activation.[49] Moreover, DNA hypomethylation seems to be a prominent epigenetic alteration in BE and EAC and has been associated with increased gene expression.[50]

DNA methylation is a normal mechanism in the mammalian genome by which cells regulate gene expression, and gene methylation patterns that are established during embryonic development are maintained in the adult to regulate gene expression. A prominent mechanism by which DNA methylation is thought to regulate gene expression is through cooperative interactions with enzymes that regulate the chromatin structure, which can induce a compacted chromatin environment that represses gene expression.[48] The interaction between DNA methylation, histone modification, and chromatin structure is complex, with abundant cross-talk. DNA methylation can impact chromatin structure, but the converse is also true. Because of the epigenetic cross-talk between DNA methylation and histone modification, aberrant DNA methylation can alter chromatin structure and gene expression, and dysregulation of histones and their modifying proteins may cause aberrant DNA methylation. There is a close association between methylated CpG islands and histones containing repressive posttranslational modifications.

Feinberg and colleagues have recently enhanced our understanding of global alterations of DNA methylation in cancer. They have proposed that in addition to CpG islands there are "CpG island shores," areas of less dense CpG dinucleotides within 2 kilobases upstream of a CpG island, that can also show abnormal methylation in cancer.[51] Methylation of CpG island shores is also associated with transcriptional inactivation and splicing alterations, tends to be tissue specific, and has been shown to be altered in colorectal cancer.[51,52] Feinberg and colleagues observed that two-thirds of cancer-associated alterations in DNA methylation can be found in large domains, termed 'large organized chromatin lysine modifications' (LOCKs), as well as in smaller regions immediately adjacent to hypermethylated DNA. Their findings suggest a close cooperation between the chromatin state and DNA methylation changes in cancer.[53]

Epigenetic Alterations in Barrett's Esophagus and Esophageal Adenocarcinoma

Global alterations in DNA methylation in Barrett's esophagus and esophageal adenocarcinoma

Microarray-based technologies have been used to interrogate global patterns of DNA methylation in BE and EAC, and to uncover candidate epigenetic drivers of BE progression. One study used Illumina HumanMethylation27 BeadChips to interrogate more than 27,000 CpG dinucleotides.[54] The authors noted that both BE (n = 77) and EAC (n = 117) samples were highly methylated compared with normal esophagus (n = 94), indicating that epigenetic alterations occurs early in the BE to EAC progression sequence. They also found numerous previously undescribed hypermethylated genes in BE and EAC tissues, including genes encoding ADAM (A Disintegrin And Metalloproteinase) peptidase proteins, cadherins and protocadherins, and potassium voltage-gated channels. Alvi and colleagues[55] also used the HumanMethylation27 BeadChips to compare methylation patterns, focusing on imprinted and X chromosome genes, from 24 BE and 22 EAC samples and validated their findings in retrospective and prospective cohorts to assess the ability of methylated genes to classify individuals as having prevalent BE, dysplastic BE, or EAC. They found 4 genes (*SLC22A18*, *PIGR*, *GJA12*, and *RIN2*) had the greatest area under curve (0.988) to distinguish between BE and dysplasia/EAC in their retrospective cohort. In the prospective cohort, this methylated gene panel was able to stratify patients into low, intermediate, or high risk groups based on the number of genes that were methylated.

Kaz and colleagues[56] utilized GoldenGate methylation microarrays (1505 CpGs in 807 genes) to compare methylation of normal squamous (n = 30), BE (n = 29), BE plus HGD (n = 8), and EAC (n = 30) cases. Distinct global methylation signatures were seen among the different tissue types, as well as specific genes demonstrating differential methylation between these groups. Within the BE and EAC cases, there were subgroups with distinct methylation signatures (high and low methylation epigenotypes), suggesting that there may be a CpG island methylator phenotype (CIMP) molecular class of BE and EAC (**Figs. 2** and **3**). Further studies are needed to confirm this observation.

In another genome-wide study, massively parallel sequencing was performed in matched BE and EAC tissues and esophageal cell lines to characterize methylation at 1.8 million CpG dinucleotides.[57] The authors found that DNA hypomethylation was more frequent than hypermethylated DNA in both BE and EAC cases and that the hypomethylated regions were found in intragenic and noncoding regions. One long noncoding RNA, *AFAP1-AS1*, was highly hypomethylated and overexpressed in BE and EAC tissues and cell lines. When *AFAP1* was silenced using small interfering RNA technologies, esophageal cells exhibited increased apoptosis and reduced proliferation and colony-forming abilities, suggesting a cancer-promoting role for this noncoding RNA in BE and EAC.

Specific epigenetic alterations in Barrett's esophagus and esophageal adenocarcinoma

Aberrant methylation of promoter CpG islands, which leads to gene silencing of a subset of genes, has been shown to occur frequently in BE, dysplastic BE, and EAC. Epigenetic changes involving the promoter regions of several dozen genes have been evaluated using candidate gene approaches based on findings seen in other types of cancers. One of the first tumor suppressor genes shown to be aberrantly methylated in BE was *CDKN2A* (*p16INK4a*), which normally blocks phosphorylation of the Rb protein and inhibits cell-cycle progression. *CDKN2A* promoter hypermethylation combined with 9p21 chromosomal loss leads to inactivation of this gene in some cases of EAC or BE with dysplasia.[58,59] CpG island hypermethylation of the *CDKN2A* promoter has been reported in 3% to 77% of BE cases, suggesting that *CDKN2A* methylation is in early event in BE pathogenesis.[60–63]

Eads and colleagues[64] evaluated methylation patterns of *APC*, *ESR1*, and *CDH1* in 6 esophagectomy specimens, which contained both BE and EAC. They analyzed 107 distinct regions of each resected specimen to create spatial methylation maps. They found an high incidence of methylation of *ESR1*, *APC*, and *CDKN2A* in BE, BE with dysplasia, and EAC in a pattern suggesting simultaneous methylation in large contiguous fields, or clonal expansion of cells that acquired methylation. Similar patterns consistent with clonal expansion in BE have been reported in studies that focused on LOH or mutations of *APC*, *TP53*, and *CDKN2A*.[61,65,66]

Aberrant methylation of *APC* and *CDH1* in BE and EAC has been evaluated by other groups as well.[67,68] One group found hypermethylated *APC* in 39.5% of BE and 92% of EAC cases, but not in matched normal esophagus. Methylated *APC* could also be detected in the plasma of 25% of EAC patients, and was associated with decreased survival.[67] Another group found high levels of methylated *APC* in greater than 95% of BE and EAC, supporting the concept that aberrant methylation of tumor suppressor genes occurs early in the BE→EAC sequence.[69]

Other genes implicated in carcinogenesis have been found to be methylated in BE/EAC, including the STAT-induced STAT inhibitors (SSIs), suppressors of cytokine signaling (*SOCS-1* and *-3*) and *Reprimo* (*RPRM*) and members of the glutathione S-transferase (GST) and glutathione peroxidase (GPX) family.[70–72] Other groups

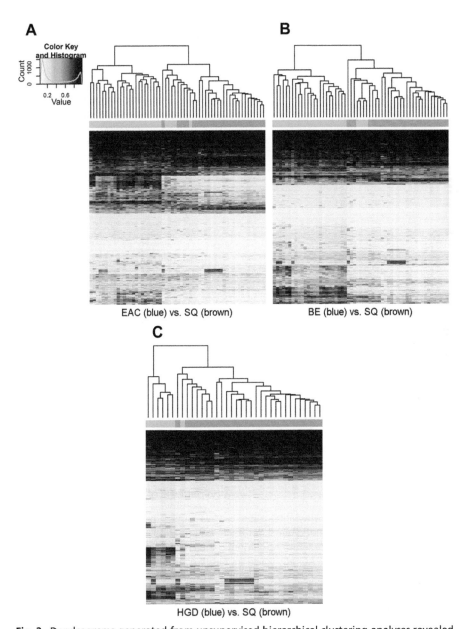

Fig. 2. Dendrograms generated from unsupervised hierarchical clustering analyses revealed distinct methylation profiles based on histologic subtype. Each column represents a single sample, and each row an individual CpG site. The darker blue colors correspond to higher β values (ie, a greater degree of methylation) at particular CpGs. (*A*) Esophageal adenocarcinoma (EAC) versus squamous (SQ) samples. (*B*) Barrett's esophagus (BE) versus SQ samples. (*C*) High-grade dysplasia (HGD) versus SQ samples. (*From* Kaz AM, Wong CJ, Luo Y, et al. DNA methylation profiling in Barrett's esophagus and esophageal adenocarcinoma reveals unique methylation signatures and molecular subclasses. Epigenetics 2011;6(12):1405; with permission.)

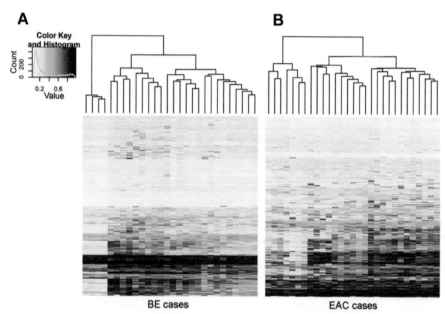

Fig. 3. Dendrograms generated from unsupervised hierarchical clustering analyses within a single histologic subtype. Each column represents a single sample and each row an individual CpG site; the darker blue colors correspond to higher β values. When analyzing the Barrett's esophagus (BE) cases independently (A) or the esophageal adenocarcinoma (EAC) cases independently (B), we noted 2 distinct methylation profiles within each of these tissue types: a high and low methylation epigenotype subgroup. (*From* Kaz AM, Wong CJ, Luo Y, et al. DNA methylation profiling in Barrett's esophagus and esophageal adenocarcinoma reveals unique methylation signatures and molecular subclasses. Epigenetics 2011;6(12):1406; with permission.)

have identified methylation of somatostatin (*SST*), tachykinin-1 (*TAC1*), *NELL1*, *CDH13*, and noted that the incidence of methylation was increased in BE, BE with dysplasia, and EAC versus normal esophageal samples.[73–77] In vitro treatment of cultured cells with the demethylating agent 5-aza resulted in increased mRNA expression levels of these hypermethylated genes, substantiating the link between aberrant methylation and gene expression. Additional genes reported to demonstrate aberrant methylation in BE and/or EAC are listed in **Table 1**. In general, hypermethylation of these genes is detectable in cases of BE without dysplasia, suggesting that many of the epigenetic alterations that occur in EAC are already present in BE.

CLINICAL IMPLICATIONS
Risk Stratification and Prognosis for Barrett's Esophagus

There remains some uncertainty regarding the histologic interpretation of BE, BE with low-grade dysplasia, and BE with HGD, and also which patients with BE are at the greatest risk for progression to EAC. Given the limitations of standard histopathology, genomic and epigenomic analysis has the potential to aid in risk stratification. Given features such as *TP53* and *SMAD4* mutations, chromosomal instability, and genetic diversity are associated with progressive disease, it is highly feasible that assays for such features could be used increasingly to aid the pathologic assessment of disease and to select patients for more careful monitoring and/or ablation of their BE. The

Table 1
Hypermethylated genes in BE, BE with dysplasia, and EAC

Gene	Precursor (M%)	Cancer (M%)	References
CDKN2A	BE (3%–77%); IND (60%); LGD (20%–56%); HGD (60%–75%)	EAC (39%–85%)	58–64,69,79–82
ESR1	BE (69%); LGD (100%); HGD (67%)	EAC (51%–100%)	64,80
APC	BE (40%–85%); LGD (83%); HGD (66%)	EAC (42%–92%; 25% M in plasma)	64,67,69,79
CDH1	BE (8%); LGD (0%); HGD (0%)	EAC (0%–84%)	64,68,79,83
SOCS-1, SOCS-3	BE SOCS-3 (13%); SOCS-1 (0%); HGD SOCS-3 (69%), SOCS-1 (21%); LGD SOCS-3 (22%), SOCS-1 (4%)	EAC SOCS-3 (74%); SOCS-1 (42%)	70
Reprimo	BE (36%); HGD (64%)	EAC (63%)	71
GPX3, GPX7, GSTM2		EAC GPX3 (62%); GPX7 (67%), GSTM2 (69%)	72
SST	BE (70%); HGD (71%)	EAC (72%)	73
TAC1	BE (56%); any dysplasia (58%)	EAC (61%)	74
NELL1	BE (42%); any dysplasia (52%)	EAC (48%)	75
AKAP12	BE (39%), any dysplasia (52%)	EAC (52%)	77
CDH13	BE (70%); any dysplasia (78%)	EAC (76%)	76
DAPK	BE (50%), any dysplasia (53%)	EAC (19%–60%)	80,84
VIM	BE (91%); HGD (100%)	EAC (81%)	85
SFRP1,2,4,5	BE SFRP1 (81%), SFRP2 (89%), SFRP4 (78%), SFRP5 (73%)	EAC SFRP1 (93%), SFRP2 (83%), SFRP4 (73%), SFRP5 (85%)	86
EYA4	BE (77%)	EAC (83%)	87
p14ARF	BE (7%)	EAC (0%–20%)	63,79
MGMT	BE (62%)	EAC (56%–64%)	80,88
TIMP-3	BE (72%)	EAC (19%–90%)	80,89

Abbreviations: BE, Barrett's esophagus; EAC, esophageal adenocarcinoma; HGD, high-grade dysplasia; IND, indefinite for dysplasia; LGD, low-grade dysplasia; M%, percent of cases demonstrating methylation of given gene.
Data from Refs.[58–64,67–77,79–89]

results from the Weaver study, showing common tumor suppressor mutations in non-dysplastic BE, demonstrate the need to carefully assess the specificity of genomic markers that might be associated with increased risk of progression.[17] Additionally, further development of techniques to optimize sampling of BE tissue is required given the likelihood of clonal diversity within fields of BE. Efforts to procure esophageal tissue samples that are more representative of the entire BE segment will likely increase the proportion of patients with positive genomic findings, making the assessment of the specificity of markers of even greater importance. Emerging noninvasive approaches for epithelial sampling of BE, such as the Cytosponge, could allow cost-effective and safe sampling across the entire field of BE.[17]

Maley,[8] Reid and colleagues[14] have conducted numerous studies describing the relationship between clonal diversity and clonal expansions and the risk of BE progression. One prospective study of 268 BE patients evaluated whether clonal expansions during the progression of BE led to homogenous cell populations or result in clonal diversity.[8] The authors found that patients with greater clonal diversity had greater risk of progression to EAC (*P*<.001). In a follow-up study, this group compared clonal diversity in 79 BE progressors and 169 nonprogressors over 20,425 person-months of follow-up, finding that nonprogressors had types of chromosomal instability (small localized deletions involving fragile sites and 9p loss/copy neutral LOH) that generated relatively little genetic diversity.[14] Individuals who progressed to EAC, meanwhile, developed chromosome instability with initial gains and losses, genomic diversity, and selection of somatic chromosomal alterations followed by catastrophic genome doublings. These data suggest that molecular testing to assess risk of progression in BE may need to incorporate assessment of structural genomic alterations and also assessment of multiple foci of BE from individual patients.

Prognostic and Predictive Markers for Esophageal Adenocarcinoma

Current histologic assessment of EAC is relatively uncomplicated, and no histologic subtype has been shown to be associated with any specific genomic alterations (in contrast with gastric adenocarcinoma, where, for example, loss of CDH1 is associated with diffuse-type tumors). Increasingly, however, as more genomic alterations are demonstrated to have utility as prognostic or predictive biomarkers, testing for these changes will become increasingly routine. Currently, the only standard tests performed in EAC measure changes in HER/ERBB2 using a combination of immunohistochemistry and fluorescent in-situ hybridization. The results of these tests are used to guide use of the anti-ERBB2 drug trastuzumab in patients with metastatic disease.[78] Clinical trials investigating other candidate gene/genomic targets are ongoing. Over time, it is likely that multiplexed cancer genomic panels will supplant the use of single gene tests. New approaches, including the use of plasma for cancer genome profiling, are under development, which may allow more comprehensive assessment of the heterogeneity of genomic markers in cancer.[21]

SUMMARY

BE is a metaplastic tissue that develops in response to chemical injury and is a major risk factor for EAC. The fact that many individuals with BE undergo periodic endoscopy with tissue biopsy means that a valuable source of material to study the molecular changes associated with BE, BE with dysplasia, and EAC is readily available. The molecular changes that have been identified to date include structural genomic alterations, DNA sequence alterations, and epigenetic modifications.

Genomic studies of BE have revealed that it is not simply a metaplastic tissue, but characterized by frequent somatic alterations, including mutations in *TP53* and other genes. BE is also characterized by aneuploidy and activation of oncogenes, both of which seem to be important precursors for progression to cancer. Newer sequencing technologies that have now been used to characterize EAC have demonstrated relatively high somatic mutation rates compared with most other epithelial cancers.

Epigenetic alterations are also frequently found in BE and EAC. Candidate gene approaches as well as genome-wide array-based studies have identified several genes with aberrant promoter DNA methylation in BE and EAC, and in many cases the epigenetic alterations that were found in EAC were also seen in BE.

In general, both genetic and epigenetic abnormalities are seen in BE before the development of dysplasia or EAC. This has important implications if these molecular alterations are to be used as assays to predict the risk of BE progression; although it may be true that certain tumor suppressor genes are inactivated in many cases of BE, most individuals with BE will not progress to dysplasia or cancer.

Given the limitations of histopathology, genomic and epigenomic analysis has the potential to improve the precision of risk stratification. Specific gene mutations, chromosomal instability, and genetic diversity are associated with neoplastic progression, and it is foreseeable that assays to detect these features could be used to support the pathologic assessment of disease and to select patients for more intensive surveillance.

REFERENCES

1. Zhang XM, Guo MZ. The value of epigenetic markers in esophageal cancer. Front Med China 2010;4(4):378–84.
2. Long E, Beales IL. The role of obesity in oesophageal cancer development. Therap Adv Gastroenterol 2014;7(6):247–68.
3. Brown LM, Devesa SS. Epidemiologic trends in esophageal and gastric cancer in the United States. Surg Oncol Clin N Am 2002;11(2):235–56.
4. Spechler SJ. Clinical practice. Barrett's Esophagus. N Engl J Med 2002;346(11): 836–42.
5. Werner M, Mueller J, Walch A, et al. The molecular pathology of Barrett's esophagus. Histol Histopathol 1999;14(2):553–9.
6. Flejou JF. Barrett's oesophagus: from metaplasia to dysplasia and cancer. Gut 2005;54(Suppl 1):i6–12.
7. Reid BJ, Levine DS, Longton G, et al. Predictors of progression to cancer in Barrett's esophagus: baseline histology and flow cytometry identify low- and high-risk patient subsets. Am J Gastroenterol 2000;95(7):1669–76.
8. Maley CC, Galipeau PC, Finley JC, et al. Genetic clonal diversity predicts progression to esophageal adenocarcinoma. Nat Genet 2006;38(4):468–73.
9. Reid BJ, Barrett MT, Galipeau PC, et al. Barrett's esophagus: ordering the events that lead to cancer. Eur J Cancer Prev 1996;5(Suppl 2):57–65.
10. Barrett MT, Galipeau PC, Sanchez CA, et al. Determination of the frequency of loss of heterozygosity in esophageal adenocarcinoma by cell sorting, whole genome amplification and microsatellite polymorphisms. Oncogene 1996;12(9):1873–8.
11. Galipeau PC, Prevo LJ, Sanchez CA, et al. Clonal expansion and loss of heterozygosity at chromosomes 9p and 17p in premalignant esophageal (Barrett's) tissue. J Natl Cancer Inst 1999;91(24):2087–95.
12. Maley CC, Galipeau PC, Li X, et al. Selectively advantageous mutations and hitchhikers in neoplasms: p16 lesions are selected in Barrett's esophagus. Cancer Res 2004;64(10):3414–27.
13. Werther M, Saure C, Pahl R, et al. Molecular genetic analysis of surveillance biopsy samples from Barrett's mucosa–significance of sampling. Pathol Res Pract 2008;204(5):285–94.
14. Li X, Galipeau PC, Paulson TG, et al. Temporal and spatial evolution of somatic chromosomal alterations: a case-cohort study of Barrett's esophagus. Cancer Prev Res (Phila) 2014;7(1):114–27.
15. Agrawal N, Jiao Y, Bettegowda C, et al. Comparative genomic analysis of esophageal adenocarcinoma and squamous cell carcinoma. Cancer Discov 2012; 2(10):899–905.
16. Streppel MM, Lata S, DelaBastide M, et al. Next-generation sequencing of endoscopic biopsies identifies ARID1A as a tumor-suppressor gene in Barrett's esophagus. Oncogene 2014;33(3):347–57.

17. Weaver JM, Ross-Innes CS, Shannon N, et al. Ordering of mutations in preinvasive disease stages of esophageal carcinogenesis. Nat Genet 2014;46(8): 837–43.
18. Nancarrow DJ, Handoko HY, Smithers BM, et al. Genome-wide copy number analysis in esophageal adenocarcinoma using high-density single-nucleotide polymorphism arrays. Cancer Res 2008;68(11):4163–72.
19. Goh XY, Rees JR, Paterson AL, et al. Integrative analysis of array-comparative genomic hybridisation and matched gene expression profiling data reveals novel genes with prognostic significance in oesophageal adenocarcinoma. Gut 2011; 60(10):1317–26.
20. Davison JM, Yee M, Krill-Burger JM, et al. The degree of segmental aneuploidy measured by total copy number abnormalities predicts survival and recurrence in superficial gastroesophageal adenocarcinoma. PLoS One 2014;9(1):e79079.
21. Haber DA, Velculescu VE. Blood-based analyses of cancer: circulating tumor cells and circulating tumor DNA. Cancer Discov 2014;4(6):650–61.
22. Mermel CH, Schumacher SE, Hill B, et al. GISTIC2.0 facilitates sensitive and confident localization of the targets of focal somatic copy-number alteration in human cancers. Genome Biol 2011;12(4):R41.
23. Dulak AM, Schumacher SE, van Lieshout J, et al. Gastrointestinal adenocarcinomas of the esophagus, stomach, and colon exhibit distinct patterns of genome instability and oncogenesis. Cancer Res 2012;72(17):4383–93.
24. Ismail A, Bandla S, Reveiller M, et al. Early G(1) cyclin-dependent kinases as prognostic markers and potential therapeutic targets in esophageal adenocarcinoma. Clin Cancer Res 2011;17(13):4513–22.
25. Lin L, Bass AJ, Lockwood WW, et al. Activation of GATA binding protein 6 (GATA6) sustains oncogenic lineage-survival in esophageal adenocarcinoma. Proc Natl Acad Sci U S A 2012;109(11):4251–6.
26. Carter SL, Cibulskis K, Helman E, et al. Absolute quantification of somatic DNA alterations in human cancer. Nat Biotechnol 2012;30(5):413–21.
27. Dulak AM, Stojanov P, Peng S, et al. Exome and whole-genome sequencing of esophageal adenocarcinoma identifies recurrent driver events and mutational complexity. Nat Genet 2013;45(5):478–86.
28. Nones K, Waddell N, Wayte N, et al. Genomic catastrophes frequently arise in esophageal adenocarcinoma and drive tumorigenesis. Nat Commun 2014;5:5224.
29. Bartel DP. MicroRNAs: genomics, biogenesis, mechanism, and function. Cell 2004;116(2):281–97.
30. Feber A, Xi L, Luketich JD, et al. MicroRNA expression profiles of esophageal cancer. J Thorac Cardiovasc Surg 2008;135(2):255–60 [discussion: 260].
31. Garman KS, Owzar K, Hauser ER, et al. MicroRNA expression differentiates squamous epithelium from Barrett's esophagus and esophageal cancer. Dig Dis Sci 2013;58(11):3178–88.
32. Revilla-Nuin B, Parrilla P, Lozano JJ, et al. Predictive value of MicroRNAs in the progression of Barrett esophagus to adenocarcinoma in a long-term follow-up study. Ann Surg 2013;257(5):886–93.
33. Suzuki H, Tokino T, Shinomura Y, et al. DNA methylation and cancer pathways in gastrointestinal tumors. Pharmacogenomics 2008;9(12):1917–28.
34. Feinberg AP. The epigenetics of cancer etiology. Semin Cancer Biol 2004;14(6): 427–32.
35. Sharma A, Heuck CJ, Fazzari MJ, et al. DNA methylation alterations in multiple myeloma as a model for epigenetic changes in cancer. Wiley Interdiscip Rev Syst Biol Med 2010;2(6):654–69.

36. Sawan C, Herceg Z. Histone modifications and cancer. Adv Genet 2010;70:57–85.
37. Ballestar E, Esteller M. Epigenetic gene regulation in cancer. Adv Genet 2008;61: 247–67.
38. Ting AH, McGarvey KM, Baylin SB. The cancer epigenome–components and functional correlates. Genes Dev 2006;20(23):3215–31.
39. van Engeland M, Derks S, Smits KM, et al. Colorectal cancer epigenetics: complex simplicity. J Clin Oncol 2011;29(10):1382–91.
40. Bestor TH. The DNA methyltransferases of mammals. Hum Mol Genet 2000; 9(16):2395–402.
41. Gardiner-Garden M, Frommer M. CpG islands in vertebrate genomes. J Mol Biol 1987;196(2):261–82.
42. Comb M, Goodman HM. CpG methylation inhibits proenkephalin gene expression and binding of the transcription factor AP-2. Nucleic Acids Res 1990; 18(13):3975–82.
43. Inamdar NM, Ehrlich KC, Ehrlich M. CpG methylation inhibits binding of several sequence-specific DNA-binding proteins from pea, wheat, soybean and cauliflower. Plant Mol Biol 1991;17(1):111–23.
44. Campanero MR, Armstrong MI, Flemington EK. CpG methylation as a mechanism for the regulation of E2F activity. Proc Natl Acad Sci U S A 2000;97(12):6481–6.
45. Deng G, Chen A, Pong E, et al. Methylation in hMLH1 promoter interferes with its binding to transcription factor CBF and inhibits gene expression. Oncogene 2001;20(48):7120–7.
46. Bednarik DP, Duckett C, Kim SU, et al. DNA CpG methylation inhibits binding of NF-kappa B proteins to the HIV-1 long terminal repeat cognate DNA motifs. New Biol 1991;3(10):969–76.
47. Hinoue T, Weisenberger DJ, Lange CP, et al. Genome-scale analysis of aberrant DNA methylation in colorectal cancer. Genome Res 2012;22(2):271–82.
48. Bird A. DNA methylation patterns and epigenetic memory. Genes Dev 2002; 16(1):6–21.
49. Hellman A, Chess A. Gene body-specific methylation on the active X chromosome. Science 2007;315(5815):1141–3.
50. Alvarez H, Opalinska J, Zhou L, et al. Widespread hypomethylation occurs early and synergizes with gene amplification during esophageal carcinogenesis. PLoS Genet 2011;7(3):e1001356.
51. Irizarry RA, Ladd-Acosta C, Wen B, et al. The human colon cancer methylome shows similar hypo- and hypermethylation at conserved tissue-specific CpG island shores. Nat Genet 2009;41(2):178–86.
52. Doi A, Park IH, Wen B, et al. Differential methylation of tissue- and cancer-specific CpG island shores distinguishes human induced pluripotent stem cells, embryonic stem cells and fibroblasts. Nat Genet 2009;41(12):1350–3.
53. Hansen KD, Timp W, Bravo HC, et al. Increased methylation variation in epigenetic domains across cancer types. Nat Genet 2011;43(8):768–75.
54. Xu E, Gu J, Hawk ET, et al. Genome-wide methylation analysis shows similar patterns in Barrett's esophagus and esophageal adenocarcinoma. Carcinogenesis 2013;34(12):2750–6.
55. Alvi MA, Liu X, O'Donovan M, et al. DNA methylation as an adjunct to histopathology to detect prevalent, inconspicuous dysplasia and early-stage neoplasia in Barrett's esophagus. Clin Cancer Res 2013;19(4):878–88.
56. Kaz AM, Wong CJ, Luo Y, et al. DNA methylation profiling in Barrett's esophagus and esophageal adenocarcinoma reveals unique methylation signatures and molecular subclasses. Epigenetics 2011;6(12):1403–12.

57. Wu W, Bhagat TD, Yang X, et al. Hypomethylation of noncoding DNA regions and overexpression of the long noncoding RNA, AFAP1-AS1, in Barrett's esophagus and esophageal adenocarcinoma. Gastroenterology 2013;144(5):956–66.e4.

58. Wong DJ, Barrett MT, Stoger R, et al. p16INK4a promoter is hypermethylated at a high frequency in esophageal adenocarcinomas. Cancer Res 1997;57(13):2619–22.

59. Klump B, Hsieh CJ, Holzmann K, et al. Hypermethylation of the CDKN2/p16 promoter during neoplastic progression in Barrett's esophagus. Gastroenterology 1998;115(6):1381–6.

60. Eads CA, Lord RV, Wickramasinghe K, et al. Epigenetic patterns in the progression of esophageal adenocarcinoma. Cancer Res 2001;61(8):3410–8.

61. Wong DJ, Paulson TG, Prevo LJ, et al. p16(INK4a) lesions are common, early abnormalities that undergo clonal expansion in Barrett's metaplastic epithelium. Cancer Res 2001;61(22):8284–9.

62. Bian YS, Osterheld MC, Fontolliet C, et al. p16 inactivation by methylation of the CDKN2A promoter occurs early during neoplastic progression in Barrett's esophagus. Gastroenterology 2002;122(4):1113–21.

63. Vieth M, Schneider-Stock R, Rohrich K, et al. INK4a-ARF alterations in Barrett's epithelium, intraepithelial neoplasia and Barrett's adenocarcinoma. Virchows Arch 2004;445(2):135–41.

64. Eads CA, Lord RV, Kurumboor SK, et al. Fields of aberrant CpG island hypermethylation in Barrett's esophagus and associated adenocarcinoma. Cancer Res 2000;60(18):5021–6.

65. Barrett MT, Sanchez CA, Prevo LJ, et al. Evolution of neoplastic cell lineages in Barrett oesophagus. Nat Genet 1999;22(1):106–9.

66. Prevo LJ, Sanchez CA, Galipeau PC, et al. p53-mutant clones and field effects in Barrett's esophagus. Cancer Res 1999;59(19):4784–7.

67. Kawakami K, Brabender J, Lord RV, et al. Hypermethylated APC DNA in plasma and prognosis of patients with esophageal adenocarcinoma. J Natl Cancer Inst 2000;92(22):1805–11.

68. Bongiorno PF, al-Kasspooles M, Lee SW, et al. E-cadherin expression in primary and metastatic thoracic neoplasms and in Barrett's oesophagus. Br J Cancer 1995;71(1):166–72.

69. Smith E, De Young NJ, Pavey SJ, et al. Similarity of aberrant DNA methylation in Barrett's esophagus and esophageal adenocarcinoma. Mol Cancer 2008;7:75.

70. Tischoff I, Hengge UR, Vieth M, et al. Methylation of SOCS-3 and SOCS-1 in the carcinogenesis of Barrett's adenocarcinoma. Gut 2007;56(8):1047–53.

71. Hamilton JP, Sato F, Jin Z, et al. Reprimo methylation is a potential biomarker of Barrett's-Associated esophageal neoplastic progression. Clin Cancer Res 2006;12(22):6637–42.

72. Peng DF, Razvi M, Chen H, et al. DNA hypermethylation regulates the expression of members of the Mu-class glutathione S-transferases and glutathione peroxidases in Barrett's adenocarcinoma. Gut 2009;58(1):5–15.

73. Jin Z, Mori Y, Hamilton JP, et al. Hypermethylation of the somatostatin promoter is a common, early event in human esophageal carcinogenesis. Cancer 2008;112(1):43–9.

74. Jin Z, Olaru A, Yang J, et al. Hypermethylation of tachykinin-1 is a potential biomarker in human esophageal cancer. Clin Cancer Res 2007;13(21):6293–300.

75. Jin Z, Mori Y, Yang J, et al. Hypermethylation of the nel-like 1 gene is a common and early event and is associated with poor prognosis in early-stage esophageal adenocarcinoma. Oncogene 2007;26(43):6332–40.

76. Jin Z, Cheng Y, Olaru A, et al. Promoter hypermethylation of CDH13 is a common, early event in human esophageal adenocarcinogenesis and correlates with clinical risk factors. Int J Cancer 2008;123(10):2331–6.

77. Jin Z, Hamilton JP, Yang J, et al. Hypermethylation of the AKAP12 promoter is a biomarker of Barrett's-associated esophageal neoplastic progression. Cancer Epidemiol Biomarkers Prev 2008;17(1):111–7.

78. Bang YJ, Van Cutsem E, Feyereislova A, et al. Trastuzumab in combination with chemotherapy versus chemotherapy alone for treatment of HER2-positive advanced gastric or gastro-oesophageal junction cancer (ToGA): a phase 3, open-label, randomised controlled trial. Lancet 2010;376(9742):687–97.

79. Sarbia M, Geddert H, Klump B, et al. Hypermethylation of tumor suppressor genes (p16INK4A, p14ARF and APC) in adenocarcinomas of the upper gastrointestinal tract. Int J Cancer 2004;111(2):224–8.

80. Brock MV, Gou M, Akiyama Y, et al. Prognostic importance of promoter hypermethylation of multiple genes in esophageal adenocarcinoma. Clin Cancer Res 2003;9(8):2912–9.

81. Wang JS, Guo M, Montgomery EA, et al. DNA promoter hypermethylation of p16 and APC predicts neoplastic progression in Barrett's esophagus. Am J Gastroenterol 2009;104(9):2153–60.

82. Hardie LJ, Darnton SJ, Wallis YL, et al. p16 expression in Barrett's esophagus and esophageal adenocarcinoma: association with genetic and epigenetic alterations. Cancer Lett 2005;217(2):221–30.

83. Corn PG, Heath EI, Heitmiller R, et al. Frequent hypermethylation of the 5' CpG island of E-cadherin in esophageal adenocarcinoma. Clin Cancer Res 2001; 7(9):2765–9.

84. Kuester D, Dar AA, Moskaluk CC, et al. Early involvement of death-associated protein kinase promoter hypermethylation in the carcinogenesis of Barrett's esophageal adenocarcinoma and its association with clinical progression. Neoplasia 2007;9(3):236–45.

85. Moinova H, Leidner RS, Ravi L, et al. Aberrant vimentin methylation is characteristic of upper gastrointestinal pathologies. Cancer Epidemiol Biomarkers Prev 2012;21(4):594–600.

86. Zou H, Molina JR, Harrington JJ, et al. Aberrant methylation of secreted frizzled-related protein genes in esophageal adenocarcinoma and Barrett's esophagus. Int J Cancer 2005;116(4):584–91.

87. Zou H, Osborn NK, Harrington JJ, et al. Frequent methylation of eyes absent 4 gene in Barrett's esophagus and esophageal adenocarcinoma. Cancer Epidemiol Biomarkers Prev 2005;14(4):830–4.

88. Baumann S, Keller G, Puhringer F, et al. The prognostic impact of O6-Methylguanine-DNA Methyltransferase (MGMT) promotor hypermethylation in esophageal adenocarcinoma. Int J Cancer 2006;119(2):264–8.

89. Darnton S, Hardie L, Muc R, et al. Tissue inhibitor of metalloproteinase-3 (TIMP-3) gene is methylated in the development of esophageal adenocarcinoma: Loss of expression correlates with poor prognosis. Int J Cancer 2005;115(3):351–8.

Index

Note: Page numbers of article titles are in **boldface** type.

A

Ablation
    Barrett's esophagus after, chemoprevention for, 393
    photodynamic, 346–347, 382–383, 433, 436
    radiofrequency. See Radiofrequency ablation.
    with freezing temperatures, 345–346, 363
Ablation of Intestinal Metaplasia dysplasia trial, 364–365
Acetic acid, for chromoendoscopy, 440, 444
Acid suppression, 405. See also Proton pump inhibitors.
    trials of, 401–402
    versus antireflux surgery, 463–465
    with mucosal resection, 328
ADAM gene, 479
Adenocarcinoma, esophageal. See Esophageal adenocarcinoma.
Adipokines, in obesity, 398–399
Adiponectin, in obesity, 255–257
Adipose tissue and adipocytes, excess of. See Obesity.
AFAP1-AS1 gene, 480
Age, as risk factor, 212–214, 304–305
AKAP12 gene, 483
Alcohol use, as risk factor, 208–209, 277
American College of Gastroenterology
    GERD guidelines of, 420–421
    surveillance guidelines of, 292–293
American College of Physicians, surveillance guidelines of, 292
American Gastroenterology Association
    endoscopic eradication therapy recommendations of, 357
    surveillance guidelines of, 292–293
American Society for Gastrointestinal Endoscopy, surveillance guidelines of, 292–293
Annexin-A6, as biomarker, 383, 385
Anterior gradient-2, as biomarker, 376
Antideath pathways, drugs targeting, 396–397
Antioxidants, for chemoprevention, 398
Antireflux surgery, 420, 459–465
AP-1 transcription factor, 397
AP-2 transcription factor, 478
APC gene, 376, 380, 480, 483
Apoptosis
    drugs targeting, 396–397
    leptin inhibiting, 256
Arachidonic metabolites, drugs targeting, 395
Argon blue laser light, in confocal laser endomicroscopy, 448–451

Gastroenterol Clin N Am 44 (2015) 491–505
http://dx.doi.org/10.1016/S0889-8553(15)00043-6
0889-8553/15/$ – see front matter © 2015 Elsevier Inc. All rights reserved.

Printed and bound by CPI Group (UK) Ltd, Croydon, CR0 4YY

03/10/2024

01040496-0012